Global Thoracic Surgery

Editor

GITA N. MODY

THORACIC SURGERY CLINICS

www.thoracic.theclinics.com

Consulting Editor
VIRGINIA R. LITLE

August 2022 • Volume 32 • Number 3

ELSEVIER

1600 John F. Kennedy Boulevard • Suite 1800 • Philadelphia, Pennsylvania, 19103-2899

http://www.thoracic.theclinics.com

THORACIC SURGERY CLINICS Volume 32, Number 3
August 2022 ISSN 1547-4127, ISBN-13: 978-0-323-84979-1

Editor: John Vassallo (j.vassallo@elsevier.com)
Developmental Editor: Jessica Nicole B. Cañaberal

Thoracic Surgery Clinics (ISSN 1547-4127) is published quarterly by Elsevier Inc., 360 Park Avenue South, New York, NY 10010-1710. Months of publication are February, May, August, and November. Business and editorial offices: 1600 John F. Kennedy Boulevard, Suite 1800, Philadelphia, PA 19103-2899. Periodicals postage paid at New York, NY, and additional mailing offices. Subscription prices are $405.00 per year (US individuals), $875.00 per year (US institutions), $100.00 per year (US students), $473.00 per year (Canadian individuals), $893.00 per year (Canadian institutions), $100.00 per year (Canadian students), $225.00 per year (international students), $494.00 per year (international individuals), and $893.00 per year (international institutions). Foreign air speed delivery is included in all Clinics' subscription prices. All prices are subject to change without notice. **POSTMASTER:** Send address changes to Thoracic Surgery Clinics, Elsevier Health Sciences Division, Subscription Customer Service, 3251 Riverport Lane, Maryland Heights, MO 63043. **Customer Service (orders, claims, online, change of address): Telephone: 1-800-654-2452 (U.S. and Canada); 314-447-8871 (outside U.S. and Canada). Fax: 314-447-8029. E-mail: journalscustomerservice-usa@elsevier.com (for print support); journalsonlinesupport-usa@elsevier.com (for online support).**

Reprints. For copies of 100 or more, of articles in this publication, please contact Commercial Rights Department, Elsevier Inc., 360 Park Avenue South, New York, NY 10010-1710. Tel: 212-633-3874; Fax: 212-633-3820; E-mail: reprints@elsevier.com.

Thoracic Surgery Clinics is covered in *MEDLINE/PubMed (Index Medicus), EMBASE/Excerpta Medica, Science Citation Index Expanded (SciSearch®), Journal Citation Reports/Science Edition,* and *Current Contents®/Clinical Medicine*.

Contributors

CONSULTING EDITOR

VIRGINIA R. LITLE, MD, FACS
Section Chief of Thoracic Surgery, Cardiovascular Surgery, Medical Director of Thoracic Surgery, Intermountain Healthcare, Murray, Utah, USA

EDITOR

GITA N. MODY, MD, MPH, FACS
Director of Thoracic Surgical Oncology, Assistant Professor of Surgery, Division of Cardiothoracic Surgery, Department of Surgery, The University of North Carolina at Chapel Hill, Chapel Hill, North Carolina, USA

AUTHORS

BARNABAS TOBI ALAYANDE, MBBS, MBA, FMCS
University of Global Health Equity Kigali Heights, Kigali, Rwanda; Program in Global Surgery and Social Change, Harvard Medical School, Boston, Massachusetts, USA

APURVA ASHOK, MS
Division of Thoracic Surgery, Department of Surgical Oncology, Tata Memorial Centre, Homi Bhabha National Institute, Tata Memorial Hospital, Mumbai, India

JUN ATSUMI, MD, PhD
Thoracic Surgeon, Section of Chest Surgery, Fukujuji Hospital, Japan Anti Tuberculosis Association, Tokyo, Japan

DANIEL R. BACON, MD
General Surgery Resident, Department of Surgery, The Ohio State University School of Medicine, Columbus, Ohio, USA

ALEMAYEHU GINBO BEDADA, MD, FACS
Department of Surgery, Faculty of Medicine, Princess Marina Hospital, University of Botswana, Gaborone, Botswana

ABEBE BEKELE, MD, FACS, FCS (ECSA)
Professor of Surgery, University of Global Health Equity Kigali Heights, Kigali, Rwanda; Addis Ababa University, Addis Ababa, Ethiopia

BENOIT JACQUES BIBAS, MD
Division of Thoracic Surgery, Instituto do Coracao, Hospital das Clinicas HCFMUSP, Faculdade de Medicina, Universidade de Sao Paulo, Hospital Israelita Albert Einstein, Hospital Municipal Vila Santa Catarina, Sao Paulo, Sao Paulo, Brazil

ANTHONY CHARLES, MD, MPH
Department of Surgery, The University of North Carolina at Chapel Hill, Chapel Hill, North Carolina, USA; Kamuzu Central Hospital, Lilongwe, Malawi

MARIANA RODRIGUES CREMONESE, MD
Division of Thoracic Surgery, Instituto do Coracao, Hospital das Clinicas HCFMUSP, Faculdade de Medicina, Universidade de Sao Paulo, Sao Paulo, Sao Paulo, Brazil

FAROUK DAKO, MD, MPH
Department of Radiology, University of Pennsylvania, University of Pennsylvania Health System, Philadelphia, Pennsylvania, USA

THOMAS M. DANIEL, MD
Professor Emeritus of Thoracic Surgery, Coordinator for International Teaching of Simulation Surgery, Department of Surgery, University of Virginia School of Medicine, Charlottesville, Virginia, USA

ABIGAIL M. FELSTED, BS
Global Surgery Education Scholar, Department of Surgery, University of Utah, Center for Global Surgery, Salt Lake City, Utah, USA

CHRIS HAIR, FRACP, MBBS, BSc, AMICDA
University Hospital, Epworth Private Hospital, Geelong, Australia; Deakin University, Waurn Ponds, Australia; ANZGITA, Melbourne, Australia

MIYAKO HIRAMATSU, MD, PhD
Thoracic Surgeon, Section of Chest Surgery, Fukujuji Hospital, Japan Anti Tuberculosis Association, Tokyo, Japan

SUDHA JAYARAMAN, MD, MSc
Professor of Surgery, Director of Center for Global Surgery, Department of Surgery, University of Utah, Center for Global Surgery, Salt Lake City, Utah, USA

SABITA JIWNANI, MCh, MRCS
Division of Thoracic Surgery, Department of Surgical Oncology, Tata Memorial Centre, Homi Bhabha National Institute, Mumbai, India

RACHEL KOCH, MD
Instructor, Department of Surgery, University of Utah, Center for Global Surgery, Salt Lake City, Utah, USA

LYNNETTE TUMWINE KYOKUNDA, MBChB, MMed Anat Path, FCPath (ECSA), PhD
Department of Pathology, Faculty of Medicine, University of Botswana, Gaborone, Botswana

CLEVERSON ALEX LEITÃO, MD, MSc
Department of Radiology, Hospital de Clínicas da Universidade Federal do Paraná, Paraná, Brazil

YIHAN LIN, MD, MPH
Division of Cardiothoracic Surgery, University of Colorado School of Medicine, Aurora, Colorado, USA

VIRGINIA LITLE, MD, FACS
Section Chief of Thoracic Surgery, Cardiovascular Surgery, Medical Director of Thoracic Surgery, Intermountain Healthcare, Murray, Utah, USA

HENRY LIZI, ACO, BSA, BAI (Bachelor of Science in Anesthesia and Intensive Care)
Kamuzu University of Health Sciences, Blantyre, Malawi

ROBERT LUKANDE, MB ChB, PGD (Computer Sc), MMed(Path), FCPath (ECSA)
Department of Pathology, College of Health Sciences, Makerere University, Kampala, Uganda

DAN A. MILNER, Jr, MD, MSc(Epi), MBA, FASCP
Chief Medical Officer, American Society for Clinical Pathology, Chicago, Illinois, USA; Adjunct Professor, Harvard T. H. Chan School of Public Health, Boston, Massachusetts, USA

MONICA MIRANDA-SCHAEUBINGER, MD, MSPH
Department of Radiology, Children's Hospital of Philadelphia, Philadelphia, Pennsylvania, USA

JOHN D. MITCHELL, MD
Division of Cardiothoracic Surgery, University of Colorado School of Medicine, Aurora, Colorado, USA

GITA N. MODY, MD, MPH, FACS
Director of Thoracic Surgical Oncology, Assistant Professor of Surgery, Division of Cardiothoracic Surgery, Department of Surgery, The University of North Carolina at Chapel Hill, Chapel Hill, North Carolina, USA

GIFT MULIMA, MBBS, FCS(ecsa)
Kamuzu Central Hospital, Lilongwe, Malawi

BRYANT A. MURPHY, MD, MBA
Professor of Anesthesiology, Senior Associate Dean for Leadership Development, Department of Anesthesiology, University of North Carolina School of Medicine, Chapel Hill, North Carolina, USA

MICHAEL MWACHIRO, MBChB, MPH
Tenwek Hospital, Bomet, Kenya

EDMOND NTAGANDA, MD, MMed, FCS (ECSA) ECSA
Consultant Pediatric Surgeon, Centre Hospitalier Universitaire de Kigali (CHUK), Kigali, Rwanda; Assistant Professor of Surgery, Loma Linda University School of Medicine, San Bernando, California, USA

EILEEN S. NATUZZI, MD, MPH
Solomon Islands Country Coordinator, ANZGITA, San Diego, California, USA

ABASS NOOR, MD
Department of Radiology, University of Pennsylvania, University of Pennsylvania Health System, Philadelphia, Pennsylvania, USA

HANSEL J. OTERO, MD
Department of Radiology, Children's Hospital of Philadelphia, Philadelphia, Pennsylvania, USA

PAULO HENRIQUE PEITL-GREGORIO, MD
Division of Thoracic Surgery, Instituto do Coracao, Hospital das Clinicas HCFMUSP, Faculdade de Medicina, Universidade de Sao Paulo, Sao Paulo, Sao Paulo, Brazil

PRASANTH PENUMADU, MS, MCh
Department of Surgical Oncology, Jawaharlal Institute of Medical Education and Research, JIPMER, Gorimedu, Pondicherry, India

JANEY R. PHELPS, MD
Professor of Anesthesiology and Pediatrics, Department of Anesthesiology, University of North Carolina School of Medicine, Chapel Hill, North Carolina, USA

SILVIA PORTILLA, MD
Department of Anesthesia, María Auxiliadora Hospital, Lima, Peru

C.S. PRAMESH, MS, FRCS
Director, Division of Thoracic Surgery, Department of Surgical Oncology, Tata Memorial Centre, Homi Bhabha National Institute, Tata Memorial Hospital, Mumbai, India

NOBHOJIT ROY, MD, MPH, PhD
Lancet Commissioner, WHO Collaborating Centre for Research on Surgical Care Delivery in LMICs, Mumbai, India; The George Institute of Global Health, New Delhi, India

RANJAN SAPKOTA, MBBS, MS, MCh
Manmohan Cardio-Thoracic Vascular and Transplant Center, Institute of Medicine, Department of Cardio-Thoracic and Vascular Surgery, Kathmandu, Nepal

YUJI SHIRAISHI, MD, PhD
Thoracic Surgeon, Section of Chest Surgery, Fukujuji Hospital, Japan Anti Tuberculosis Association, Tokyo, Japan

ALFREDO SOTOMAYOR, MD
Department of Thoracic and Cardiovascular Surgery, Hipólito Unanue National Hospital, Lima, Peru

ROBINSON SSEBUUFU, MB, ChB, MMed (Surgery), FCS (ECSA)
Uganda Medical and Dental Practitioners Council (UMDPC), Kampala, Uganda

RICARDO MINGARINI TERRA, MD, PhD
Division of Thoracic Surgery, Instituto do Coracao, Hospital das Clinicas HCFMUSP, Faculdade de Medicina, Universidade de Sao Paulo, Hospital Israelita Albert Einstein, Sao Paulo, Sao Paulo, Brazil

BIBHUSAL THAPA, MBBS, MS, PhD
Thoracic Surgery Unit, Division of Surgery, Northern Hospital, Melbourne, Australia

DOMINIQUE VERVOORT, MD, MPH, MBA
Institute of Health Policy, Management and Evaluation, University of Toronto, Toronto, Ontario, Canada

SARGUN VIRK, MBBS
Global Surgery Fellow, Sri Guru Ram Das Institute of Medical Sciences and Research, Amritsar, India; WHO Collaborating Centre for Research on Surgical Care Delivery in LMICs, Mumbai, India

RUSSELL WHITE, MD, MPH
Tenwek Hospital, Bomet, Kenya; Warren Alpert School of Medicine, Brown University, Providence, Rhode Island, USA

BRITTNEY M. WILLIAMS, MD, MPH
Department of Surgery, The University of North Carolina at Chapel Hill, Chapel Hill, North Carolina, USA

ELIZABETH HA'UPALA WORE, MD, MBBS/MMED
Internal Medicine Consultant, Co-chair of Solomon Islands Endoscopy Program, National Referral Hospital, Honiara, Solomon Islands

Contents

Foreword: Think Globally, Act Globally xiii

Virginia R. Litle

Preface: Global Health Equity: A Vision for Engaging Thoracic Surgeons xv

Gita N. Mody

Surgical Capacity Building in Low- and Middle-Income Countries: Lessons for Thoracic Surgery 269

Rachel Koch, Abigail M. Felsted, Sargun Virk, Nobhojit Roy, and Sudha Jayaraman

There is great need for intentional investment in capacity building for thoracic surgical conditions. This article provides a brief overview of thoracic surgical capacity building for low- and middle-income countries using the Lancet framework of infrastructure, workforce, financing, and information management. The authors highlight the needs, opportunities, and challenges that are relevant for the thoracic surgical community, as it aims to increase care for patients with these conditions globally.

Teaching Thoracic Surgery in a Low-Resource Setting: Creation of a Simulation Curriculum in Rwanda 279

Edmond Ntaganda, Robinson Ssebuufu, Daniel R. Bacon, and Thomas M. Daniel

Surgical education and global health partnerships have evolved over the years. There is growing recognition of the importance of in-country training of surgeons and surgeon specialists in low-resource settings to support the local health care system. There are numerous ways in which high-income partners can support local training programs. The Human Resources for Health program was initiated in 2012 to advance in-country training of health care professionals in Rwanda. As there was a limited in-country operative experience for teaching general thoracic surgery, simulation models were developed, influenced by a prior course developed for American cardiothoracic trainees. Local Rwandan faculty were engaged. Adaptations from the American version included constructing models from inexpensive materials to make the simulation more feasible in the Rwanda setting.

Radiology for Thoracic Conditions in Low- and Middle-Income Countries 289

Monica Miranda-Schaeubinger, Abass Noor, Cleverson Alex Leitão, Hansel J. Otero, and Farouk Dako

With a disproportionately high burden of global morbidity and mortality caused by chronic respiratory diseases (CRDs) in low and middle-income countries (LMICs), access to radiological services is of critical importance for screening, diagnosis, and treatment guidance.

Pathology for Thoracic Conditions in Low- and Middle-Income Countries 299

Robert Lukande, Lynnette Tumwine Kyokunda, Alemayehu Ginbo Bedada, and Dan Milner Jr.

Pulmonary disease in low- and middle-income countries is highly diverse and dependent on the population, background epidemiology, environmental exposures, and smoking status. Credible evaluation of lung diseases requires skilled clinicians, imaging infrastructure, microbiology, and pathologic diagnostics, including imaging-guided cytology and biopsy. When these tools are available, improvement in patient outcomes is feasible. Pathologic diagnostics of lung lesions, including histology, immunohistochemistry, and molecular testing, are critical to properly stratify patient risk and determine exact therapies for each patient. A critical focus on research and directed interventions in lung cancer treatment specifically is needed to downstage this disease and improve patient outcome.

Anesthesia for Global General Thoracic Surgery **307**

Janey R. Phelps, Henry Lizi, and Bryant A. Murphy

Anesthesia in low-to-middle income countries (LMICs) is often provided by nonphysician anesthetists. The training and resources for anesthesia in LMICs are limited, and this must be evaluated when starting or expanding a thoracic surgery program in LMICs. The ability to access a patient's baseline pulmonary and cardiovascular status is often based on rudimentary studies and a thorough history and physical. Advance studies, such as echocardiograms, cardiovascular stress test, cardiac catherizations, pulmonary function tests, and MRIs, are often not available. Careful assessment of both preoperative patient selection, intraoperative ability to provide one-lung ventilation, and postoperative critical care management must be considered when surgical planning is occurring.

Development of an Endoscopy Training Partnership in a Developing Country **317**

Eileen S. Natuzzi, Chris Hair, Elizabeth Ha'upala Wore, and Virginia Litle

Gastrointestinal and pulmonary disease is prevalent in many developing countries. Establishing an endoscopy training partnership can transfer skills that can influence policy and stakeholder support to address disease morbidity and mortality. Any new program needs to consider the environmental services that will be delivered and give consideration to the sustainability of the program over time. This article outlines what we have learned from our training partnership in the Pacific Islands Region.

Chest Trauma Management in Low- and Middle-Income Countries **329**

Brittney M. Williams, Gift Mulima, and Anthony Charles

Trauma is a leading cause of death and disability worldwide and disproportionately affects those in low- and middle-income countries (LMICs). Globally, two-thirds of injured patients sustain trauma to the thoracic cavity. Further research, capacity building, and increased awareness are needed to limit the high thoracic trauma-associated morbidity and mortality in LMICs.

Surgical Management of Mycobacterial Infections and Related Complex Pleural Space Problems: From History to Modern Day **337**

Miyako Hiramatsu, Jun Atsumi, and Yuji Shiraishi

Owing to the advent of effective drugs for tuberculosis in the mid-twentieth century, few cases require surgery for active tuberculosis in the present day in areas where effective drugs are available. However, surgical techniques developed to combat tuberculosis in the predrug era are still useful to manage the challenging chest pathology of our time surgically, such as destroyed lung or postresectional empyema. Thoracoplasty and open window thoracostomy are representative procedures and discussed in detail in this review.

Management of Pulmonary Hydatidosis and Lung Abscess in Low-Resource Settings **349**

Alfredo Sotomayor, Silvia Portilla, and Gita N. Mody

In the modern era, infections of the lung are typically managed medically. However, all pulmonary hydatid cysts require surgery with rare exceptions, and bacterial abscesses require surgery if they are complicated, resistant to treatment, and/or large. Surgical treatment of these pulmonary conditions requires clinical knowledge of tests for causative organisms, perioperative antimicrobial therapies, options for surgical management, and postoperative care.

Management of Empyema Thoracis in Low-Resource Settings **361**

Abebe Bekele and Barnabas Tobi Alayande

Most cases of empyema thoracis are sequelae of severe pneumonia, but chest trauma and complications of chest tube insertion as cause are not uncommon in low-resource settings. Diagnosis is usually delayed due to delayed presentation to health care facilities, low index of suspicion among health care professionals, and inability to properly stage the disease with the available diagnostic tools. Early use of antibiotics and appropriate-sized and well-placed chest tube drainage is associated with good outcomes at a decreased cost. Surgical management of empyema thoracis is indicated when chest tube drainage and antibiotic treatment fail to achieve complete resolution.

Tracheobronchial Surgery in Emerging Countries **373**

Benoit Jacques Bibas, Paulo Henrique Peitl-Gregorio, Mariana Rodrigues Cremonese, and Ricardo Mingarini Terra

Tracheobronchial surgery is widely performed in emerging countries mainly as a consequence of the high number of airway-related complications and poor management in intensive care units. This has led to great expertise in the surgical management of postintubation tracheal stenosis, and opportunity for advancing scientific knowledge. Nonetheless, tracheal stenosis has a severe impact on a patient's quality of life, is a major burden to the health system, and should be prevented. Incorporation of innovative techniques, technologies, and prospective databases should prompt earlier diagnosis and lead to fewer complications.

Lung Cancer Management in Low and Middle-Income Countries **383**

Sabita Jiwnani, Prasanth Penumadu, Apurva Ashok, and C.S. Pramesh

Lung cancer is an increasing problem in the developing world due to rising trends in smoking, high incidence of air pollution, lack of awareness and screening, delayed presentation, and diagnosis at the advanced stage. Even after diagnosis, there are disparities in access to health care facilities and inequitable distribution of resources and treatment options. In addition, the shortage of trained personnel and infrastructure adds to the challenges faced by patients with lung cancer in these regions. A multi-pronged effort targeting tobacco cessation, health promotion and awareness, capacity building, and value-based care are the need of the hour.

Management of Esophageal Cancer Treatment in Resource-Limited Settings **397**

Michael Mwachiro and Russell White

Due to the luminal nature of the disease, esophageal cancer diagnosis and treatment is challenging. Majority of the patients usually present with dysphagia, at which point the disease is often locally advanced. Diagnosis and treatment need a multidisciplinary approach which often involves endoscopy, imaging services, oncology services, surgical services, and critical care services. Surgery is associated with significant morbidity and mortality and care should be domiciled in high-volume centers. Training and mentorship are key to building capacity for esophageal cancer care.

Minimally Invasive Thoracic Surgery for Low- and Middle-Income Countries **405**

Yihan Lin, Dominique Vervoort, Bibhusal Thapa, Ranjan Sapkota, and John D. Mitchell

The burden of respiratory and upper-gastrointestinal diseases especially affects low- and middle-income countries. Five billion people lack access to safe, timely, and affordable surgical care, including thoracic surgical care. Minimally invasive thoracic surgery (MITS) has been shown to reduce complications, shorten hospital lengths of stay, and minimize health care costs, thereby enabling patients to pay less out-of-pocket and/or limit time away from work and families. Experiences with MITS exist but are limited in low- and middle-income countries; professional societies, academic institutions, policymakers, and industry can facilitate scale-up of MITS by increasing financing, expanding surgical training, and optimizing surgical supply chains.

THORACIC SURGERY CLINICS

FORTHCOMING ISSUES

November 2022
Esophageal Cancer
Jonathan Yeung and Elena Elimova, *Editors*

February 2023
Robotic Thoracic Surgery
Elliott L. Servais and Peter J. Smit, *Editors*

May 2023
Controversies in Thoracic Surgery
Lana Y. Schumacher and David C. Griffin, *Editors*

RECENT ISSUES

May 2022
Lung Transplantation
Jasleen Kukreja and Aida Venado, *Editors*

February 2022
Social Disparities in Thoracic Surgery
Cherie P. Erkmen, *Editor*

November 2021
Lung Cancer 2021, Part 2
Farid Shamji and Gilles Beauchamp, *Editors*

Foreword
Think Globally, Act Globally

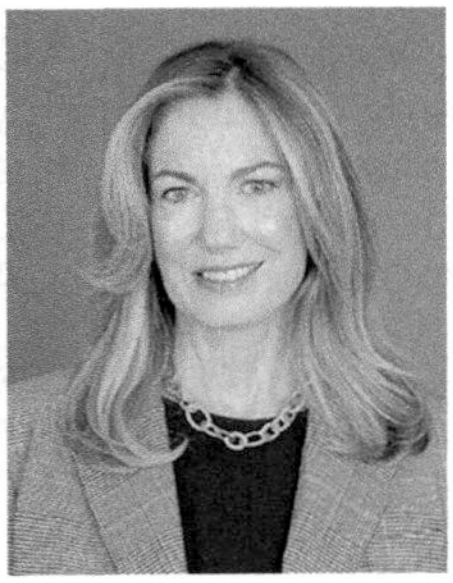

Virginia R. Litle, MD
Consulting Editor

The February 2022 issue of *Thoracic Surgery Clinics* addressed social disparities in Thoracic Surgery and covered our national diversity gaps in multiple areas, including lung cancer screening, recruitment to clinical trials, and lung transplantation donor and recipient pools. This issue of *Thoracic Surgery Clinics* concerns "Global Thoracic Surgery" and reminds us of the global disparities and needs gaps, including quite significantly a workforce shortage. Per the Lancet Commissions on Global Surgery 2030, more than 2 million surgeons, anesthetists, and obstetric providers will be needed worldwide. Global workforce disparities spill over into other integral clinicians, such as pathologists and radiologists, and aspects of infrastructure, including critical care and imaging equipment. So, we are excited to share with you the global perspective of our invited guest editor, UNC Thoracic Surgeon Gita Mody, MD, MPH. Dr Mody has brought together a diverse set of topics and international representation in authorship. Even before graduating from medical school, Dr Mody showed interest in global health with her receipt of an International Health and Tropical Medicine fellowship from Washington University. Her global passion has blossomed, and as an academic surgeon, she currently continues outreach in Malawi and Peru, where she facilitates bidirectional learning and exchange with a network of thoracic surgeons in low-resource settings.

The predominant global surgical problem is trauma; however, as thoracic surgeons, many of us certainly manage trauma, but the majority of our practices involve lung and esophagus cancer and intrathoracic infections. Although globally 40% of lung cancer is not attributable to a smoking history, for smokers, lung cancer screening is a logistical nightmare in low- to middle-income countries (LMIC). Staging a lung cancer with appropriate imaging and endobronchial ultrasound is not feasible, but if they were available, the radiologists and pathologists are not.

What are three take-home messages from the content of this monograph? (1) Surgical capacity building with education of the local providers and institution of infrastructure is considered more sustainable than medical service trips and large donations of supplies; (2) Twinning programs with high-income-country hospitals allow for

Thorac Surg Clin 32 (2022) xiii–xiv
https://doi.org/10.1016/j.thorsurg.2022.06.001
1547-4127/22/© 2022 Published by Elsevier Inc.

more availability of subspecialty training; (3) Telepresence for histology and imaging interpretation, peer-to-peer consultations, and continued education of LMIC surgical providers can provide a significant service as Internet access allows. As educators, we can support the engagement of our trainees and faculty in outreach trips and publications with local surgeons to provide a voice to those with boots on the ground.

Thank you to all the contributors and to guest editor, Dr Mody. Please enjoy the content and use it as a compendium for addressing global differences in thoracic care beyond all that came to light with the novel coronavirus pandemic. Think globally, and in the ever-evolving complex environment of health care delivery, act globally as well. We hope you will enjoy this issue!

Sincerely,

Virginia R. Litle, MD
Cardiovascular Surgery
Intermountain Healthcare
5169 So. Cottonwood St., Ste 640
84107 Murray, UT, USA

E-mail address:
vlitle@gmail.com

Preface
Global Health Equity: A Vision for Engaging Thoracic Surgeons

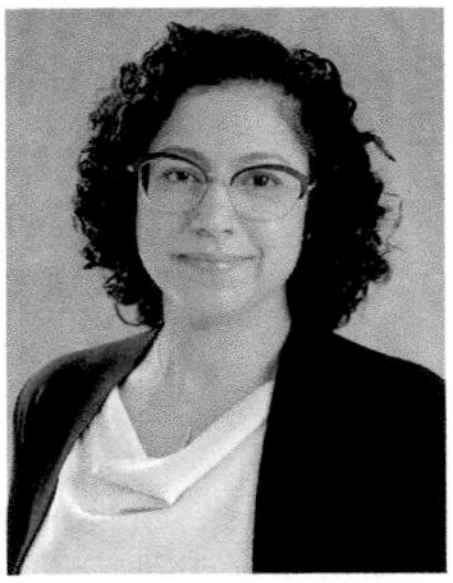

Gita N. Mody, MD, MPH, FACS
Editor

Public health priorities are evolving as increased aging populations, injuries, and mental health disorders have led to an urgent need for programs to address chronic and noncommunicable diseases.[1] Built on the infrastructure of traditional international priorities (eg, maternal and child health; infectious diseases prevention and treatment), comprehensive health system strengthening has proven fundamental to improved care delivery globally.[2] Equity in health regardless of race, income, or geography demands access to surgeons to provide more complete preventative, diagnostic, and therapeutic services. As the recent pandemic demonstrated, investments in establishing personnel and supply chains for procedural work also are crucial to global security.[3] Therefore, surgeons have an important role in leading advocacy efforts for expansion of universal health coverage and ensuring surgical care access for all.[4]

Historically, the surgical community has been deeply engaged in efforts to build, equip, and staff operating theaters that provide emergency and essential surgery. Academic faculty are increasingly involved in partnerships to improve access to surgical care, training, and innovation. Trauma surgeons have been at the forefront of several notable twinning programs given the predominance of road traffic accidents and violence as emerging countries move from low- to middle-income status.[5] Successful engagements range from short-term missions to long-term partnerships, though always with an emphasis on respectful and meaningful collaboration with the local health system and workforce.[6] These partnerships have led to important gains influencing policy and strategy at national and international levels, which are necessary to promote cost-effectiveness and sustainability.[7]

Advances in technology have led to a revolution in the approach to surgical capacity building globally. These include reliable supply chains for essential medications,[8] novel affordable medical device designs,[9] and digital health solutions including telemedicine for procedural support.[10] While the COVID-19 pandemic curtailed travel, increased support for virtual meetings has facilitated partnerships previously limited by distance and finances, including multinational collaborations.[11] Such improvements set the stage for subspecialty surgeons to contribute to developing local multidisciplinary expertise in ancillary services for diagnostics (radiology, pathology), intraoperative care (anesthesia, transfusion medicine, hybrid ORs), and postoperative management (acute critical and long-term care). Old hurdles are now supplanted by new challenges, including retention of skilled human resources, electronic data management, and developing systems-based approaches for efficiency, quality assurance, and research.[12]

Thorac Surg Clin 32 (2022) xv–xvii
https://doi.org/10.1016/j.thorsurg.2022.05.002
1547-4127/22/© 2022 Published by Elsevier Inc.

The delivery of thoracic surgical care in less-resourced areas is explored in this landmark series of articles. There is a notable diversity across the settings in which the authors work (South Asia, East Asia, Sub-Saharan Africa, Pacific Islands, South America). Common themes include the need for human resources to deliver care and train surgeons resourcefully (Koch and colleagues, Ntaganda and colleagues) and the importance of collaborations with radiology (Miranda-Schaeubinger and colleagues), pathology (Lukande and colleagues), anesthesia (Phelps and colleagues), and endoscopy services (Natuzzi and colleagues). Articles on benign conditions, including chest trauma (Williams and colleagues), mycobacterial diseases (Hiramatsu and colleagues), parasitic infections (Sotomayor and colleagues), pleural problems (Bekele and Alayande), and airway stenosis (Bibas and colleagues), provide an outstanding review of management and technique and are a testament to the long history of thoracic surgeons' leadership. Thoracic surgical oncology services for the high-burden conditions of lung cancer (Jiwnani and colleagues) and esophageal cancer (Mwachiro and White) are the next priority in these settings. Finally, the potential of minimally invasive thoracic surgery to rapidly improve outcomes will serve as a cornerstone for future learning collaboratives between our professional societies across continents (Lin and colleagues).

This vision for thoracic surgeons' engagement in global health equity is driven by a deep sense of service to our patients across the world. I am inspired by the authors, many of whom I have met through my international humanitarian and academic work. I am extremely thankful to Virginia Litle, who is a champion for disparities reduction domestically and internationally as well as to Jessica Cañaberal at Elsevier for her tremendous support of this issue. I would like to specifically acknowledge my trainees both locally and globally (Danielle O'Hara, University of North Carolina, USA; Diego La Torre Rodriguez, Universidad Peruana Cayetano Heredia, Peru; Benson Khobidi, Kamuzu Central Hospital, Malawi) for their assistance with editing the submissions. They are the future of global thoracic surgery, and their energy and drive are endless. Finally, I am humbled by the legacy of two men. My father was a physician in Uganda before immigrating, and his work alongside community leaders was deeply formative to him and by extension to me. Later, reading notable books by Paul Farmer on his mission and methods inspired me to work in Rwanda, Haiti, and Peru. As Dr. Farmer once told me, "*A chance to cut is a chance to cure.*" Now is the chance for thoracic surgeons to expand their borders and share their unique contributions to the discipline of surgery with the broader global community.

Gita N. Mody, MD, MPH, FACS
Division of Cardiothoracic Surgery
Department of Surgery
Department of Cardiothoracic Surgery
The University of North Carolina at Chapel Hill
Burnett-Womack Building
Suite 3041, Campus Box 7065
Chapel Hill, NC 27599-7065, USA

E-mail address:
gita_mody@med.unc.edu

REFERENCES

1. GBD 2019 Diseases and Injuries Collaborators. Global burden of 369 diseases and injuries in 204 countries and territories, 1990-2019: a systematic analysis for the Global Burden of Disease Study 2019. Lancet 2020;396(10258):1204–22. https://doi.org/10.1016/S0140-6736(20)30925-9 Erratum in: Lancet 2020;396(10262):1562. PMID: 33069326; PMCID: PMC7567026.
2. Hemingway CD, Bella Jalloh M, Silumbe R, et al. Pursuing health systems strengthening through disease-specific programme grants: experiences in Tanzania and Sierra Leone. BMJ Glob Health 2021; 6(10):e006615. https://doi.org/10.1136/bmjgh-2021-006615 PMID: 34615662; PMCID: PMC8496380.
3. Saha A, Alleyne G. Recognizing noncommunicable diseases as a global health security threat. Bull World Health Organ 2018;96(11):792–3. https://doi.org/10.2471/BLT.17.205732 Epub 2018 Oct 1. PMID: 30455534; PMCID: PMC6239014.
4. Reddy CL, Vervoort D, Meara JG, et al. Surgery and universal health coverage: designing an essential package for surgical care expansion and scale-up. J Glob Health 2020;10(2):020341. https://doi.org/10.7189/jogh.10.02034.
5. Riviello R, Ozgediz D, Hsia RY, et al. Role of collaborative academic partnerships in surgical training, education, and provision. World J Surg 2010;34(3): 459–65. https://doi.org/10.1007/s00268-009-0360-4.
6. Jedrzejko N, Margolick J, Nguyen JH, et al. A systematic review of global surgery partnerships and a proposed framework for sustainability. Can J Surg 2021;64(3):E280–8. https://doi.org/10.1503/cjs.010719 PMID: 33908733; PMCID: PMC8327986.
7. Peters AW, Roa L, Rwamasirabo E, et al. National surgical, obstetric, and anesthesia plans supporting the vision of universal health coverage. Glob Health Sci Pract 2020;8(1):1–9. https://doi.org/10.9745/GHSP-D-19-00314 Published 2020 Mar 31.
8. Shafiq N, Pandey AK, Malhotra S, et al. Shortage of essential antimicrobials: a major challenge to global

health security. BMJ Glob Health 2021;6(11):e006961. https://doi.org/10.1136/bmjgh-2021-006961 PMID: 34728479; PMCID: PMC8565534.

9. Mody GN, Mutabazi V, Zurovcik DR, et al. Design, testing, and scale-up of medical devices for global health: negative pressure wound therapy and non-surgical male circumcision in Rwanda. Global Health 2015;11:20. https://doi.org/10.1186/s12992-015-0101-4 PMID: 25963175; PMCID: PMC4446067.
10. Mbunge E, Batani J, Gaobotse G, et al. Virtual healthcare services and digital health technologies deployed during coronavirus disease 2019 (COVID-19) pandemic in South Africa: a systematic review. Glob Health J 2022. https://doi.org/10.1016/j.glohj.2022.03.001. Epub ahead of print. PMID: 35282399; PMCID: PMC8897959.
11. Goh S, Wong RSM, Quah ELY, et al. Mentoring in palliative medicine in the time of COVID-19: a systematic scoping review: mentoring programs during COVID-19. BMC Med Educ 2022;22(1):359. https://doi.org/10.1186/s12909-022-03409-4 PMID: 35545787; PMCID: PMC9094135.
12. Sawe HR, Reynolds TA, Weber EJ, et al. Development and pilot implementation of a standardised trauma documentation form to inform a national trauma registry in a low-resource setting: lessons from Tanzania. BMJ Open 2020;10(10):e038022. https://doi.org/10.1136/bmjopen-2020-038022 PMID: 33033093; PMCID: PMC7545631.

Surgical Capacity Building in Low- and Middle-Income Countries: Lessons for Thoracic Surgery

Rachel Koch, MD[a,b,*], Abigail M. Felsted, BS[a,b], Sargun Virk, MBBS[c,d], Nobhojit Roy, MD, MPH, PhD[d,e], Sudha Jayaraman, MD, MSc[a,b]

KEYWORDS

• Capacity building • Thoracic surgery • Partnerships

KEY POINTS

- The paradigm of global surgical activities has changed from a focus on service delivery to one that aims to strengthen surgical systems and improve access to high-quality care at the population level.
- Capacity building for thoracic surgical services requires investments in service delivery, workforce, financing, and information management.
- COVID-19 pandemic has highlighted challenges and encouraged locally relevant solutions that can enable availability of thoracic surgical care.
- Partnerships can lead to effective strategies to build surgical capacity through education, research, and innovation.

TRIBUTE TO NORMAN BETHUNE

Norman Bethune was a pioneering thoracic surgeon and member of the American Association for Thoracic Surgery in the 1930s.[1] He also could be considered a pioneer in surgical capacity building. During the Spanish civil war, he invented the first front-line mobile blood transfusion unit in military medical history, which delivered blood to every military sector along a 1000 km front.[2] As Commander of the Chinese medical troops for the communist party's military force in the second Sino-Japanese conflict, he renovated existing hospital facilities and created a model hospital in a Buddhist temple. After witnessing the shortage of health care personnel in rural areas, he established "Barefoot physicians": young peasants and laborers to whom he taught basic anatomy and physiology.[3] These workers became a necessary component of China's health care system and promoted health care equity and universal health. No article on global surgery and thoracic care would be complete without acknowledging the immense worldwide impact he had, and thus the authors dedicate this article to Dr Bethune in an attempt to recognize his accomplishments at building infrastructure, health care delivery systems, and workforce nearly a century before global surgery became an academic field.

INTRODUCTION

Strategies for surgical capacity building in low- and middle-income countries (LMICs) have changed over time to focus on strengthening surgical systems instead of service delivery. Historically, visiting teams or the occasional full-time expatriate have sporadically provided surgical care in LMICs and sometimes using donated equipment. Such short-term mission trips focused

[a] Department of Surgery, University of Utah, 30 North 1900 East, Room 3C344, Salt Lake City, UT 84132, USA; [b] University of Utah, Center for Global Surgery, Salt Lake City, UT, USA; [c] Sri Guru Ram Das Institute of Medical Sciences and Research, 18- A Tagore Nagar, Civil Lines, Ludhiana, Punjab 141001, India; [d] WHO Collaborating Centre for Research on Surgical Care Delivery in LMICs, Mumbai, India; [e] The George Institute for Global Health, 308, Third Floor, Elegance Tower, Plot No. 8, Jasola District Centre, New Delhi 110025, India
* Corresponding author. University of Utah, 30 North 1900 East, Room 3C344, Salt Lake City, UT 84132.
E-mail address: Rachel.koch@hsc.utah.edu

Thorac Surg Clin 32 (2022) 269–278
https://doi.org/10.1016/j.thorsurg.2022.02.003
1547-4127/22/

on addressing a backlog of surgical cases in one locale[4] but are not cost-effective, often lack follow-up, and create a form of dependency without building local capacity.[5,6] Those who formed longer term relationships offered greater reliability but were limited to a specific location.[7]

In 2014, the Lancet Commission on Global Surgery in 2014 found that 143 million additional surgical procedures per year were needed in order to meet the surgical burden of disease and that investing in surgical services is affordable and in fact promotes economic growth[8]; this encouraged a philosophic transition to promote sustainable surgical systems across partnerships between institutions in LMICs and high-income countries (HICs)—instead of service delivery.[9–11] The Lancet Commission recommended work in several areas to strengthen surgical systems—health care delivery and management, education and training of the workforce, information management and financing—and proposed 6 key indicators (**Fig. 1**) to assess a country's capability to deliver surgical services, ensure high quality of care, and support financial risk protection. These data, once collected, can be used to inform national plans to deliver essential and emergency surgical care.[12]

In this article, the authors discuss thoracic surgical capacity-building using the Lancet framework and discuss opportunities and challenges to support delivery of thoracic surgical care globally.

SCOPE AND NEEDS IN THORACIC SURGICAL CARE IN LOW- AND MIDDLE-INCOME COUNTRIES

To deliver high-quality thoracic surgical care, policy makers in LMICs must understand the disease priorities in their specific settings. Cancer, infections, and trauma are all common causes of operative thoracic pathology but differ in epidemiologic characteristics in various contexts. Lung cancer, the most common type of cancer worldwide, causes significantly higher mortality in LMICs compared with HICs due to delays in presentation, little access to diagnostic technology, and lack of systems for treatment.[13–15] Similarly, patients with esophageal cancer that is endemic in southern and eastern Africa and eastern Asia often present late and at an advanced stage. Mesothelioma from asbestos exposure remains a threat particularly in resource-limited countries without strict asbestos bans. Infectious complications of tuberculosis and pneumonia such as hemoptysis and empyema and chest trauma form the remaining burden of thoracic surgical disease in LMICs.[16,17] Clinicians and policy makers who recognize these unique factors and barriers to the standard care offered in HICs, but not yet available consistently across LMICs, can develop appropriate context-specific guidelines and pathways for early detection, diagnosis, treatment and surveillance as well as policies to address the epidemiologic factors. Local and regional needs assessments thus lay a critical foundation for optimal care delivery through systematic planning between stakeholders.[18] Several multidisciplinary collaborations on lung cancer and chronic obstructive pulmonary disease have already outlined strategies to improve access to thoracic care, which could be excellent models for the thoracic community to follow, as it works to address the massive, inequitable burden of thoracic surgical diseases worldwide.[14,19]

HEALTH CARE INFRASTRUCTURE FOR THORACIC SURGICAL SERVICES

High-quality surgical care requires substantial but basic infrastructure. Hospitals need well-equipped operating theaters and intensive care units (ICU)[20,21] and reliable water, electricity, and sanitation services.[22] Most thoracic procedures must be performed under general anesthesia, which requires sufficient medical gas supply, anesthesia machines, and ventilators for postoperative care. However, the COVID-19 pandemic has highlighted that more than half of LMICs lack a constant supply of oxygen, never mind staff skilled in intubation and ventilator management or adequate ICU capacity.[23,24] There are many causes of this shortage—faulty or absent equipment, lack of protocols to ensure safety, and technical handling of such equipment among other reasons.[24,25] These deficiencies have led the World Health Organization (WHO) and other major global entities to advocate for and invest in innovative solutions to build this critical infrastructure.[26,27] Efforts by donors and policy organizations have led Air Liquide and Linde, 2 of the world's leading medical oxygen providers, to commit to tackling the shortage in oxygen demand and supply in LMICs.[28] Another project in Gambia and Fiji created an innovative solar power storage system to enable reliable oxygen services.[26] Innovation has also led to development of cost-effective ventilators.[27,29] Such increases in physical infrastructure will transform the ability of health systems to deliver care for thoracic surgical diseases as well as other communicable respiratory conditions in the future.

Radiology, pathology, and laboratory services and a blood bank are essential clinical adjuncts for thoracic surgical care. A Lancet Commission on Diagnostics found that 47% of the global population has little to no access to diagnostics, and in

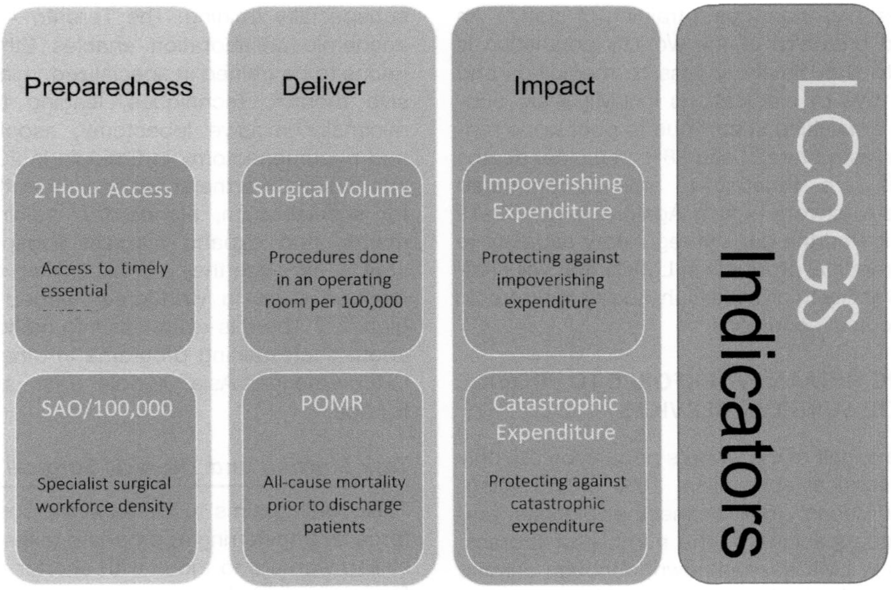

Fig. 1. 2014 lancet commission on global surgery indicators. (*Courtesy of* John G. Meara, MD, DMD, MBA, Boston, MA.)

LMICs only 19% of the population has access to basic essential diagnostic tests such as complete blood count, radiography, and ultrasound.[30] Expensive diagnostics such as high-resolution computed tomography (CT) scans and MRI are often unavailable, inaccessible, or unreliable across public and private health facilities. For example, there is less than one CT scanner per million people in LMICs.[31] Point-of-care ultrasound units provide a low-cost diagnostic alternative for some conditions but are inadequate for evaluating many thoracic conditions. A reliable supply chain to obtain pathology and laboratory consumables can be a challenge.[32] Blood banking capabilities are essential to thoracic surgical services—both elective (cardiothoracic) and emergency (trauma)—but major challenges to blood availability, quality, transfusion safety, and appropriate usage exist worldwide.[33,34] Missing or unreliable clinical adjuncts represent major limitations to diagnosing and treating thoracic conditions such as diaphragmatic injuries and malignancies.[31]

Many solutions have been proposed to address these fundamental infrastructure deficits, but investment has been sporadic. Donated imaging equipment is not a sustainable solution: one study found that almost 47% of donated imaging equipment is nonfunctional,[24,35] and frequently, there are no trained experts to maintain or repair them. The WHO has encouraged development of the WHIS-RAD radiography equipment specifically for LMICs, which can be operated where power is unreliable for extended periods of time, but it has not yet been widely adopted worldwide. Countries that have focused on addressing these needs serve as models for LMICs. In 2007, the Ethiopian government built a uniform national laboratory logistics system to meet the needs of individual laboratories, resulting in a decrease in patients' test wait times from 2 to 3 months to less than a day after the program began, addressing a well-known delay in diagnosis.[36] The Indian government has built an Internet portal called e-Rakt Kosh, which consolidates blood availability into a single online window, to ensure enough supply in blood banks,[37] and the Ministry of Health of Rwanda has increased blood availability nationwide, thanks to drone-based blood delivery.[38] Kamuzu Central Hospital in Malawi has recently established the country's first pathology laboratory in collaboration with the University of North Carolina.[39] These examples of slow but real progress in infrastructure development highlight potential opportunities for multidisciplinary partnerships between surgeons, radiologists, pathologists, and pharmacists as well as supply chain and health system leaders to build capacity for thoracic surgical care.

Lastly, treatment of thoracic surgical conditions requires reliable supply chains for medications. Access to essential drugs for pain relief are limited for many reasons including regulatory and legal constraints, cultural restrictions, procurement difficulties, and inadequate training of staff.[40] An estimated one-third of the world's population is thought to lack timely access to medicines and at least 10% of medications in LMICs are substandard or falsified in part due to poor or no regulatory infrastructure,[41] and 88% of cancer deaths worldwide are thought to involve untreated moderate-to-severe pain.[40] Again, the COVID-19 has highlighted the gaps in regulatory capacity to approve medical products in LMICs that will challenge the ability to provide high-quality for thoracic or any medical conditions.[42]

TRAINING HUMAN WORKFORCE TO PROVIDE THORACIC SURGICAL SERVICES

LMICs have half of the world's population but only 20% of surgical specialists: 19% of physician-trained surgeons, 15% of anesthesiologists, and 29% of obstetricians.[43] The number of thoracic surgeons in LMICs is unknown; although cardiac surgery is slowly becoming a subspecialty in many countries.[44] Thoracic surgeons are not separately trained or counted. Global initiatives following the Lancet Commission call to action have sought to collect data on surgical workforce and develop strategies to increase it in LMICs.[45] The shortage is likely severe. For example, the surgical training capacity in Ethiopia has increased from 1 to 8 programs from 2004 to 2014,[46] yet there are only 4 thoracic surgeons in the country[47] for a population of 92 million. By comparison, there are 1.42 thoracic surgeons per 100,000 in the United States (2005 figures[48]).

Training Thoracic Surgeons Through Partnerships

Residency programs such as the Pan-African Academy of Christian Surgeons (PAACS) and the College of Surgeons of East, Central and Southern Africa (COSECSA) have made great strides in training surgeons and have achieved retention of 79% to 100% of their graduates returning to their home countries.[49,50] However, the number of funded positions in these programs remains inadequate to cover the volume of surgeons needed. There are only 0.53 surgeons per 100,000 in the COSECSA region currently, and there are no data on thoracic surgeons in the area.[50,51] There are few thoracic surgical training positions in LMICs so surgeons often must seek subspecialty training outside their home country. One of the few fellowships in Eastern Africa was established in 2018 at Tenwek hospital in Nairobi to address the regional burden of thoracic disease.[52]

Twinning programs, which link hospitals in HICs with those in LMICs,[53] can increase availability of subspecialty training. The Toronto Addis Ababa academic collaboration enables Ethiopian surgeons to be trained in specialized, minimally invasive thoracic techniques, leading to the first minimally invasive lobectomy, esophagectomy, and pneumonectomy in Ethiopia in 2016.[47] Such international partnerships can meet the demand for specialization, standardize training environments, and expand surgical subspecialties in LMICs, although they are still unlikely to meet the massive gaps in workforce needed in the region.[50,54] There is even less information available about such training programs in other regions—Latin America, Asia, Middle East, and Eastern Europe.

Task Shifting and Thoracic Surgical Care

Task shifting aims to increase the surgical workforce by transferring appropriate tasks from highly skilled workers to those with shorter training and fewer credentials who are educated through procedural-based instruction.[55] For example, nonphysician staff may be trained how to perform certain life-saving procedures such as tube thoracostomy.[56] The authors outline a hypothetical example of applying task-shifting to thoracic surgery in **Table 1**. Such transfer of labor is already common throughout many LMICs due to massive staffing shortages.[57] However, more formal definition of tasks, training, and roles are needed.[53]

Multidisciplinary Care and Thoracic Surgical Services

Treating thoracic surgical conditions involves a variety of clinical specialties and professions including anesthesia, respiratory therapy, pulmonology, radiology, pediatrics, and oncology. These specialties may not be routinely available across LMICs. Therefore, it is imperative to collaborate with, train, and advocate for these related specialists.

Advanced anesthesia training is valuable to provide single lung ventilation as well as regional anesthesia in thoracic patients. At this time, there is a massive shortage of trained anesthetic staff based on the World Federation of Societies of Anaesthesiologists Global Anesthesia Workforce Survey[58] and no information on specialty cardiothoracic anesthesia training in LMICs. The need for pediatric- and thoracic-trained anesthesia staff to provide pediatric thoracic surgical care is particularly challenging.[59] Furthermore, there are little data on allied health professionals such as nonphysician and nonnurse anesthetists as well as respiratory therapists (including respiratory nurses or respiratory physiotherapists) in LMICs.

Table 1
An example of thoracic surgical task shifting

Health Cadre	Level of Care	Procedures Performed
Thoracic surgeon + thoracic specialty–trained physician anesthesiologist	Referral hospital	Airway reconstruction, chest and chest wall reconstruction, tracheal resection, lung transplant
General surgeon + anesthesiologist without thoracic specialty training	Tertiary hospital	Thoracotomy,[81] hiatal hernia repair, esophagectomy, resection of tuberculomas, Nissen fundoplication, pneumonectomy, lobectomy with mediastinal lymphadenectomy, bleb resection
Nonsurgical physicians including pulmonologists, ICU specialists, medical officers + nonphysician anesthetists	District hospital	Thoracostomy,[56] treatment of tuberculous pleural empyema, fiber-optic bronchoscopy, mediastinoscopy, regional thoracic nerve blocks for chest drains
Nonphysician clinicians including respiratory nurses/physiotherapists	Pre- and posthospital care at primary care facility	Tracheostomy care management, lung cancer screening,[82] referral of surgical disease,[82] intubation, handling respiratory depression or oxygen saturation <80%

Pulmonologists or physicians specializing in respiratory medicine and/or critical care are also rare worldwide.[60] One survey from Nigeria assessed the quality, capacity, and resources available for respiratory care and found only 76 registered respiratory physicians in the country and unreasonably high cost of training in respiratory medicine limiting workforce development and low capacity for inpatient, outpatient, and diagnostic respiratory services in the tertiary hospitals compared with the standard established by the British Thoracic Society. These needs were unmet before the COVID-19 pandemic and much more so in this post-COVID era. However, the COVID-19 pandemic has opened up virtual training, which may be useful to support capacity for thoracic surgical services through multidisciplinary virtual collaborations whether for trauma care or management of cancer through tumor board meetings.[61,62]

ECONOMICS AND FINANCING TO PROVIDE THORACIC SURGICAL SERVICES

Thoracic surgical care can seem prohibitively expensive. However, the economic costs of not having thoracic surgical care is likely to be substantial, although not well defined.[63,64] Surgical care is needed for roughly one-third of the global burden of all diseases and has been shown to be cost-effective by the third edition of the Disease Control Priorities Project—a collaboration of health economists, epidemiologists, and policy makers.[65] Although the Lancet Commission demonstrated that surgical care is economically feasible and beneficial to society in LMICs, the global disease burden, cost of care, and economic impact of thoracic surgical conditions have not been quantified.[7] One survey in Sierra Leone found that 14.8% of patients had a chest, breast, or back complaint in their lifetime that merited surgical consultation but nearly 40% had never sought any care for it, largely due to inability to pay.[66] An estimated 5% of patients with tuberculosis require surgical management but there is inadequate expertise, imaging, and equipment to perform indicated procedures in the places where this disease is still relevant.[67] Outcomes for patients undergoing esophagectomy are notably worse in LMICs as well,[68] thus suggesting potential socioeconomic ramifications of poor care.

The thoracic surgical community and related specialists are well positioned to study the needs and costs of care for thoracic conditions and advocate for the systems needed to provide it. The COVID-19 pandemic has forced countries to make substantial investments in health care services, workforce, equipment, infrastructure, and other technologies, which are likely to benefit patients with thoracic surgical conditions as well.[69] However, there are many unanswered questions. Which operations offer the biggest reduction in morbidity or mortality, and which are most financially and technically possible in a given context? What is the economic impact of the lack of availability of thoracic surgical care? How can we offset the high costs of care to those patients and provide the most appropriate perioperative care? These questions need to be discussed across stakeholders in every region to develop models to provide thoracic surgical services that are responsive to local needs.

INFORMATION MANAGEMENT TO PROVIDE THORACIC SURGICAL SERVICES

Data collection systems are essential. Establishing registries can help form a baseline to facilitate implementation research. Participation in Can-Reg,[70,71] an open-source platform to create a cancer registry, or IRTEC,[72] the WHO's trauma registry platform, may be a step in the right direction to understand specific local needs. These registries can help standardize language of thoracic operations and procedures and coding for conditions and injuries to allow comparisons across hospitals or even countries.

Surgical capacity assessments have been conducted across LMICs using the WHO Tool for Situational Analysis to Assess Emergency and Essential Surgical Care and the Surgeon OverSeas' Personnel Infrastructure Procedure Equipment and Supplies (PIPES) survey tool.[73–75] However, no tool specifically assesses thoracic surgical capacity nor have the results of the WHO and PIPES surveys been analyzed to determine the existing thoracic surgical infrastructure in LMICs; this is an opportunity for the thoracic surgical community to embrace.

In addition, gathering data in itself is not enough. Investment in research capacity is critical for developing effective policy and improving the care and outcomes of surgical patients in LMICs. Groups such as the American Thoracic Society Methods in Epidemiologic, Clinical, and Operations Research (MECOR) have built research capacity in LMICs for thoracic conditions and are good examples for the thoracic surgical community.[76] Incorporating these skills into clinical training can produce clinicians who can address quality improvement and develop evidence-based practice in thoracic surgical care.

Lastly, establishing metrics of high-quality care delivery is essential. The Lancet Commission developed 6 indicators to assess the capacity of a system to provide emergency and essential surgical care (see **Fig. 1**). Whether these are applicable to thoracic surgery remains to be seen. The indicators were assessed for 3 bellwether procedures—laparotomy, fracture repair, and cesarean section—but the surgical community has yet to codify key procedures for subspecialties such as thoracic surgery to guide next steps in surgical capacity building. The thoracic surgical community and policy makers will need to develop consensus-based metrics to evaluate care delivery and bench-mark within and across countries.

INNOVATION AND THORACIC SURGICAL SERVICES

Capacity building for service delivery in LMICs does not need to rely on the same stepwise progression that HICs have undergone. Leapfrogging is a process where development steps thought to be mandatory previously in one context may be skipped in another context to allow more rapid and efficient progress.[77] A nonmedical example involves skipping landline infrastructure and progressing directly to mobile phones. Minimally invasive operations have similar potential in LMICs. The countrywide implementation of laparoscopy for gallbladder operations in Mongolia transformed the standard of care.[78,79] Similarly, video-assisted thoracoscopic surgery, which has allowed advances in the treatment of a variety of thoracic surgical conditions in HICs, could be used for decortication of fibrothorax and lobectomy for cancer or infection in LMICs, and this could offer surgeons and patients the opportunity to leapfrog from the morbid and expensive thoracotomy operation and decrease hospital stay and improve functional outcomes for patients with thoracic surgical conditions.[80]

NATIONAL SURGICAL, OBSTETRIC, AND ANESTHESIA PLANS AND THORACIC SURGICAL SERVICES

National surgical obstetric and anesthesia plans (NSOAP) are being created by Ministries across LMICs to intentionally address the need for surgical services within their populations. The NSOAP development process follows a standardized process of stakeholder engagement and consensus building to develop goals and targets to improve access and quality of care. The thoracic surgical community has an opportunity to advocate for ensuring adequate infrastructure, workforce, financing, and data systems related to thoracic surgical care are incorporated in the policy and implementation.[12]

SUMMARY

Thoracic surgical services are an essential aspect of surgical systems. Building thoracic surgical capacity in LMICs requires the infrastructure to deliver thoracic surgery operative and perioperative care, training programs to develop specialists who can perform thoracic procedures and manage diseases of the thoracic cavity, as well as data systems to track the outcomes, costs, and socioeconomic impact of thoracic surgical care. Research, innovation, and advocacy are essential components to improving thoracic surgical services. Partnerships across institutions and countries to promote sustainable surgical systems have potential for substantial impact on thoracic surgical needs worldwide.

DISCLOSURE

All authors have no financial or commercial disclosures. S. Jayaraman is funded by NIH Fogarty International Center grant 1 R21 TW011636-01.

REFERENCES

1. Walt AJ. The world's best-known surgeon. Surgery 1983;94(4):582–90.
2. Franco A, Cortes J, Alvarez J, et al. The development of blood transfusion: the contributions of Norman Bethune in the Spanish Civil War (1936-1939). Can J Anaesth 1996;43(10):1076–8.
3. Deslauriers FRCSC J, Goulet D. The medical life of Henry Norman Bethune. vol. 22. Available at: http://www.hindawi.com.
4. Aliu O, Corlew SD, Heisler ME, et al. Building surgical capacity in low-resource countries. Ann Plast Surg 2014;72(1):108–12. https://doi.org/10.1097/sap.0b013e31826aefc7.
5. Shrime MG, Sleemi A, Ravilla TD. Charitable platforms in global surgery: a systematic review of their effectiveness, cost-effectiveness, sustainability, and role training. World J Surg 2015;39(1):10–20. https://doi.org/10.1007/s00268-014-2516-0.
6. Wall LL, Arrowsmith SD, Lassey AT, et al. Humanitarian ventures or "fistula tourism?": the ethical perils of pelvic surgery in the developing world. Int Urogynecol J 2006;17(6):559–62. https://doi.org/10.1007/s00192-005-0056-8.
7. Weiser TG, Regenbogen SE, Thompson KD, et al. An estimation of the global volume of surgery: a modelling strategy based on available data. Lancet 2008;372:139. https://doi.org/10.1016/S0140. Available at: www.thelancet.com.
8. Meara JG, Leather AJM, Hagander L, et al. Global surgery 2030: evidence and solutions for achieving health, welfare, and economic development. Lancet 2015;386(9993):569–624. https://doi.org/10.1016/S0140-6736(15)60160-X.
9. Finlayson SRG. How should academic surgeons respond to enthusiasts of global surgery? Surgery (United States) 2013;153(6):871–2. https://doi.org/10.1016/j.surg.2013.02.020.
10. deVries CR, Rosenberg JS. Global surgical ecosystems: a need for systems strengthening. Ann Glob Health 2016;82(4):605–13. https://doi.org/10.1016/j.aogh.2016.09.011.
11. Sabatino ME, Alkire BC, Corley J. Financial investment in global surgery - codevelopment as an accretive evolution of the field. JAMA Surg 2019;154(6):475–6. https://doi.org/10.1001/jamasurg.2019.0044.
12. Surgical care systems strengthening developing national surgical, obstetric and anaesthesia plans. 2017. Available at: http://apps.who.int/bookorders.
13. Kanavos P. The rising burden of cancer in the developing world. Ann Oncol 2006;17(Suppl. 8). https://doi.org/10.1093/annonc/mdl983.
14. Lubuzo B, Ginindza T, Hlongwana K. The barriers to initiating lung cancer care in low-and middle-income countries. Pan Afr Med J 2020;35. https://doi.org/10.11604/pamj.2020.35.38.17333.
15. Nwagbara UI, Ginindza TG, Hlongwana KW. Health systems influence on the pathways of care for lung cancer in low- and middle-income countries: a scoping review. Global Health 2020;16(1). https://doi.org/10.1186/s12992-020-00553-8.
16. Yendamuri S. Thoracic surgery in India: challenges and opportunities. J Thorac Dis 2016;8:S596–600. https://doi.org/10.21037/jtd.2016.05.08.
17. World Health Organization. Global tuberculosis report 2016.
18. Peter S, Triraganon R, IUCN Forest Conservation Programme, Regional Community Forestry Training Center for Asia-Pacific (Bangkok T). Strengthening voices for better choices: a capacity needs assessment process. IUCN, Forest Conservation Programme; 2009.
19. Hurst JR, Buist AS, Gaga M, et al. Challenges in the implementation of chronic obstructive pulmonary disease guidelines in low- and middle-income countries an official American thoracic society workshop report. Ann Am Thorac Soc 2021;18(8):1269–77. https://doi.org/10.1513/AnnalsATS.202103-284ST.
20. Papali A, Adhikari NKJ, Diaz JV, et al. Infrastructure and organization of adult intensive care units in resource-limited settings. In: Dondorp Arjen M, Schultz Marcus J, Martin W, editors. Sepsis management in resource-limited settings. Switzerland: Dünserpublisher; 2019. p. 31–68.
21. Irwin BR, Hoxha K, Grépin KA. Conceptualising the effect of access to electricity on health in low- and middle-income countries: a systematic review. Glob Public Health 2020;15(3):452–73. https://doi.org/10.1080/17441692.2019.1695873.
22. Murthy S, Leligdowicz A, Adhikari NKJ. Intensive care unit capacity in low-income countries: a systematic review. PLoS One 2015;10(1). https://doi.org/10.1371/journal.pone.0116949.
23. World Health Organization. COVID-19 oxygen emergency impacting more than half a million people in

low- and middle-income countries every day, as demand surges 2021.
24. Perry L, Malkin R. Effectiveness of medical equipment donations to improve health systems: how much medical equipment is broken in the developing world? Med Biol Eng Comput 2011;49(7): 719–22. https://doi.org/10.1007/s11517-011-0786-3.
25. Graham HR, Bagayana SM, Bakare AA, et al. Improving hospital oxygen systems for COVID-19 in low-resource settings: lessons from the field. 2020. Available at: www.ghspjournal.org.
26. Howie SR, Ebruke BE, Gil M, et al. The development and implementation of an oxygen treatment solution for health facilities in low and middle-income countries. J Glob Health 2020;10(2):020425. https://doi.org/10.7189/JOGH.10.020425.
27. el Majid B, el Hammoumi A, Motahhir S, et al. Preliminary design of an innovative, simple, and easy-to-build portable ventilator for COVID-19 patients. EuroMediterr J Environ Integr 2020;5(2). https://doi.org/10.1007/s41207-020-00163-1.
28. Access to Medicine Foundation. Global oxygen suppliers commit to closing oxygen gaps in low- and middle-income countries.
29. Madekurozwa M, Bonneuil WV, Frattolin J, et al. A novel ventilator design for COVID-19 and resource-limited settings. Front Med Technol 2021; 3. https://doi.org/10.3389/fmedt.2021.707826.
30. Fleming KA, Horton S, Wilson ML, et al. The Lancet Commission on diagnostics: transforming access to diagnostics. Lancet 2021. https://doi.org/10.1016/s0140-6736(21)00673-5.
31. Frija G, Blažić I, Frush DP, et al. How to improve access to medical imaging in low- and middle-income countries? EClinicalMedicine 2021;38. https://doi.org/10.1016/j.eclinm.2021.101034.
32. Sayed S, Cherniak W, Lawler M, et al. Improving pathology and laboratory medicine in low-income and middle-income countries: roadmap to solutions. Lancet 2018;391(10133):1939–52. https://doi.org/10.1016/S0140-6736(18)30459-8.
33. Custer B, Zou S, Glynn SA, et al. Addressing gaps in international blood availability and transfusion safety in low-and middle-income countries: a NHLBI workshop. Transfusion 2018;58(5):1307–17. https://doi.org/10.1111/trf.14598.
34. Smit Sibinga CT, Abdella YE. Availability and safety of blood transfusion in low- and middle-income countries. Transfusion 2019;59(6):2155–7. https://doi.org/10.1111/trf.15224.
35. DeStigter K, Horton S, Atalabi OM, et al. Equipment in the global radiology environment: why we fail, how we could succeed. J Glob Radiol 2019;5(1):e1079. https://doi.org/10.7191/jgr.2019.1079.
36. Allen Hamilton B. SCMS project team case study: impact of the Ethiopian national laboratory logistics system on the Harmonization of laboratory commodities. Available at: https://www.who.int/hiv/amds/amds_impact_ethiopian_lab.pdf
37. E-RaktKosh. E-rakt Kosh: centralized lood bank management system. Available at: https://www.eraktkosh.in/BLDAHIMS/bloodbank/transactions/bbpublicindex.html Accessed 30 March 2022.
38. WHO. Drones take Rwanda's national blood service to new heights. Available at: https://www.who.int/news-room/feature-stories/detail/drones-take-rwandas-national-blood-service-to-new-heights#:~:text=In%20the%20deep%20rural%20areas,rates%20between%202000%20and%202018. Accessed June 12, 2019.
39. Gopal S, Krysiak R, Liomba G. Building a pathology laboratory in Malawi. Lancet Oncol 2013;14(4): 291–2.
40. O'brien M, Mwangi-Powell F, Adewole IF, et al. Cancer control in Africa 5 improving access to analgesic drugs for patients with cancer in Sub-Saharan Africa. Lancet Oncol 2013;14:e176–82. Available at: www.thelancet.com/oncology.
41. Roth L, Bempong D, Babigumira JB, et al. Expanding global access to essential medicines: investment priorities for sustainably strengthening medical product regulatory systems. Global Health 2018;14(1). https://doi.org/10.1186/s12992-018-0421-2.
42. Worldwide assessment of low- and middle-income countries' regulatory preparedness to approve medical products during public health emergencies _ enhanced reader.
43. Holmer H, Lantz A, Kunjumen T, et al. Global distribution of surgeons, anaesthesiologists, and obstetricians. Lancet Glob Health 2015;3. https://doi.org/10.1016/S2214-109X(14)70349-3.
44. Pezzella T. Global cardiothoracic surgery advances and challenges in developing countries and emerging economies. CTS Net Dataset; 2018.
45. Raykar NP, Yorlets RR, Liu C, et al. The How Project: understanding contextual challenges to global surgical care provision in low-resource settings. BMJ Glob Health 2016;1(4). https://doi.org/10.1136/bmjgh-2016-000075.
46. Derbew M, Laytin AD, Dicker RA. The surgical workforce shortage and successes in retaining surgical trainees in Ethiopia: a professional survey. Hum Resour Health 2016;14(S1). https://doi.org/10.1186/s12960-016-0126-7.
47. Wondimagegn D, Pain C, Baheretibeb Y, et al. Toronto Addis Ababa Academic Collaboration. Acad Med 2018;93(12). https://doi.org/10.1097/ACM.0000000000002352.
48. Williams TE, Sun B, Ross P, et al. A formidable task: population analysis predicts a deficit of 2000 cardiothoracic surgeons by 2030. J Thorac Cardiovasc Surg 2010;139(4):835–40. https://doi.org/10.1016/j.jtcvs.2009.12.004.

49. van Essen C, Steffes BC, Thelander K, et al. Increasing and retaining african surgeons working in rural hospitals: an analysis of PAACS surgeons with twenty-year program follow-up. World J Surg 2019;43(1):75–86. https://doi.org/10.1007/s00268-018-4781-9.
50. O'Flynn E, Andrew J, Hutch A, et al. The specialist surgeon workforce in east, central and southern africa: a situation analysis. World J Surg 2016; 40(11). https://doi.org/10.1007/s00268-016-3601-3.
51. Charles Y, Habib T, Henning T, et al. Developing an African cardiothoracic surgery database. Niger J Cardiovasc Thorac Surg 2020;5(1).
52. Vervoort D. Moving the needle: a guide to solving the global cardiac surgery puzzle for surgeons, Societies, students, and researchers. CTS Net; 2020.
53. Farmer PE, Kim JY. Surgery and global health: a view from beyond the OR. World J Surg 2008; 32(4). https://doi.org/10.1007/s00268-008-9525-9.
54. Ajao OG, Alao A. Surgical residency training in developing countries: West African College of Surgeons as a case study. J Natl Med Assoc 2016;3(108):173–9.
55. World Health Organization. Task shifting: global recommendations and guidelinesd. Geneva, Switzerland: World Health Organization; 2008.
56. Chu K, Rosseel P, Gielis P, et al. Surgical task shifting in Sub-Saharan Africa. PLoS Med 2009;6(5). https://doi.org/10.1371/journal.pmed.1000078.
57. Falk R, Taylor R, Kornelsen J, et al. Surgical task-sharing to non-specialist physicians in low-resource settings globally: a systematic review of the literature. World J Surg 2020;44(5). https://doi.org/10.1007/s00268-019-05363-7.
58. Kempthorne P, Morriss WW, Mellin-Olsen J, et al. The WFSA global anesthesia workforce survey. Anesth Analgesia 2017;125(3):981–90. https://doi.org/10.1213/ANE.0000000000002258.
59. Jacob R. Anesthesia for thoracic surgery in children in developing countries. Paediatr. Anaesth 2009; 19(1):19–22. https://doi.org/10.1111/j.1460-9592.2008.02865.x.
60. Obaseki D, Adeniyi B, Kolawole T, et al. Gaps in capacity for respiratory care in developing countries Nigeria as a case study. Ann Am Thorac Soc 2015;12(4):591–8. https://doi.org/10.1513/AnnalsATS.201410-443AR.
61. Brandão M, Guisseve A, Bata G, et al. Survival impact and <scp>Cost-effectiveness of a multidisciplinary tumor board for breast cancer in Mozambique, Sub-Saharan Africa. Oncologist 2021;26(6). https://doi.org/10.1002/onco.13643.
62. Dyer L, Llerena L, Brannick M, et al. Advanced trauma life support course delivery: comparison of outcomes from modifications during covid-19. Cureus 2021. https://doi.org/10.7759/cureus.16811.
63. Cardarelli M, Vaikunth S, Mills K, et al. Cost-effectiveness of humanitarian pediatric cardiac surgery programs in low- and middle-income countries. JAMA Netw Open 2018;1(7):e184707. https://doi.org/10.1001/jamanetworkopen.2018.4707.
64. Chao TE, Sharma K, Mandigo M, et al. Cost-effectiveness of surgery and its policy implications for global health: a systematic review and analysis. Lancet Glob Health 2014 Jun;2(6):e334–45.
65. Debas HT, Peter D, Gawande A, et al. Disease control priorities 3rd edition - essential surgery. vol. 1. 2015. Available at: https://openknowledge.worldbank.org/handle/10986/21568.
66. Zogg CK, Kamara TB, Groen RS, et al. Prevalence of thoracic surgical care need in a developing country: results of a cluster-randomized, cross-sectional nationwide survey. Int J Surg 2015;13:1–7. https://doi.org/10.1016/j.ijsu.2014.11.026.
67. Dewan RK, Pezzella AT. Surgical aspects of pulmonary tuberculosis: an update. Asian Cardiovasc Thorac Ann 2016;24(8):835–46. https://doi.org/10.1177/0218492316661958.
68. Kamarajah SK, Nepogodiev D, Bekele A, et al. Mortality from esophagectomy for esophageal cancer across low, middle, and high-income countries: an international cohort study. Eur J Surg Oncol 2021;47(6): 1481–8. https://doi.org/10.1016/j.ejso.2020.12.006.
69. Deloitte insights. 2021 Global Health Care Outlook. 2021. Available at: https://documents.deloitte.com/insights/Globalhealthcareoutlook. Accessed December 9, 2021.
70. International Association of Cancer Registries. Software - CanReg5. Available at: http://www.iacr.com.fr/index.php?option=com_content&view=article&id=9:canreg5&catid=68&Itemid=445. Accessed March 30, 2022.
71. Fatunmbi M, Saunders A, Chugani B, et al. Cancer registration in resource limited environments—experience in Lagos, Nigeria. J Surg Res 2019;235: 167–70. https://doi.org/10.1016/j.jss.2018.09.021.
72. WHO Emergencies Preparedness, WHO International registry for trauma and emergency care. WHO, October, 12, 2020.
73. Choo S, Perry H, Hesse AAJ, et al. Assessment of capacity for surgery, obstetrics and anaesthesia in 17 Ghanaian hospitals using a WHO assessment tool. Trop Med Int Health 2010;15(9):1109–15. https://doi.org/10.1111/j.1365-3156.2010.02589.x.
74. Bhatia MB, Mohan SC, Blair KJ, et al. Surgical and trauma capacity assessment in Rural Haryana, India. Ann Glob Health 2021;87(1):1–11. https://doi.org/10.5334/aogh.3173.
75. Osen H, Chang D, Choo S, et al. Validation of the world health organization tool for situational analysis to assess emergency and essential surgical care at district hospitals in Ghana. World J Surg 2011;35(3): 500–4. https://doi.org/10.1007/s00268-010-0918-1.
76. Buist AS, Parry V. The american thoracic society methods in epidemiologic, clinical, and operations

research program a research capacity-building program in low- and middle-income countries. Ann Am Thorac Soc 2013;10(4):281–9. https://doi.org/10.1513/AnnalsATS.201304-081OT.

77. Industry agenda health systems leapfrogging in emerging economies project paper.
78. Wells KM, Shalabi H, Sergelen O, et al. Patient and physician perceptions of changes in surgical care in mongolia 9 years after roll-out of a national training program for laparoscopy. World J Surg 2016;40(8): 1859–64. https://doi.org/10.1007/s00268-016-3498-x.
79. Wells KM, Lee YJ, Erdene S, et al. Building operative care capacity in a resource limited setting: the Mongolian model of the expansion of sustainable laparoscopic cholecystectomy. Surgery (United States) 2016;160(2):509–17. https://doi.org/10.1016/j.surg.2016.04.001.
80. Vargas G, Price RR, Sergelen O, et al. A successful model for laparoscopic training in Mongolia. Int Surg 2012;97(4):363–71.
81. Hassan M, Elmi A, Baldan M. Experience of thoracic surgery performed under difficult conditions in Somalia. East Cent Afr J Surg 2004.
82. Lester L, Njuguna B, Vedanthan R. Team-based care along the cardiac surgical care cascade. Cham, Switzerland: Springer Nature; 2022. https://doi.org/10.1007/978-3-030-83864-5_13.

Teaching Thoracic Surgery in a Low-Resource Setting: Creation of a Simulation Curriculum in Rwanda

Edmond Ntaganda, MD, MMed, FCS (ECSA) ECSA[a,b], Robinson Ssebuufu, MB, ChB, MMed (Surgery), FCS (ECSA)[c], Daniel R. Bacon, MD[d], Thomas M. Daniel, MD[e,*]

KEYWORDS

• Simulation • Training • Education • Low Resource Settings • Low- and Middle-Income Countries • Human Resources For Health • Thoracic Surgery

KEY POINTS

- Trauma, infectious etiologies, and malignancy are common clinical situations in less-resourced settings that may require thoracic surgery. Preoperative assessment and subsequent performance of thoracic surgery procedures require adaptation and improvisation in a setting whereby there are limited resources.
- Simulation courses allow the teaching of thoracic surgery in these settings, particularly when presenting case volume is low and inadequate to transfer skills.
- Simulation models should be designed to match the resources of the setting (eg,.it is important to design models both with and without animal mediastinal and lung tissue).
- There are several internet-based resources for teaching simulation general thoracic surgery.
- Developing professional relationships with the host institution is fundamental to teaching thoracic surgery in Low- and Middle-Income Countries (LMICs).

INTRODUCTION

Surgery in Africa has been likened to the "neglected stepchild" of global public health.[1] Historically, much greater emphasis has been placed on infectious diseases than has been afforded on surgical capacity building. More recently, it has been recognized that surgically treatable conditions account for almost one-third of the global burden of disease, and more deaths occur from diseases needing surgical care (16.9 million) than HIV (1.46 million), tuberculosis (1.2 million), and malaria (1.17 million) combined.[2] Thus, surgery is an essential component of global health care, as endorsed by the World Bank 3rd edition of Disease Control Priorities,[3] the Lancet Commission on Global Surgery,[4] and the World Health Assembly.[5] For these reasons, organizations such as the College of Surgeons of East Central and Southern Africa (COSECSA), and the Pan-African Academy of Christian Surgeons (PAACS) are continuing to augment surgical training capacity with a focus on surgeon retention.[6,7]

In this article, we review the scope of surgical education in Low- and Middle-Income Countries

[a] Consultant Pediatric Surgeon, Centre Hospitalier Universitaire de Kigali (CHUK), KN 4th Avenue, Kigali City, P.O. Box 655, Kigali, Rwanda; [b] Loma Linda University School of Medicine, San Bernando, California, USA; [c] Uganda Medical and Dental Practitioners Council (UMDPC), P.O. Box 1594, Kampala, Uganda; [d] Department of Surgery, The Ohio State University School of Medicine, Columbus, OH, USA; [e] Department of Surgery, University of Virginia School of Medicine, P.O. Box 800709, Charlottesville, VA 22908, USA

* Corresponding author.

E-mail address: tmdanielm144@gmail.com

Thorac Surg Clin 32 (2022) 279–287
https://doi.org/10.1016/j.thorsurg.2022.05.001

(LMICs), surgical education challenges unique to low-resource settings, and discuss applications of surgical simulation and other alternative educational methods in LMICs such as Rwanda.

SCOPE OF SURGICAL EDUCATION INITIATIVES IN LMICS

A recent systematic review of postgraduate surgical education in LMICs describes significant heterogeneity in scope, duration, curricula, and requirements across 34 countries.[8] Sub-Saharan African (SSA) physicians currently can pursue surgical training through university programs typically resulting in a Master of Medicine (MMED) degree or through regional bodies such as the West African College of Surgeons (WACS) or College of Surgeons from East, Central, and Southern Africa (COSECSA), resulting in a Fellowship of the College of Surgeons (FCS). Alternatively, SSA medical graduates can pursue training abroad. In addition, the Pan-African Academy of Christian Surgeons (PAACS) is a faith-based nongovernmental organization (NGO), which collaborates with WACS, COSECSA, and Loma Linda University to provide accredited surgical residency training to graduates of African medical schools. PAACS has established 12 training programs in 8 counties in general surgery, orthopedics, head and neck surgery, and pediatric surgery.[7] As of 2017, PAACS has graduated 63 general surgeons and 4 pediatric surgeons, all of whom practice in Africa in 20 different countries, and with a 35% long-term rural retention (5 years).[7]

Despite these remarkable achievements in surgical training over the past 2 decades, there remains a persistently vast shortage of surgeons in LMICs.[4] In response, many organizations including academic institutions, faith-based organizations, and philanthropic individuals have made strides to close this the gap in surgical skill transfer with varying levels of sustainability.

One example of a surgical skill transfer is via short-term missions. Nthumba outlines many benefits and pitfalls of such missions including the provision of needed surgical care, but at times with high complication rates and variable follow-up.[9–11] Sustainable short-term efforts emphasize education and skill transfer.[12] For example, Team Heart is a collaboration between the Rwanda Ministry of Health, the Rwanda Heart Foundation, and a humanitarian cardiac surgery program that emphasized training local team members on peri- and intraoperative care for patients with rheumatic heart disease.[13]

Academic institutional partnerships have also played a substantial role in augmenting surgical education efforts in LMICs. These partnerships emphasize the same aims characteristic of academic surgery in high-income countries (HICs) which include education, research, patient care, and quality improvement.[14] Examples individual partnerships of academic surgery departments with LMIC partners include Brown University and Tenwek Hospital,[15] University of North Carolina at Chapel Hill and the Malawi Ministry of Health,[16] and Weill Cornell Medical College with Weill Bugando University College of Health Sciences in Mwanza, Tanzania.[17] Due to a tendency for these relationships to disproportionately benefit the academic careers of HIC physicians, the American Surgical Association Working Group on Global Surgery has outlined principles for effective and bilateral partnerships with LMIC institutions.[18,40] In an effort to synchronize the goals of various academic partners with the in-country goals, the Human Resource for Health (HRH) program led by the Ministry of Health of Rwanda–in partnership with 23 American institutions–is a robust example of how to address health care workforce shortages with coordinated, intensive educational and training initiatives. [19,20] source for Health (HRH) program led by the Ministry of Health of Rwanda, in partnership with 23 American institutions is a robust example of how to address health care workforce shortages with intensive educational and training initiatives. (ed, 2017).

CHALLENGES IN SURGICAL EDUCATION FOR LMICs

Many challenges in surgical education in LMICs are rooted in resource shortages including attending surgeons themselves,[21,22] as well as nurses,[23] allied health staff,[23] equipment,[24] electricity,[25] diagnostic and educational resources,[22] operative case volumes.[26]

Currently, there is a global maldistribution of surgeons available to train new surgeons; LMICs account for 48% of the world population, but only 19% of world surgeons.[21] This amounts to 0.13 to 1.57 surgeons per 100,000 population,[22] which is an inadequate number to develop properly distributed training programs.

Intuitively, this maldistribution and its attendant educational challenges are compounded for surgical subspecialty training. General surgeons and general practitioners provide most of the surgical care in LMICs.[27,28] Even when local and visiting subspecialty surgeons are accessible, speciality case volumes become an educational rate-limiting factor. Ramirez and colleagues[29] found that major thoracic cases accounted for only 1.76% of surgical procedures at 3 Rwandan referral centers. Low case volumes are not purely a function of regional epidemiology, but rather attributable to many factors including surgeon availability, cost, and travel barriers. Regardless, low case volumes beget obvious challenges for surgical trainees, particularly for urgent or emergent surgical indications. Kang and colleagues[30] experience implementing laparoscopic training in Ghana demonstrate how educational interventions may ultimately facilitate increased referrals and certainly has generalizable applications to thoracic surgery training.

DIGITAL EDUCATION AND SIMULATION

Given the cited barriers to surgical training, alternative education delivery methods are increasingly used to bridge gaps and supplement bedside clinical training. Raigani and colleagues[31] review many innovative examples including virtual symposiums, synchronous and asynchronous webinars, and resource libraries. Other methods include web-based modules,[32] teleconferences,[31] surgical video atlases,[33] online forums and webinars,[34] and simulation-based curriculum such as our experience in thoracic surgery education in Rwanda.[35] Okrainec and colleagues[36] have demonstrated success with remote telesimulation for a Fundamentals of Laparoscopic Surgery (FLS) course. There are of course limitations in LMICs with access to reliable Internet, and thus downloadable prerecorded content has proved useful.[37]

Box 1
Case Report

- *Presentation:* 11-year-old girl presents with gunshot wound (entry: subxiphoid; exit: left posterolateral chest wall)
- *Injuries:* partial tear of distal esophagus
- *Initial management:* Chest tube thoracostomy only x 2 months (no thoracic surgeon available).
- *Complications*: Inadequate drainage leading to an esophago-pleural fistula and associated empyema, sepsis, and malnourishment.
- *Resource limitations:* Lack of radiologic expertise to define the inferior border of the empyema critical for Eloesser flap for preoperative planning.
- *Low Resource Improvisation:* Coin localization and Barium swallow to delineate inferior border (**Fig. 1**).
- *Outcome:* Successful Eloesser flap (see **Figs. 1** and **2**) with a follow-up barium swallow showing closure of fistula without stenosis or distal obstruction.

THORACIC SURGERY TEACHING EXPERIENCE IN RWANDA ILLUSTRATES THE UTILITY OF SIMULATION

As previously discussed, major thoracic surgery was found to account for less than 2% of case volume at 3 Rwandan referral centers.[29] In this context, the senior author's (T.D.) experience in performing and teaching thoracic surgery in Rwanda provides insight into the challenges to training based on presenting case volume in resource-limited settings. Teaching visits were conducted at the Center Hospitalier Universitaire de Kigali (CHUK), King Faisal Hospital in Kigali and at the Center Hospitalier Universitaire de Butare (CHUB). During the first visit, 20 thoracic cases were performed over an 8-week period (<3/wk), with 3 of the total cases being lung resections (pneumonectomy, lobectomy, and lung biopsy). The remaining cases included decortications

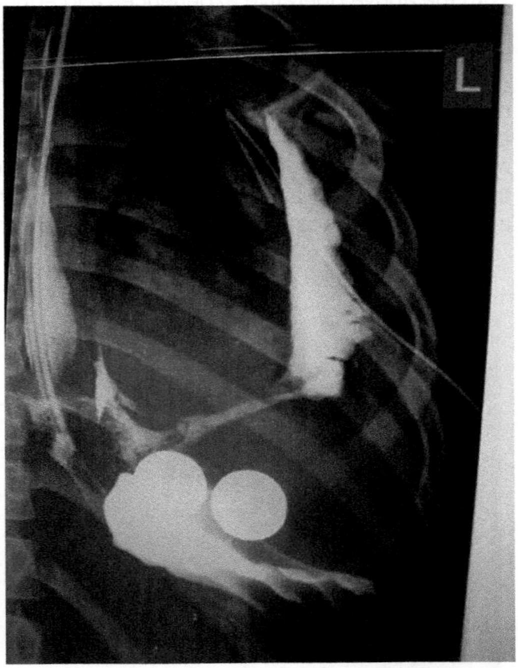

Fig. 1. A barium swallow from **Box 1** case presentation showing the chronic esophago-pleural fistula. Note the high placement of the chest tube and the 2 coins secured to the patient's back to assist subsequent surgical localization of the inferior-most portion of the empyema. This image was used to plan the site for Eloesser flap creation for adequate drainage and subsequent spontaneous fistula closure.

(n = 7) biopsies or excisions of mediastinal masses (n = 6) and creation of Eloesser flap (open window thoracotomy) (n = 4) for drainage of organized empyemas. In the authors' experience, low case volume-combined with late presentations and associated case complexity–created a challenging educational environment in which simulation-based supplementation was greatly needed. **Box 1** and **Fig. 1 and 2** demonstrate a clinical case presentation that required clinical improvisation to solve. The case was one of a delayed presentation of an 11-year-old girl who suffered a gunshot wound to the chest, which was managed initially with chest tube insertion only. She developed a chronic esophago-pleural fistula that required a surgical repair with a good outcome. Importantly, the delayed presentation precluded teaching acute esophageal perforation repair, for which simulation models were later used as described later in discussion.

CREATION OF SIMULATION THORACIC SURGERY MODELS AND WEBSITE VIDEO ARCHIVE

With the above operative experiences and educational challenges in mind, the senior author (T.D)–with the added perspective of the Rwandan surgical faculty he had worked within the operating room–developed several thoracic surgery simulation models before returning to Rwanda to address the needs of Rwandan surgical resident trainees.[38] **Table 1** and associated figures outline a sampling of procedures, materials needed, and

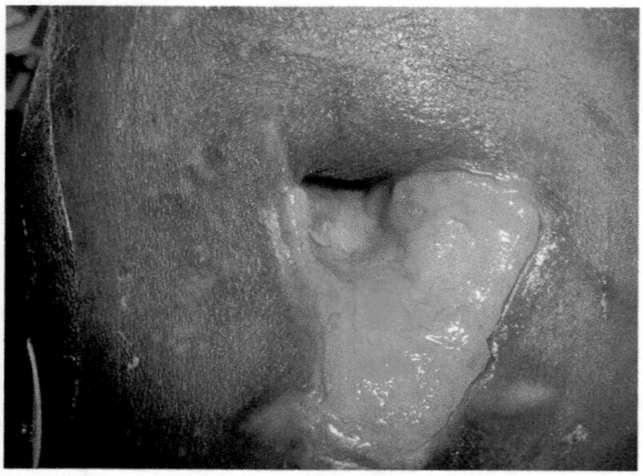

Fig. 2. View of patient's left postero-lateral chest wall picturing an Eloesser flap in left chest wall that allowed adequate full drainage of the empyema cavity and resultant closure of the fistula at the esophageal level. Note the red/pink granulation tissue at the inferior edge of the flap and the skin flap at the superior edge of the incision.

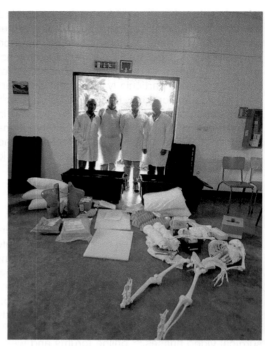

Fig. 3. Rwandan surgery residents viewing simulation thoracic surgery equipment on its arrival at the teaching facility at the Center Hospitalier Universitaire de Kigali (CHUK).

set up instructions. One of the models-the hemithorax models (Fig 5) created from a human manakin donated by a men's store in the USA was copied from a model in a cardiothoracic surgery simulation course given by Feins and colleagues.[39]

To make simulation interventions sustainable and accessible to faculty and surgical residents worldwide, a free thoracic surgery education website[35] (thoracicsurgeryeducation.com) was also created to archive a video library and a comprehensive manual for a select set of procedures. The website was intended to augment the training of LMICs surgeons after their initial exposure to an in-country onsite simulation thoracic surgery course and serves as a sustainable educational platform. Each simulation exercise includes: (1) learning objectives, (2) necessary equipment, (3) surgical instruments needed, (4) assembly instructions, and (5) step-by-step video recordings of simulation procedures. In all, the website contains: 37 video demonstrations, 10 operative procedures with associated learning objectives, a list of equipment, preparation details, and a 44-page comprehensive manual with pictures of each operative step.

Table 1
Creation of thoracic surgery simulation models for transportation and teaching in Rwanda

Case/Technique	Materials Needed	Set up and Procedural Steps
Basic surgical skills	Surgical board, pickups and suture holders. (**Fig 4**).	Practice suture placement and knot tying. (**Fig 4**).
Posterolateral thoracotomy positioning	A life-size skeletal model of the entire human body was used along with pillows, stabilizing tape, padded arm boards, and an operating room table. (**Fig. 3**)	Demonstrate proper positioning of the chest over an upward bend of the OR table.
Posterolateral thoractomy		The life-sized skeletal model described above was placed in proper positioning for the passage of the surgeon's hand under the left scapula to identify the first rib and then count down to the desired intercostal space for the optimum exposure of the planned lung, diaphragm, or mediastinal procedure.
Pulmonary decortication	American football, modeling clay, (**Fig 6**) clear plastic tape, and thick plastic foam tape.	1. Wrap one layer of clear plastic tape around football simulating the visceral pleura. 2. Wrap 3 layers of thick plastic foam tape simulating the organized thickened peel lying on top of the plastic layer simulating the hyalinized pleural thickening seen in organized empyema. 3. Incise the "pleural peel" using the belly of a scalpel with a shallow incision. 4. Spread the pleural edges with a small gauze sponge set in a curved hemostat after each deepening incision to avoid incising the pleural layer. 5. Use the blunt dissector with a small sponge to advance the plane of dissection.

(*continued on next page*)

Table 1
(*continued*)

Case/Technique	Materials Needed	Set up and Procedural Steps
Esophageal stenosis (graduated bougie dilation)	Locally acquired mediastinal tissue (goat or porcine).	The esophagus was narrowed externally with an expandible material to simulate stenosis and then esophageal bougies of increasing size were then passed.
Acute Esophageal perforation	Locally acquired mediastinal tissue (goat or porcine).	Locally acquired goat mediastinal and lung tissue was placed inside the left half-chest model. The distal esophagus was then longitudinally incised. Further opening of the mucosal and submucosal layers, proximally and distally underneath the intact esophageal muscle layers, was then performed to simulate the type of tear seen in human esophageal rupture.

Simulation models were designed by the author (T.D.) except for the chest manakin thoracotomy model, which was created by Feins and colleagues.[39] Materials were transported to Rwanda in 2 trunks (each 34″ long; 19″ wide; and 20″ tall), which were maximally packed with simulation surgery teaching equipment (**Fig. 3**). Mediastinal tissue was acquired locally. The models were used to demonstrate various surgical techniques and maneuvers.

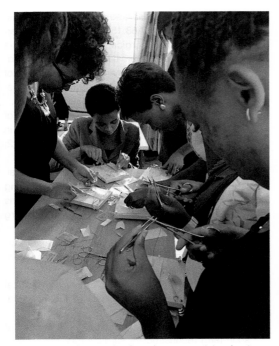

Fig. 4. Rwandan medical students practicing basic surgical skills of surgical knot tying and suturing. This course was designed to expose female medical students to a hands-on surgical experience in order to familiarize them with the option of considering a surgical career.

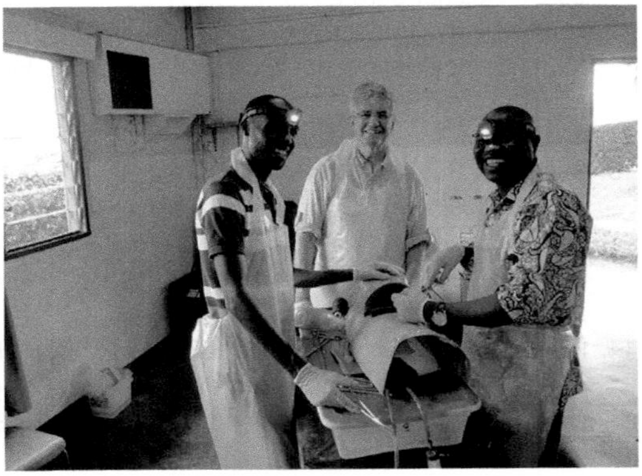

Fig. 5. Dr Edmond Ntaganda (on the left)–current Chief of Pediatric Surgery at Center Hospitalier Universitaire de Kigali (CHUK)–is shown teaching simulation lung surgery to a surgical resident (on the right) in 2014. Total cost for all the simulation surgery created was $800 US dollars. The chest model was a chest manikin obtained from an American Men's store and divided in half vertically. Note the simulation "blood" (ie, ketchup) in the tubing within the chest model (in foreground) that was used to perfuse and to expand the pulmonary vessels. The diamond-shaped black hole (in the rear, later in discussion Dr Ntaganda's left hand) cut into the chest model simulates the thoracotomy incision. Dr Daniel is pictured in the center.

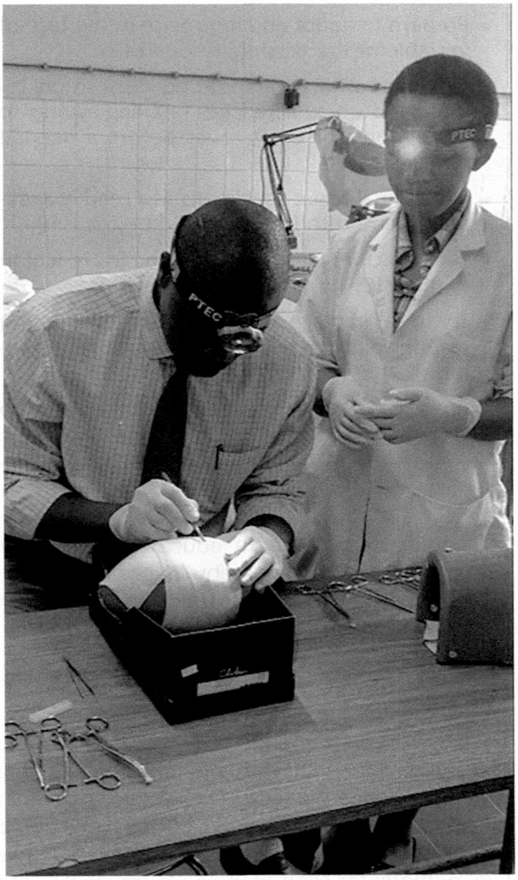

Fig. 6. Dr Ssebuufu is shown teaching pulmonary decortication to a surgery resident at Center Hospitalier Universitaire de Butare (CHUB).

PRINCIPLES FOR EQUITABLE, BILATERAL, AND SUSTAINABLE PARTNERSHIPS

Adhering to and building on the framework by Mock and colleagues,[18] the authors engaged local

Box 2
Important Lessons Learned

- Plan to visit the low-resource setting for at least several weeks-ideally as a separate initial visit-before implementing educational or clinical initiatives.
- Earnestly hear the perspectives of local physicians and staff about their teaching needs.
- Be wary of having preconceived ideas regarding what will work in a new context or culture before visiting and spending time in the country.
- Observe the operative and teaching facilities.

- Prepare to adapt and improvise in the face of variable or inaccessible resources.
- Cultivate an accommodating disposition toward the unexpected (ie, families having to raise funds for chest tubes before a needed operation).
- Use animal tissue specimens as a readily available method to increase validity (realism).
- Seek reciprocal collaboration in teaching with LMICs surgical faculty and staff.
- Try to set in place a full transition of teaching responsibility to the local faculty before leaving the host country.
- Consider developing a patient registry to facilitate needs and gap assessment.

stakeholders to cocreate educational initiatives, using improvisation whereby necessary. **Box 2** lists important lessons learned in establishing effective and bilateral partnerships.

SUMMARY

There has been tremendous growth and evolution of surgical education partnerships over the years with more focus placed on capacity building and sustainability in recent years. Challenges for in-country training still remain, but there are innovative methods for High-Income Countries (HICs) to support this training. Simulation provides an opportunity to teach critical surgical skills regardless of the patient volume.

DISCLOSURE

All authors have no current financial or commercial disclosures. .

REFERENCES

1. Farmer PE, Kim JY. Surgery and global health: a view from beyond the OR. World J Surg 2008; 32(4):533–6.
2. Shrime MG, Bickler SW, Alkire BC, et al. Global burden of disease: na estimation from the provider perspective. Lancet Glob Health 2015;3(suppl 2): S8–9.
3. Mock CN, Donkor P, Gawande A, et al. Essential surgery: key messages from Disease Control Priorities. Lancet 2015;385(9983):2209–19.
4. Meara JG, Leather AJM, Hagander L, et al. Global Surgery 2030: evidence and solutions for achieving health, welfare, and economic development. Lancet 2015;386(9993):569–624.
5. Price RR, Makasa E, Hollands M. World Health Assembly resolution WHA68.15: "Strengthening Emergency and Essential Surgical Care and Anesthesia as a Component of Universal Health Coverage" - addressing the public health gaps arising from lack of safe, affordable and accessible surgical and anesthetic services. World J Surg 2015;39(9):2115–25.
6. Mulwafu W, Fualal J, Bekele A, et al. The impact of COSECSA in developing the surgical workforce in East Central and Southern Africa. Surgeon 2022; 20(1):2–8.
7. Van Essen C, Steffes BC, Thelander K, et al. Increasing and retaining african surgeons working in rural hospitals: an analysis of PAACS surgeons with twenty-year program follow-up. World J Surg 2019;43(1):75–86.
8. Rickard J. Systematic Review of Postgraduate Surgical Education in Low- and Middle-Income Countries. World J Surg 2016;40(6):1324–35.
9. Nthumba PM. "Blitz surgery": redefining surgical needs, training, and practice in sub-Saharan Africa. World J Surg 2010;34(3):433–7.
10. Hendriks T, Botman M, Rahmee C, et al. Impact of short-term reconstructive surgical missions: a systematic review. BMJ Glob Health 2019;4(2): e001176.
11. Honeyman C, Patel V, Yonis E, et al. Long-term outcomes associated with short-term surgical missions treating complex head and neck disfigurement in Ethiopia: A retrospective cohort study. J Plast Reconstr Aesthet Surg 2020;73(5):951–8.
12. Mitchell KB, Kotecha DB, Said SA, et al. Short-term surgical missions: joining hands with local providers to ensure sustainability. S Afr J Surg 2012;50(1):2.
13. Swain JD, Pugliese DN, Mucumbitsi J, et al. Partnership for sustainability in cardiac surgery to address critical rheumatic heart disease in sub-Saharan Africa: the experience from Rwanda. World J Surg 2014;38(9):2205–11.
14. Riviello R, Ozgediz D, Hsia RY, et al. Role of collaborative academic partnerships in surgical training, education, and provision. World J Surg 2010;34(3): 459–65.
15. Parker RK, Mwachiro MM, Ranketi SS, et al. Curative surgery improves survival for colorectal cancer in rural kenya. World J Surg 2020;44(1):30–6.
16. Qureshi JS, Samuel J, Lee C, et al. Surgery and global public health: the UNC-Malawi surgical initiative as a model for sustainable collaboration. World J Surg 2011;35(1):17–21.
17. Mitchell KB, Giiti G, Kotecha V, et al. Surgical education at Weill Bugando Medical Centre: supplementing surgical training and investing in local health care providers. Can J Surg 2013;56(3):199–203.
18. Mock C, Debas HT, Balch CM, et al. Global surgery: effective involvement of US academic surgery.

Report of the American Surgical Association Working Group on Global Surgery. Ann Surg 2018;268: 557–63.
19. Binagwaho A, Kyamanywa P, Farmer PE, et al. The Human Resources for Health Program in Rwanda - A New Partnership. N Engl J Med 2013;369(21): 2054–9.
20. Cancedda C, Riviello R, Wilson K, et al. Building Workforce Capacity Abroad While Strengthening Global Health Programs at Home: Participation of Seven Harvard-Affiliated Institutions in a Health Professional Training Initiative in Rwanda. Acad Med 2017;92(5):649–58.
21. Holmer H, Lantz A, Kunjumen T, et al. Global distribution of surgeons, anaesthesiologists, and obstetricians. Lancet Glob Health 2015;(3 Suppl 2):S9–11.
22. Hoyler M, Finlayson SRG, McClain CD, et al. Shortage of doctors, shortage of data: a review of the global surgery, obstetrics, and anesthesia workforce literature. World J Surg 2014;38(2):269–80.
23. Scheffler R, Cometto G, Tulenko K, et al. Health workforce requirements for universal health coverage and the sustainable development goals. Background paper N.1. Human resources for health observer series No 17. World Health Organization; 2016. Available at: https://apps.who.int/iris/bitstream/handle/10665/250330/9789241511407-eng.pdf.
24. Talib Z, Narayan L, Harrod T. Postgraduate medical education in sub-saharan africa: a scoping review spanning 26 years and lessons learned. J Grad Med Educ 2019;11(4 Suppl):34–46.
25. Apenteng BA, Opoku ST, Ansong D, et al. The effect of power outages on in-facility mortality in healthcare facilities: Evidence from Ghana. Glob Public Health 2018;13(5):545–55.
26. Rajaguru PP, Jusabani MA, Massawe H, et al. Understanding surgical care delivery in Sub-Saharan Africa: a cross-sectional analysis of surgical volume, operations, and financing at a tertiary referral hospital in rural Tanzania. Glob Health Res Policy 2019;4: 30.
27. O'Flynn E, Andrew J, Hutch A, et al. The specialist surgeon workforce in east, central and southern africa: a situation analysis. World J Surg 2016; 40(11):2620–7.
28. Hoyler M, Hagander L, Gillies R, et al. Surgical care by non-surgeons in low-income and middle-income countries: a systematic review. Lancet 2015; 385(Suppl 2):S42.
29. Ramirez AG, Nuradin N, Byiringiro F, et al. General thoracic surgery in rwanda: an assessment of surgical volume and of workforce and material resource deficits. World J Surg 2019;43(1):36–43.
30. Kang MJ, Apea-Kubi KB, Apea-Kubi KAK, et al. Establishing a sustainable training program for laparoscopy in resource-limited settings: experience in ghana. Ann Glob Health 2020;86(1):89.
31. Raigani S, Numanoglu A, Schwachter M, et al. Online resources in pediatric surgery: the new era of medical information. Eur J Pediatr Surg 2014;24(4): 308–12.
32. College of surgeons of East, Central and Southern Africa (COSECSA). Accessed April 30, 2022. https://www.schoolforsurgeons.net/
33. Jotwani P, Srivastav V, Tripathi M, et al. Free-access open-source e-learning in comprehensive neurosurgery skills training. Neurol India 2014;62(4):352–61.
34. GlobalCastMD website. Available at: https://globalcastmd.com/. Accessed April 30, 2022.
35. Daniel TM. General and Thoracic Surgery Education website. Available at: https://thoracicsurgeryeducation.com/. Accessed April 30, 2022.
36. Okrainec A, Henao O, Azzie G. Telesimulation: an effective method for teaching the fundamentals of laparoscopic surgery in resource-restricted countries. Surg Endosc 2010;24(2):417–22.
37. Hadley GP. Mars M. e-Education in paediatric surgery: a role for recorded seminars in areas of low bandwidth in sub-Saharan Africa. Pediatr Surg Int 2011;27(4):407–10.
38. Ramirez AG, Nuradin N, Byiringiro F, et al. Creation, implementation, and assessment of a general thoracic surgery simulation course in rwanda. Ann Thorac Surg 2018;105:1842–50.
39. Feins RH, Burkhart HM, Conte JV, et al. Simulation-based training in cardiac surgery. Ann Thorac Surg 2017;103(1):312–21.
40. Debas H, Alatise OI, Balch CM, et al. Academic partnerships in global surgery: an overview american surgical association working group on academic global surgery. Ann Surg 2020;271(3):460–9.

Radiology for Thoracic Conditions in Low- and Middle-Income Countries

Monica Miranda-Schaeubinger, MD, MSPH[a], Abass Noor, MD[b], Cleverson Alex Leitão, MD, MSc[c], Hansel J. Otero, MD[a], Farouk Dako, MD, MPH[b,*]

KEYWORDS

• Thoracic imaging • Imaging in LMICs • Thoracic conditions in LMICs • Global radiology

KEY POINTS

- Adequate access to thoracic medical imaging has a high potential impact to reduce morbidity and mortality in low resource settings, which bear a disproportionately high burden of worldwide disease.
- Current epidemiology of thoracic diseases in low and middle-income countries (LMICs) highlights the importance of thoracic imaging in the diagnosis and management of both communicable and noncommunicable diseases.
- Limited access to health care exacerbated by the shortage of staff could be alleviated by technology advances including teleradiology and artificial intelligence. However, investment in local infrastructure is needed particularly for those targeting the diseases with highest burden such as COPD and lung cancer.

INTRODUCTION

Nature of the Problem

There are approximately 3 to 4 billion people in the world currently lacking adequate access to radiology services.[1] The absence of diagnostic imaging creates the downstream effect of delayed diagnosis and treatment resulting in poor health outcomes and the continued spread of disease. The disparity in imaging infrastructure is highlighted by the fact that the CT scanner density is 65 times greater in high-income countries (HICs) compared with low- and middle-income countries (LMICs).[1] There is also a significant shortage of radiologists and an even greater shortage of medical imaging technologists in many LMICs.[2] The personnel shortage is further exacerbated by the migration of health care personnel from LMICs to HICs. The reason for the "brain drain" is multifactorial, partly due to the absence of imaging infrastructure, and results in a vicious cycle that leads to weak health care systems and poor health outcomes.[3]

There is a disproportionate high burden of global morbidity and mortality caused by chronic respiratory diseases (CRDs) in LMICs due to socioeconomic determinants of health and limited availability of high-quality health services.[4] LMICs are undergoing a rapid epidemiologic transition to noncommunicable diseases (NCDs). More than 70% of all NCD deaths are in LMICs.[5] In referral centers, the shift has resulted in radiologists having to diagnose increasingly complex cases of congenital anomalies, cancer,

[a] Department of Radiology, Children's Hospital of Philadelphia, 3401 Civic Center Boulevard, Philadelphia, PA 19104, USA; [b] Department of Radiology, University of Pennsylvania, University of Pennsylvania Health System, 3400 Spruce Street, Philadelphia, PA 19104, USA; [c] Department of Radiology, Hospital de Clínicas da Universidade Federal do Paraná, Paraná, Brazil
* Corresponding author.
E-mail address: farouk.dako@pennmedicine.upenn.edu
Twitter: @MonicaMirandaSc (M.M.-S.); @ceelwaaq (A.N.); @oterocobo (H.J.O.); @farouk_dako (F.D.)

Thorac Surg Clin 32 (2022) 289–298
https://doi.org/10.1016/j.thorsurg.2022.03.001

cardiovascular and neurologic conditions.[6–8] Although an increase in Internet connectivity has allowed for remote technical support and teleradiology and artificial intelligence have the potential to limit the impact of the shortage of radiologists,[9,10] sustainable and scalable solutions to strengthen health care systems and improve health outcomes in LMICs are needed. Locoregional disease patterns and available imaging modalities should be considered when developing solutions to build local health care capacity.

Burden of Disease in Low and Middle-Income Countries

While the classic portrayal of disease in LMICs is infectious and parasitic diseases, these countries also bear the burden of noncommunicable diseases (NCDs).[11] Pneumonia, diarrhea, and malaria for example, remain some of the leading causes of mortality in LMIC. However, other conditions including cancer, road injuries, and cardiovascular diseases are becoming more prevalent. LMICs have been undergoing a rapid epidemiologic transition with a rising burden of NCDs in recent years.[12] When using the age-standardization of the weighted average of age-specific death rates, NCDs have higher death rates in LMICs than high-income countries (HICs).[13] This epidemiologic shift requires special attention when planning health care interventions and services, including the need for medical imaging.

Due to ease of performance and interpretation, chest radiography is the main imaging modality used in the diagnosis of thoracic diseases. CT and to a lesser degree MRI are often performed for complication detection in infections and trauma or for cancer staging.[14,15] More recently, ultrasonography has become increasingly available and could likely yield important survival gains in low-income settings. Major advantages of ultrasound include its low cost, safety, ability to be performed at bedside and repeated without radiation dose consideration.[16] One notable form of task-shifting is the performance of point of care ultrasound (POCUS) by nonradiologists (physicians and nonphysicians providers).[17]

COMMUNICABLE DISEASES

Despite the described epidemiologic shift, infections remain a serious cause of morbidity and mortality in LMICs.[18] The term "Infectious Diseases of Poverty" (IDoP) is used to describe those infectious diseases that are most prevalent among poor and vulnerable populations. They comprise HIV/AIDS, tuberculosis (TB), malaria, and neglected tropical diseases (a group of diverse communicable diseases that prevail in tropical and subtropical conditions).[19] Additionally note should be made of fungal diseases endemic to various LMIC regions such as Paracoccidioidomycosis in parts of Central and South America (**Fig. 1**) and those associated with immunocompromised hosts such as *Pneumocystics jiroveci* pneumonia (PJP) in patients with HIV.[20,21]

Human Immunodeficiency Virus Infection

While the availability of testing and treatment of combination antiretroviral treatment (cART) and prevention programs for maternal-to-child transmission have decreased the rates of perinatal infection, there are approximately 37.7 million people living with HIV, with over two-thirds of them living in the World Health Organization's African Region.[22] HIV exposure in utero affects even uninfected infants with reduced lung function, particularly in children born to mothers with poorly controlled HIV during pregnancy.[4]

Imaging plays a significant role in the management of HIV such as in the detection of opportunistic infections and associated neoplasms. By 2018, around 2.8 million children globally were living with HIV, of whom 9 out of 10 were from sub-Saharan Africa.[23] Absent or delayed diagnosis and treatment could result in mortality in more than 50% of children with congenitally acquired infection before they reach 3 years of age.[24]

Pneumonia

Pneumonia has a considerable impact on morbidity and mortality worldwide. While in HICs, community-acquired pneumonia (CAP) mostly affects the elderly, it predominantly affects the working-age group in LMICs.[25] Furthermore, TB, gram-negative bacteria, and HIV-associated infectious agents predominate in LMICs, whereby a staggering 90% of the global deaths from pneumonia occur.[26] The diagnosis of pneumonia is usually made without routine medical imaging. Medical imaging is usually reserved for patients that require hospitalization, those with suspected complications, immunosuppression, and those that exhibit persistent or recurrent symptoms despite initial empiric treatment. More recently, ultrasound has gained interest as the equipment becomes cheaper and more accessible at a time when there is particular interest in clinician-led POCUS.[27–29]

Tuberculosis

Tuberculosis is still a major health problem with around 10 million new cases in 2019,[30] and most cases occurring in LMICs. While the incidence is

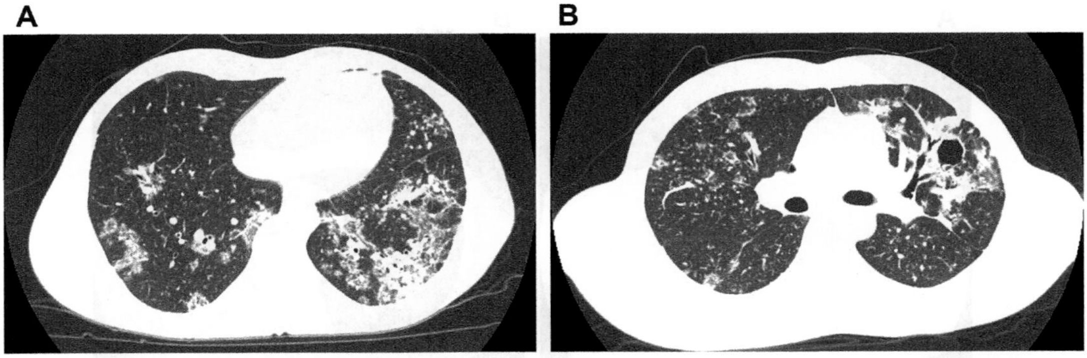

Fig. 1. CT of the lung at the level of lower lobes (*A*) shows multifocal ground-glass opacities, some of them with peripheral consolidations (reversed halo sign). Upper lobe images of the same patient (*B*) revealed associated centrilobular nodules (*right upper lobe*) and cavitation (*left upper lobe*). Bronchoalveolar lavage was positive for *Paracoccidioides brasiliensis*.

slowly declining, TB remains one of the top 10 causes of death, and the leading cause from a single infectious agent (above HIV/AIDS).[31] Case finding and diagnosis remain one of the TB's biggest challenges.[32] In patients with presumptive TB in whom smears and Xpert MTB/RIF results are negative, management decisions are usually made with the results of chest radiograph, which is challenging given that there are various imaging patterns defined in TB (**Figs. 2 and 3**).[32] This is especially challenging in patients with HIV associated TB, in which imaging patterns vary significantly.[33]

COVID-19

The COVID-19 pandemic has highlighted the role of thoracic imaging in the management of thoracic conditions through surveillance and diagnosis. Chest CT continues to be used for diagnosis of COVID-19 pneumonia in symptomatic patients in some middle-income settings with established imaging capacity despite reports of inferior accuracy to RT-PCR and professional societies recommendations.[33–38] The discrepancy between recommendations and continuous use of chest imaging is likely due to preexisting infrastructure for rapid access and results from CT compared with limited availability of RT-PCR tests early in the pandemic as well as issues around the supply chain of needed materials for testing.[39] Typical, indeterminate, or atypical patterns for COVID-19 can be described in hospitalized patients, with ground-glass opacities without consolidation being the most commonly described findings. However, no finding is exclusive to COVID-19 and there is an overlap of findings with other viral low respiratory tract infections and organizing pneumonia.

Chest radiography is usually the initial imaging test in the evaluation of COVID-19 pneumonia due to its ubiquity and portability. This also allows it to be used to monitor disease progression in admitted patients without the need for patient transportation. Imaging findings on chest radiograph mirror those on chest CT although with less accuracy in detection. For some settings in which CT or radiographs are not available, POCUS can be an option with relatively high sensitivity. Caution must be held with POCUS, however, given its low specificity.[40–42]

NONCOMMUNICABLE DISEASES

More than two-thirds of global deaths are attributable to NCDs.[43,44] Numerous chest-related conditions drive the increasing burden reported in the Global Burden of Disease report of 2020.[45] Chronic obstructive pulmonary disease (COPD) and lung cancer are among the top 10 leading causes of disability-adjusted life years in the ≥50 age group.[44,45] CRDs such as asthma, COPD, bronchiectasis, and post-TB lung disease (PTLD) span the life course and are commonly neglected.[4]

ENVIRONMENTAL EXPOSURES

In-utero and early childhood exposures can lead to increased risks of CRDs later in life.[4] In-utero exposure to tobacco smoke affects lung structure and function, and is associated with lower tidal volumes and higher lung clearance indices.[46,47] Other forms of air pollution such as atmospheric pollution are associated with similar outcomes.[48] There is strong evidence of an association between air pollution and lung cancer incidence across the world[49–52] and the International Agency for Research on Cancer has labeled outdoor air

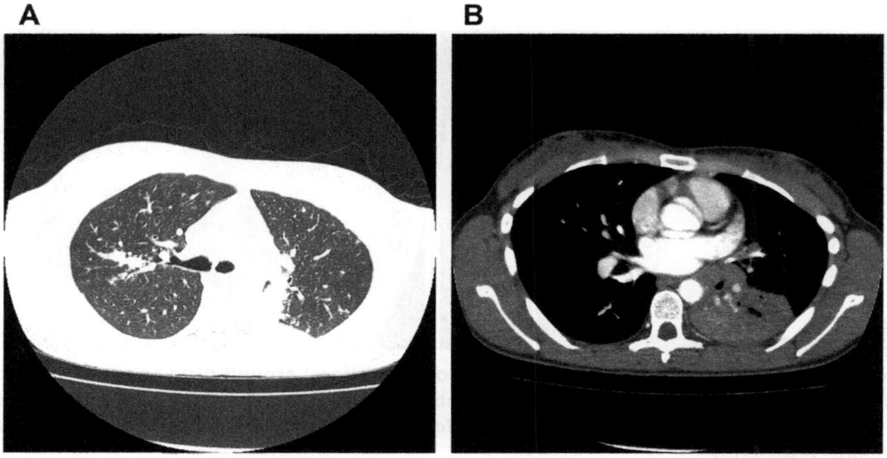

Fig. 2. CT of the lung at the level of upper lobes (*A*) in a 25-year-old female from South Brazil with primary tuberculosis shows centrilobular and acinar nodules along the bronchovascular bundle in the right upper lobe. CT of the same patient (*B*) also showed left lower lobe collapse and left hilar lymphadenopathy.

pollution as a leading environmental cause of cancer death.[53,54]

Some households in LMICs reach high indoor house pollution due to indoor cooking with traditional cookstoves, dependence on fossil-fuel-powered generators for electric supply, poor ventilation, and overcrowding.[55–59] Furthermore, exposure to indoor air pollution increases the susceptibility to pneumonia, the leading cause of death in children less than 5 years.

CHRONIC OBSTRUCTIVE PULMONARY DISEASE IN LOW AND MIDDLE-INCOME COUNTRIES

The third leading cause of death worldwide in 2017 was COPD.[60] More than 90% of COPD deaths occur in LMICs.[60] Guidelines for appropriate diagnosis and management of COPD are only available for 21.9% of LMIC countries.[61] Unfortunately, COPD often goes underdiagnosed, depriving patients of timely management with nonpharmacologic, cost-saving management.[62,63] Diagnosis and subsequently, management of COPD in LMICs is limited as spirometry is not widely available.[64] Furthermore, while imaging is not required to diagnose COPD, CT and radiography play an important supportive diagnostic role and in excluding complications and alternative diagnoses.

LUNG CANCER IN LOW AND MIDDLE-INCOME COUNTRIES

Lung cancer is known as a silent killer due to difficulty with early detection which is exacerbated in LMICs by inadequate imaging infrastructure and shortage of radiologists results in underdiagnosis and poor surveillance. The increasing burden of cancer in LMICs is a major threat to achieving

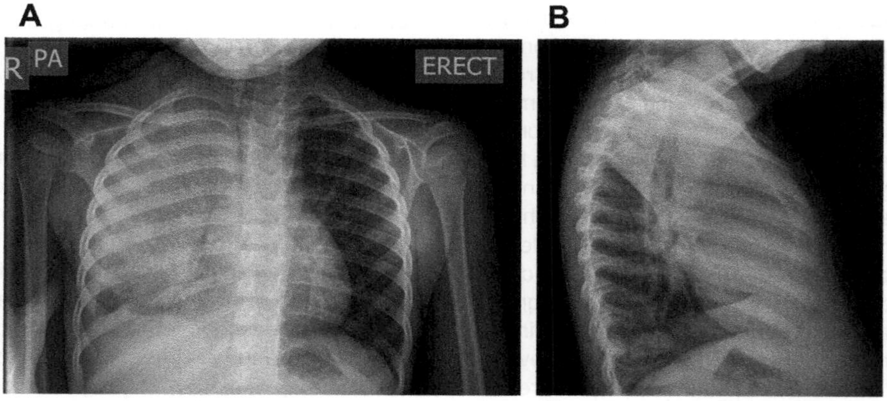

Fig. 3. Frontal (*A*) and lateral (*B*) chest radiographs in a 2-year-old patient front South Sudan demonstrate right upper lobe opacities and moderate right pleural effusion also diagnosed with primary tuberculosis.

the SDGs.[65] Lung cancer continues to be the largest cause of cancer mortality worldwide with an increasing proportion noted among never smokers and in LMICs.[65–67] About every 3 in five cases are now diagnosed in LMICs, often in advanced stages of disease, resulting in a poor prognosis.[65] Early detection of lung cancer has been shown to dramatically improve patient prognosis with a 5-year survival rate of 70% to 90% versus 15% when diagnosis is delayed. The critical role and shortage of medical imaging in LMICs for cancer management are increasingly being recognized—a 2021 report by the Lancet Oncology Commission showed that the scale-up of imaging alone globally would avert 2.46 million of all 76 million deaths caused by the modeled cancers worldwide between 2020 and 2030 with a net benefit of $209.46 billion and net return of $31.61 per $1 invested.[68]

Lung cancer screening with low dose computed tomography (LDCT) compared with chest radiography demonstrated a 20% mortality reduction in the National Lung Screening Trial (NLST) performed in the United States[69]—an even greater reduction in mortality (24%) was shown in the European NELSON trial.[70] These trials demonstrated smoking and age as the major risk factors for lung cancer and emphasized that lung cancer screening using LDCT should select high-risk groups for lung cancer and measuring cost-effectiveness.[71,72]

Lung cancer screening with LDCT has demonstrated cost-effectiveness in high-income countries (HICs)[73–75]; however, reports on its performance from limited data in LMICs are inconclusive.[76] A current limitation in defining high-risk groups for lung cancer, highlighted in the Surveillance, Epidemiology, and End Result (SEER) database, is evidenced by the fact that only 27% of subjects diagnosed with lung cancer in the US met the NLST inclusion criteria.[77] This limitation is likely greater in LMICs due to demographic differences compared with the US. and Europe, a higher proportion of lung cancer in never smokers (LCINS), and the presence of not well-known local risk factors contributing to lung cancer.[78]

There is no LDCT lung cancer screening study reported in the continent of Africa which will be home to more than 25% of the world's population by 2050.[76] Barriers to lung cancer screening programs in LMICs include a shortage of trained radiologists for the interpretation of LDCT scans, lack of required infrastructure, public awareness and policies, and absence of defined high-risk groups.[76] The higher incidence of granulomatous infections in LMICs can lead to increased detection of lung nodules in screening LDCTs which supports the need for more studies assessing the effectiveness of screening in these settings.[79]

IMAGE-GUIDED PROCEDURES

While HIC have greater than 1 interventional radiologist per 100,0000 people, those in LMICs have access to less than 1 interventional radiologist per 800,000 to 36 million people, or even a complete lack of services at the national level.[80]

Thoracic Ultrasound

Ultrasound is a safe, efficient, and cost-effective imaging modality that, in the hands of an experienced sonographer, can be a powerful tool at the point of care in both diagnostic and therapeutic procedures. Ultrasound is widely available and used in LMICs. The use of thoracic ultrasound in diagnosing pneumonia, pulmonary edema, and pneumothorax has been described.[81] Thoracic ultrasound has also been shown to decrease complications when performing thoracentesis and pleural tube placement for drainage or decompression of pneumothorax.[82] Additionally, thoracic ultrasound has been used to guide closed pleural and peripheral lung nodule biopsy, and intraoperatively during video-assisted thoracoscopic surgery to aid in identifying the location of pulmonary nodules.[83–85]

Computed Tomography Guided Thoracic Biopsy

As thoracic surgery, clinical pathology, and surgical pathology become more available in low-LMICs, radiology groups are increasingly offering CT-guided fine-needle aspiration and core biopsy services (**Fig. 4**).[86–89] CT-guided tissue sampling has been proven to be a safe and effective method with adequate diagnostic yield across thoracic diseases.[90–92] Challenges presented in offering these services are primarily in the availability of imaging technology and medical supplies, as well as education and training programs.[93] For example, according to the World Health Organization's 2017 Global Atlas of Medical Equipment, a survey of member states found that only 24% of respondent countries in Africa have at least one CT scanner per 1 million people.[94] Despite barriers to availability in imaging technology, over the last decade we have seen significant progress in establishing radiology residency programs in LMICs.[95] In time, particularly with the development of interventional radiology training programs in LMICs,[96] it is expected that services can be expanded to include therapeutic CT-guided procedures.

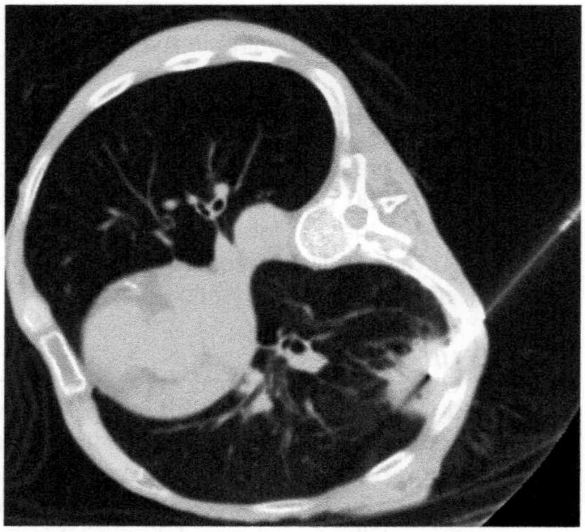

Fig. 4. CT-guided biopsy of a peripheral right lower lobe mass in a patient with weight loss and hemoptysis performed in a Tertiary Hospital in Paraná, Brazil. Histology revealed lung adenocarcinoma.

THE PROMISE OF ARTIFICIAL INTELLIGENCE

Computer-aided detection (CAD) is becoming an increasingly important tool in image interpretation.[97–99] This is reflected in the WHO 2021 TB screening updates which for the first time recommended CAD with Artificial Intelligence (AI) technology as an alternative to human interpretation of digital chest radiograph TB screening and triage.[100] CAD techniques have for long shown great potential in the detection of pulmonary nodules on chest CT.[97,99] The incorporation of AI in CAD has resulted in deep learning algorithms for the detection and classification of pulmonary nodules on CT that in some cases comparable to that of a trained radiologist.[101] Multiple studies have demonstrated the feasibility of automated pulmonary nodule detection on CT using AI algorithms.[102–105]

The introduction of AI in LMICs requires special considerations due to differences in personnel, clinical experience, disease patterns, demographics, digital infrastructure, and radiology equipment.[9] It has the potential to revolutionize medical imaging and reduce disparities in quality of care and yet could also act to widen health inequities between HICs and LMICs without a global health implementation strategy. A three-pronged approach emphasizing clinical radiology education, infrastructure implementation, and phased AI introduction has been recommended.[9]

SUMMARY

Radiology has an important role in reducing the burden of thoracic diseases in LMICs through early diagnosis as well as treatment and procedure guidance. NCDs such as COPD and lung cancer require special attention and targeted programmatic solutions due to their high morbidity and mortality. Teleradiology and AI provide additional opportunities to mitigate radiology personnel shortages. However, there is a need to develop sustainable and scalable solutions to strengthen local health care imaging infrastructure.

DISCLOSURE

The authors declare that they have no relevant or material financial interests that relate to the research described in this article.

REFERENCES

1. Human Health Campus - Database & Statistics. Available at: https://humanhealth.iaea.org/HHW/DBStatistics/IMAGINE.html. Accessed December 14, 2021.
2. Tanzania faces acute shortage of radiology, imaging experts - the Citizen. Available at: https://www.thecitizen.co.tz/news/Tanzania-faces-acute-shortage-of-radiology–imaging-experts/1840340-3818168-ccwvk9/index.html. Accessed December 14, 2021.
3. Saluja S, Rudolfson N, Massenburg BB, et al. The impact of physician migration on mortality in low and middle-income countries: an economic modelling study. BMJ Glob Health 2020;5(1):e001535.
4. Meghji J, Mortimer K, Agusti A, et al. Improving lung health in low-income and middle-income countries: from challenges to solutions. Lancet 2021;397(10277):928–40.
5. Marten R, Mikkelsen B, Shao R, et al. Committing to implementation research for health systems to manage and control non-communicable diseases. Lancet Glob Health 2021;9(2):e108–9.
6. Bhakta N, Force LM, Allemani C, et al. Childhood cancer burden: a review of global estimates. Lancet Oncol 2019;20(1):e42–53.
7. Zühlke L, Lawrenson J, Comitis G, et al. Congenital Heart Disease in Low- and Lower-Middle-Income Countries: Current Status and New Opportunities. Curr Cardiol Rep 2019;21(12):163.
8. Dewan MC, Rattani A, Mekary R, et al. Global hydrocephalus epidemiology and incidence: systematic review and meta-analysis. *J Neurosurg* April 2018;1–15.
9. Mollura DJ, Culp MP, Pollack E, et al. Artificial Intelligence in Low- and Middle-Income Countries: Innovating Global Health Radiology. Radiology 2020;297(3):513–20.
10. Haleem A, Javaid M, Singh RP, et al. Telemedicine for healthcare: Capabilities, features, barriers, and

applications. Sensors Int 2021;2:100117. https://doi.org/10.1016/j.sintl.2021.100117.
11. Achwoka D, Mutave R, Oyugi JO, et al. Tackling an emerging epidemic: the burden of non-communicable diseases among people living with HIV/AIDS in sub-Saharan Africa. Pan Afr Med J 2020;36:271. https://doi.org/10.11604/pamj.2020.36.271.22810.
12. Oni T, McGrath N, BeLue R, et al. Chronic diseases and multi-morbidity–a conceptual modification to the WHO ICCC model for countries in health transition. BMC Public Health 2014;14:575. https://doi.org/10.1186/1471-2458-14-575.
13. Coates MM, Ezzati M, Robles Aguilar G, et al. Burden of disease among the world's poorest billion people: An expert-informed secondary analysis of Global Burden of Disease estimates. PLoS One 2021;16(8):e0253073.
14. Maru DS-R, Schwarz R, Jason A, et al. Turning a blind eye: the mobilization of radiology services in resource-poor regions. Glob Health 2010;6:18. https://doi.org/10.1186/1744-8603-6-18.
15. Mehta AC, Chua A-P, Gleeson F, et al. The debate on CXR utilization and interpretation is only just beginning: a Pro/Con debate. Respirology 2010; 15(8):1152–6.
16. Dudink J, Jeanne Steggerda S, Horsch S, eurUS.-brain group. State-of-the-art neonatal cerebral ultrasound: technique and reporting. Pediatr Res 2020;87(Suppl 1):3–12.
17. Ward ZJ, Scott AM, Hricak H, et al. Estimating the impact of treatment and imaging modalities on 5-year net survival of 11 cancers in 200 countries: a simulation-based analysis. Lancet Oncol 2020; 21(8):1077–88.
18. Holmes KK, Bertozzi S, Bloom BR, et al. Major Infectious Diseases: Key Messages from Disease Control Priorities, Third Edition. In: Holmes KK, Bertozzi S, Bloom BR, et al, editors. Major infectious diseases. 3rd edition. Washington (DC): The International Bank for Reconstruction and Development/The World Bank; 2017. https://doi.org/10.1596/978-1-4648-0524-0_ch1.
19. Bhutta ZA, Sommerfeld J, Lassi ZS, et al. Global burden, distribution, and interventions for infectious diseases of poverty. Infect Dis Poverty 2014; 3:21. https://doi.org/10.1186/2049-9957-3-21.
20. Paracoccidioidomycosis | Fungal Diseases | CDC. Available at: https://www.cdc.gov/fungal/diseases/other/paracoccidioidomycosis.html. Accessed December 14, 2021.
21. Hansen C, Paintsil E. Infectious diseases of poverty in children: A tale of two worlds. Pediatr Clin North Am 2016;63(1):37–66.
22. HIV/AIDS. Available at: https://www.who.int/data/gho/data/themes/hiv-aids. Accessed November 18, 2021.
23. HIV Statistics - Global and Regional Trends - UNICEF DATA. Available at: https://data.unicef.org/topic/hivaids/global-regional-trends/. Accessed November 30, 2021.
24. Moreira-Silva SF, Zandonade E, Miranda AE. Mortality in children and adolescents vertically infected by HIV receiving care at a referral hospital in Vitoria, Brazil. BMC Infect Dis 2015;15:155. https://doi.org/10.1186/s12879-015-0893-0.
25. Aston SJ. Pneumonia in the developing world: Characteristic features and approach to management. Respirology 2017;22(7):1276–87.
26. Adaji EE, Ekezie W, Clifford M, et al. Understanding the effect of indoor air pollution on pneumonia in children under 5 in low- and middle-income countries: a systematic review of evidence. Environ Sci Pollut Res Int 2019;26(4):3208–25.
27. Pervaiz F, Chavez MA, Ellington LE, et al. Building a prediction model for radiographically confirmed pneumonia in peruvian children: from symptoms to imaging. Chest 2018;154(6):1385–94.
28. Lenahan JL, Volpicelli G, Lamorte A, et al. Multicentre pilot study evaluation of lung ultrasound for the management of paediatric pneumonia in low-resource settings: a study protocol. BMJ Open Respir Res 2018;5(1):e000340. https://doi.org/10.1136/bmjresp-2018-000340.
29. Nadimpalli A, Tsung JW, Sanchez R, et al. Feasibility of Training Clinical Officers in Point-of-Care Ultrasound for Pediatric Respiratory Diseases in Aweil, South Sudan. Am J Trop Med Hyg 2019; 101(3):689–95.
30. Tuberculosis. Available at: https://www.who.int/news-room/fact-sheets/detail/tuberculosis. Accessed November 30, 2021.
31. Organization WH. Global tuberculosis report 2018. World Health Organization; 2018.
32. Harries AD, Kumar AMV. Challenges and Progress with Diagnosing Pulmonary Tuberculosis in Low- and Middle-Income Countries. Diagnostics (Basel) 2018; 8(4). https://doi.org/10.3390/diagnostics8040078.
33. Chamie G, Luetkemeyer A, Walusimbi-Nanteza M, et al. Significant variation in presentation of pulmonary tuberculosis across a high resolution of CD4 strata. Int J Tuberc Lung Dis 2010;14(10):1295–302.
34. Ai T, Yang Z, Hou H, et al. Correlation of Chest CT and RT-PCR Testing for Coronavirus Disease 2019 (COVID-19) in China: A Report of 1014 Cases. Radiology 2020;296(2):E32–40.
35. Bai HX, Hsieh B, Xiong Z, et al. Performance of Radiologists in Differentiating COVID-19 from Non-COVID-19 Viral Pneumonia at Chest CT. Radiology 2020;296(2):E46–54.
36. Bernheim A, Mei X, Huang M, et al. Chest CT Findings in Coronavirus Disease-19 (COVID-19): Relationship to Duration of Infection. Radiology 2020; 295(3):200463.

37. Xie X, Zhong Z, Zhao W, et al. Chest CT for Typical Coronavirus Disease 2019 (COVID-19) Pneumonia: Relationship to Negative RT-PCR Testing. Radiology 2020;296(2):E41–5.
38. Han X, Cao Y, Jiang N, et al. Novel Coronavirus Disease 2019 (COVID-19) Pneumonia Progression Course in 17 Discharged Patients: Comparison of Clinical and Thin-Section Computed Tomography Features During Recovery. Clin Infect Dis 2020; 71(15):723–31.
39. ACR Recommendations for the use of Chest Radiography and Computed Tomography (CT) for Suspected COVID-19 Infection | Am Coll Radiol. Available at: https://www.acr.org/Advocacy-and-Economics/ACR-Position-Statements/Recommendations-for-Chest-Radiography-and-CT-for-Suspected-COVID19-Infection. Accessed December 1, 2021.
40. Bar S, Lecourtois A, Diouf M, et al. The association of lung ultrasound images with COVID-19 infection in an emergency room cohort. Anaesthesia 2020; 75(12):1620–5.
41. Abrams ER, Rose G, Fields JM, et al. Point-of-Care Ultrasound in the Evaluation of COVID-19. J Emerg Med 2020;59(3):403–8.
42. Islam N, Salameh J-P, Leeflang MM, et al. Thoracic imaging tests for the diagnosis of COVID-19. Cochrane Database Syst Rev 2020; 11:CD013639. https://doi.org/10.1002/14651858.CD013639.pub3.
43. Lozano R, Naghavi M, Foreman K, et al. Global and regional mortality from 235 causes of death for 20 age groups in 1990 and 2010: a systematic analysis for the Global Burden of Disease Study 2010. Lancet 2012;380(9859):2095–128.
44. NCD Countdown 2030 collaborators. NCD Countdown 2030: worldwide trends in non-communicable disease mortality and progress towards Sustainable Development Goal target 3.4. Lancet 2018;392(10152):1072–88.
45. GBD 2019 Diseases, Injuries Collaborators. Global burden of 369 diseases and injuries in 204 countries and territories, 1990-2019: a systematic analysis for the Global Burden of Disease Study 2019. Lancet 2020;396(10258):1204–22.
46. Bush A. Lung development and aging. Ann Am Thorac Soc 2016;13(Suppl 5):S438–46.
47. Gray DM, Turkovic L, Willemse L, et al. Lung function in african infants in the drakenstein child health study. impact of lower respiratory tract illness. Am J Respir Crit Care Med 2017;195(2): 212–20.
48. Lee AG, Kaali S, Quinn A, et al. Prenatal Household Air Pollution Is Associated with Impaired Infant Lung Function with Sex-Specific Effects. Evidence from GRAPHS, a Cluster Randomized Cookstove Intervention Trial. Am J Respir Crit Care Med 2019;199(6):738–46.
49. Hystad P, Demers PA, Johnson KC, et al. Long-term residential exposure to air pollution and lung cancer risk. Epidemiology 2013;24(5):762–72.
50. Wong CM, Tsang H, Lai HK, et al. Cancer Mortality Risks from Long-term Exposure to Ambient Fine Particle. Cancer Epidemiol Biomarkers Prev 2016; 25(5):839–45.
51. Hughes BD, Maharsi S, Obiarinze RN, et al. Correlation between air quality and lung cancer incidence: A county by county analysis. Surgery 2019;166(6):1099–104.
52. Loomis D, Grosse Y, Lauby-Secretan B, et al. The carcinogenicity of outdoor air pollution. Lancet Oncol 2013;14(13):1262–3.
53. Loomis D, Huang W, Chen G. The International Agency for Research on Cancer (IARC) evaluation of the carcinogenicity of outdoor air pollution: focus on China. Chin J Cancer 2014;33(4):189–96.
54. IARC: Outdoor air pollution a leading environmental cause of cancer deaths – IARC. Available at: https://www.iarc.who.int/news-events/iarc-outdoor-air-pollution-a-leading-environmental-cause-of-cancer-deaths/. Accessed November 24, 2021.
55. Isara AR, Aigbokhaode AQ. Household Cooking Fuel Use among Residents of a Sub-Urban Community in Nigeria: Implications for Indoor Air Pollution. Eurasian J Med 2014;46(3):203–8.
56. Checkley W, Ghannem H, Irazola V, et al. Management of NCD in low- and middle-income countries. Glob Heart 2014;9(4):431–43.
57. Akintan O, Jewitt S, Clifford M. Culture, tradition, and taboo: Understanding the social shaping of fuel choices and cooking practices in Nigeria. Energy Res Social Sci 2018;40:14–22. https://doi.org/10.1016/j.erss.2017.11.019.
58. Agbo KE, Walgraeve C, Eze JI, et al. A review on ambient and indoor air pollution status in Africa. Atmos Pollut Res 2021;12(2):243–60.
59. Godson Rowland A, Mayowa MO, Adekunle FG. Indoor air quality and risk factors associated with respiratory conditions in Nigeria. In: Nejadkoorki F, editor. Current air quality issues. InTech; 2015. https://doi.org/10.5772/59864.
60. GBD 2015 Chronic Respiratory Disease Collaborators. Global, regional, and national deaths, prevalence, disability-adjusted life years, and years lived with disability for chronic obstructive pulmonary disease and asthma, 1990-2015: a systematic analysis for the Global Burden of Disease Study 2015. Lancet Respir Med 2017;5(9):691–706.
61. Tabyshova A, Hurst JR, Soriano JB, et al. Gaps in COPD Guidelines of Low- and Middle-Income Countries: A Systematic Scoping Review. Chest 2021;159(2):575–84.
62. Brakema EA, van Gemert FA, van der Kleij RMJJ, et al. COPD's early origins in low-and-middle income countries: what are the implications of a false

start? NPJ Prim Care Respir Med 2019;29(1):6. https://doi.org/10.1038/s41533-019-0117-y.
63. Landry MD, Hamdan E, Al Mazeedi S, et al. The precarious balance between "supply" and "demand" for health care: the increasing global demand for rehabilitation service for individuals living with chronic obstructive pulmonary disease. Int J Chron Obstruct Pulmon Dis 2008; 3(3):393–6.
64. Halpin DMG, Celli BR, Criner GJ, et al. The GOLD Summit on chronic obstructive pulmonary disease in low- and middle-income countries. Int J Tuberc Lung Dis 2019;23(11):1131–41.
65. Shah SC, Kayamba V, Peek RM, et al. Cancer Control in Low- and Middle-Income Countries: Is It Time to Consider Screening? J Glob Oncol 2019; 5:1–8. https://doi.org/10.1200/JGO.18.00200.
66. Shankar A, Saini D, Dubey A, et al. Feasibility of lung cancer screening in developing countries: challenges, opportunities and way forward. Transl Lung Cancer Res 2019;8(Suppl 1):S106–21.
67. Sung H, Ferlay J, Siegel RL, et al. Global cancer statistics 2020: GLOBOCAN estimates of incidence and mortality worldwide for 36 cancers in 185 countries. CA Cancer J Clin 2021;71(3): 209–49.
68. Hricak H, Abdel-Wahab M, Atun R, et al. Medical imaging and nuclear medicine: a Lancet Oncology Commission. Lancet Oncol 2021;22(4):e136–72.
69. National Lung Screening Trial Research Team, Aberle DR, Adams AM, et al. Reduced lung-cancer mortality with low-dose computed tomographic screening. N Engl J Med 2011;365(5): 395–409.
70. de Koning HJ, van der Aalst CM, de Jong PA, et al. Reduced Lung-Cancer Mortality with Volume CT Screening in a Randomized Trial. N Engl J Med 2020;382(6):503–13.
71. Black WC, Gareen IF, Soneji SS, et al. Cost-effectiveness of CT screening in the National Lung Screening Trial. N Engl J Med 2014;371(19): 1793–802.
72. Duffy SW, Field JK. Mortality Reduction with Low-Dose CT Screening for Lung Cancer. N Engl J Med 2020;382(6):572–3.
73. Goffin JR, Flanagan WM, Miller AB, et al. Cost-effectiveness of Lung Cancer Screening in Canada. JAMA Oncol 2015;1(6):807–13.
74. Ten Haaf K, Tammemägi MC, Bondy SJ, et al. Performance and Cost-Effectiveness of Computed Tomography Lung Cancer Screening Scenarios in a Population-Based Setting: A Microsimulation Modeling Analysis in Ontario, Canada. Plos Med 2017;14(2):e1002225.
75. Pyenson BS, Tomicki SM. Lung Cancer Screening: A Cost-Effective Public Health Imperative. Am J Public Health 2018;108(10):1292–3.
76. Edelman Saul E, Guerra RB, Edelman Saul M, et al. The challenges of implementing low-dose computed tomography for lung cancer screening in low- and middle-income countries. Nat Cancer 2020. https://doi.org/10.1038/s43018-020-00142-z.
77. Pinsky PF, Berg CD. Applying the National Lung Screening Trial eligibility criteria to the US population: what percent of the population and of incident lung cancers would be covered? J Med Screen 2012;19(3):154–6.
78. Gaafar R. SC17.05 lung cancer in africa: challenges and perspectives. J Thorac Oncol 2017; 12(1):S115–6.
79. dos Santos RS, Franceschini JP, Chate RC, et al. Do current lung cancer screening guidelines apply for populations with high prevalence of granulomatous disease? results from the first brazilian lung cancer screening trial (BRELT1). Ann Thorac Surg 2016;101(2):481–6.
80. England RW, Gage D, Kesselman A, et al. To New Heights: Interventional Radiology Outreach to Underserved Regions via Aircraft-Delivered Mobile Health Units. Cardiovasc Intervent Radiol 2021; 44(9):1478–80.
81. Hendin A, Koenig S, Millington SJ. Better with ultrasound: thoracic ultrasound. Chest 2020;158(5): 2082–9.
82. Thiboutot J, Bramley KT. Ultrasound-Guided Pleural Investigations: Fluid, Air, and Biopsy. Clin Chest Med 2021;42(4):591–7.
83. Hou Y-L, Wang Y-D, Guo H-Q, et al. Ultrasound location of pulmonary nodules in video-assisted thoracoscopic surgery for precise sublobectomy. Thorac Cancer 2020;11(5):1354–60.
84. Scisca C, Rizzo M, Maisano R, et al. The role of ultrasound-guided aspiration biopsy of peripheral pulmonary nodules: our experience. Anticancer Res 2002;22(4):2521–3.
85. Koegelenberg CFN, Dorfman S, Schewitz I, et al. Recommendations for lung cancer screening in Southern Africa. J Thorac Dis 2019;11(9): 3696–703.
86. Ogbole GI, Adeoye PO, Okolo CA, et al. CT-guided percutaneous transthoracic lung biopsy: first experience in Ibadan, Nigeria. Niger J Clin Pract 2013; 16(4):544–7.
87. Niang A, Bonnichon A, Ba-Fall K, et al. [Lung cancer in Senegal]. Med Trop (Mars) 2007;67(6): 651–6.
88. Rai DK. Role of image-guided fine needle aspiration cytology of lung lesions in diagnosis and primary care of patients: Experience in a Government Medical College of Eastern India. J Fam Med Prim Care 2020;9(10):5386–7.
89. Eklund MJ, Hudgins PA, Kebede T, et al. Introduction of Thoracic CT-Guided Fine-Needle Aspiration to a Resource-Limited Radiology Department in

Addis Ababa, Ethiopia. J Am Coll Radiol 2016;13(1):98–103.
90. Watane GV, Hammer MM, Barile MF. CT-guided Core-Needle Biopsy of the Lung Is Safe and More Effective than Fine-Needle Aspiration Biopsy in Patients with Hematologic Malignancies. Radiol Cardiothorac Imaging 2019;1(5):e180030.
91. Hsu JL, Kuschner WG, Paik J, et al. The diagnostic yield of CT-guided percutaneous lung biopsy in solid organ transplant recipients. Clin Transpl 2012;26(4):615–21.
92. Schneider F, Smith MA, Lane MC, et al. Adequacy of core needle biopsy specimens and fine-needle aspirates for molecular testing of lung adenocarcinomas. Am J Clin Pathol 2015;143(2):193–200. quiz 306.
93. Morris MA, Saboury B. Access to imaging technology in global health. In: Mollura DJ, Culp MP, Lungren MP, editors. Radiology in global health: strategies, implementation, and applications. Cham: Springer International Publishing; 2019. p. 15–33. https://doi.org/10.1007/978-3-319-98485-8_3.
94. Organization WH. Global atlas of medical devices. World Health Organization; 2017.
95. Rehani B, Brown I, Dandekar S, et al. Radiology Education in Africa: Analysis of Results From 13 African Countries. J Am Coll Radiol 2017;14(2):247–52.
96. Laage Gaupp FM, Solomon N, Rukundo I, et al. Tanzania IR initiative: training the first generation of interventional radiologists. J Vasc Interv Radiol 2019;30(12):2036–40.
97. Yuan R, Vos PM, Cooperberg PL. Computer-aided detection in screening CT for pulmonary nodules. AJR Am J Roentgenol 2006;186(5):1280–7.
98. Onega T, Aiello Bowles EJ, Miglioretti DL, et al. Radiologists' perceptions of computer aided detection versus double reading for mammography interpretation. Acad Radiol 2010;17(10):1217–26.
99. Way TW, Sahiner B, Chan H-P, et al. Computer-aided diagnosis of pulmonary nodules on CT scans: improvement of classification performance with nodule surface features. Med Phys 2009;36(7):3086–98.
100. WHO announces updated guidance on the systematic screening for tuberculosis. Available at: https://www.who.int/news/item/22-03-2021-who-announces-updated-guidance-on-the-systematic-screening-for-tuberculosis. Accessed November 30, 2021.
101. Ahn Y, Lee SM, Noh HN, et al. Use of a Commercially Available Deep Learning Algorithm to Measure the Solid Portions of Lung Cancer Manifesting as Subsolid Lesions at CT: Comparisons with Radiologists and Invasive Component Size at Pathologic Examination. Radiology 2021;299(1):202–10.
102. Cui S, Ming S, Lin Y, et al. Development and clinical application of deep learning model for lung nodules screening on CT images. Sci Rep 2020;10(1):13657.
103. Murphy A, Skalski M, Gaillard F. The utilisation of convolutional neural networks in detecting pulmonary nodules: a review. Br J Radiol 2018;91(1090):20180028.
104. Ciompi F, Chung K, van Riel SJ, et al. Towards automatic pulmonary nodule management in lung cancer screening with deep learning. Sci Rep 2017;7:46479.
105. Liu K, Li Q, Ma J, et al. Evaluating a fully automated pulmonary nodule detection approach and its impact on radiologist performance. Radiol Artif Intell 2019;1(3):e180084.

Pathology for Thoracic Conditions in Low- and Middle-Income Countries

Robert Lukande, MB ChB, PGD (Computer Sc), MMed(Path), FCPath (ECSA)[a], Lynnette Tumwine Kyokunda, MBChB, MMed Anat Path, FCPath (ECSA), PhD[b], Alemayehu Ginbo Bedada, MD[c], Dan Milner Jr, MD, MSc(Epi), MBA[d,e,*]

KEYWORDS

• Pathology • Thoracic • Africa • Pulmonary • Diagnostics • Histopathology

KEY POINTS

- Thoracic diseases are difficult to evaluate in LMICs because of lack of infrastructure, equipment, diagnosis-treatment axes, and patient awareness.
- Lung cancer is a common disease in LMICs that, in the current situation, presents late, has few available treatment options, and is highly fatal.
- Interventions that focus on lung cancer diagnosis and treatment have demonstrated impact and should be expanded and supported with additional research in LMICs.
- Infectious diseases and chronic conditions of the lung remain challenges in LMICs, which require increased clinical acumen and access to diagnostic tools to parse from other conditions.

INTRODUCTION

Thoracic pathology encompasses conditions that involve the lungs, pleura, and mediastinal space. Based on etiology, these conditions are categorized under two large groups: neoplastic and nonneoplastic (including trauma). Further subcategorization of the neoplastic conditions gives benign and malignant conditions, and the latter is primary or secondary. The nonneoplastic group includes the infectious and noninfectious conditions. The occupation-related conditions straddle across the two large groups.

The literature is sparse on the pathology of thoracic conditions in low- and middle-income countries (LMICs). The epidemiology, diagnosis, and management of these directly depend on the availability and access to thoracic surgery, pulmonology, radiology, anesthesia, oncology, and pathology services. The availability and quality of these services remain a challenge in LMICs and vary from country to country and between public and private sector within a country. Several common challenges include absent or limited availability of funding, specialized staffing for chest clinics and thoracic surgical centers, lack of specialized radiographic services, postprocedure pulmonary support (chest tubes, suction machines, ventilators), and equipment for diagnostic pathology laboratories.[1–4] Therefore, the journey from initial assessment to referral for diagnosis and treatment is difficult and translates into delayed diagnosis in which advanced stages of disease confer poorer outcomes. However, in some LMICs, these services are totally lacking, and some diagnoses are made only at autopsy.

[a] Department of Pathology, College of Health Sciences, Makerere University, Mulago Hill Road, Room B24 Pathology Building, Kampala, Uganda; [b] Department of Pathology, Faculty of Medicine, Sir Ketumile Masire Teaching Hospital, University of Botswana, 2nd Floor F2013, Gaborone, Botswana; [c] Department of Surgery, Faculty of Medicine, Princess Marina Hospital, University of Botswana, River Walk, Village, PO Box 45759, Gaborone, Botswana; [d] American Society for Clinical Pathology, 33 West Monroe Street, Suite 1600, Chicago, IL 60603, USA; [e] Harvard T. H. Chan School of Public Health, Boston, MA, USA
* Corresponding author. American Society for Clinical Pathology, 33 West Monroe Street, Suite 1600, Chicago, IL 60603.
E-mail address: dan.milner@ascp.org

Thorac Surg Clin 32 (2022) 299–306
https://doi.org/10.1016/j.thorsurg.2022.04.006
1547-4127/22/

thoracic.theclinics.com

In the developed world, improved awareness of the risk factors for cancer with well-established preventive measures, and widespread availability of screening services and quality, timely health care provide a greater chance of a good outcome and survival.[4] Lung cancer is a leading cause of cancer death in males and the second leading cause of death in females in LMICs.[4] This is largely a consequence of late presentation and diagnosis. Poor socioeconomic status, weak health care system, and poor knowledge about disease risk factors complicates the diagnosis, effectiveness of treatment, and overall outcome.[4] Clinically, lung cancer in LMICs may be misdiagnosed for long periods of time as tuberculosis or other chronic conditions resulting in late-stage diagnosis or never diagnosed.

Patient-level risk factors for late presentation include lack of recognition and knowledge of symptoms, which are shared by other common diseases that seem to be not serious at early stage (eg, cough).[4] Educational level and knowledge of the patient about lung cancer regarding potential prevention strategies (eg, avoiding some risk factors) and treatability of the disease are other factors that affect the outcome in lung cancer treatment.[4] The socioeconomic status and place of residence (eg, repeated travel for cancer care) has a significant impact in lung cancer care.[4] Culture and societal differences play an important part in cancer care. In LMICs culture influences the attitude and beliefs of understanding disease and cure that includes considering alternative medicine.[4] Patients may have impaired thoughts that originate from the stress of their cancer and it is important to communicate with the language they can understand easily.[4] Stigmatization, an attribute associated with negative evaluation, can lead to negative treatment acceptance or discrimination and identity threat.[4] Another important factor that affects cancer care in most LMICs is the existing poor health services: absence of screening services to detect early cancers; inconsistent, poor, delayed, and incomplete referral procedures; and absence of clinical staff training in health facilities.[4] Skilled clinicians with the required laboratory and imaging services are critical to reduce misdiagnosis of lung cancer where there is a high pulmonary tuberculosis rate.[4]

In this article, we explore published literature on the pathology of common thoracic conditions (neoplastic, nonneoplastic, and occupation-related), focusing on the epidemiology, current state of health services, health system challenges to diagnosis and management, and research toward improving services. We focus on the epidemiology and diagnosis of thoracic conditions in Africa primarily given our expertise in this region. Additionally, we suggest a way forward to call for support and strategize for improving the support services for understanding thoracic pathology in LMICs.

EPIDEMIOLOGY

Pulmonary Conditions

In Africa, pulmonary infections are the most common cause of death seen in autopsy specimens.[5,6,7,8] In HIV-associated adult deaths, pulmonary and extrapulmonary tuberculosis are seen in up to 69% of the cases.[5] In childhood deaths, coinfection with multiple pathologies were seen in up to 66% of HIV infections.[5]

Chronic respiratory diseases include asthma and respiratory allergies, chronic obstructive pulmonary disease (COPD), other occupation-related diseases, pulmonary hypertension, and lung cancer.[9] COPD is the fourth leading cause of death globally.[10,11] Smoking is a major risk factor for COPD, although a large number of patients with COPD have no smoking history.[10] Other factors associated with COPD are age older than 40, indoor and outdoor air pollution (eg, cooking fire practices, exposure to biomass, exposure to certain gases), low socioeconomic status, genetic factors, history of pulmonary tuberculosis, and HIV infection.[10] COPD is rare in the African population where there are low rates of smoking but with evidence that tobacco use prevalence increases with advancing age.[10] Chronic respiratory disease contributed 9.0% of the admissions and 9.8% of mortality in Uganda, with asthma and COPD as the commonest identified diagnoses.[9] This may be an underestimation of the burden of chronic respiratory diseases in Uganda because of limited diagnostic equipment and lack of awareness of the condition.[9]

Lung cancer is the fourth most common cancer among men in Africa.[4] In both sexes combined lung cancer is the most commonly diagnosed cancer and the leading cause of cancer-related death.[4] However, true incidence and prevalence of lung cancer for men and women in LMICs are underreported for lack of diagnostic tools and misdiagnosing lung cancer for other lung pathologies that mimic lung cancer. Recent data from Tanzania have demonstrated that without proper diagnostic tools, all the following conditions were misdiagnosed in patients who ultimately had evidence of lung cancer when the appropriate tools were used: posttuberculosis cavitation, pleural effusions of tuberculosis, active tuberculosis, chronic inflammatory lung disease, lung abscess, and lung fibrosis (Nestory Masalu, AORTIC 2021 and personal communication). Moreover, the addition of lung cancer to the differential along with the tools to evaluate lung cancer (eg, chest radiograph, computed tomography [CT] scans, endobronchial and core tissue biopsy, pathology services, specialized testing) properly led to a migration of patients from predominantly stage 4 (87%) to stage 2 or 3 (69%) with a remarkable 11% stage 4 after only 2 years (Nestory Masalu, AORTIC 2021 and personal communication). Although a single experience, these data support that, with proper training, tools, and treatment, lung cancer is effectively identified/diagnosed at early stages and treated with a better outcome in LMICs.

Intrathoracic Nonpulmonary Conditions

Achalasia is an idiopathic primary motility disorder of the esophagus with poor relaxation of the lower esophageal sphincter that results in progressive dysphasia, esophageal dilatation, and subsequent complete loss of primary peristalsis and stasis.[3] Although the cause is largely unknown in most settings, multifactorial models have been proposed with etiologic agents including viral infections, genetic and/or autoimmune components, and inflammatory changes.[12]

High-grade Barrett esophagus, a disease progressively increasing in LMICs, has a 1% risk progression to invasive cancer.[2] Esophageal cancer is an aggressive neoplasm more common in older age groups and results in progressive esophageal obstruction and nutritional abnormality.[2] Esophageal cancer spreads easily via direct extension, through the lymphatic system, and hematogenously, mimicking a primary lung or thoracic lesion.[2] It has higher incidence and mortality in Southern and Eastern Africa, Central Asia, Turkey, Iran, and China because of variable factors (discussed later).[2] It is rare in West Africa.[2] It is the eighth most common cancer and sixth leading cause of cancer-related death worldwide.[2] It is three to four times more common in males.[2] Esophageal cancer is usually diagnosed at a late stage in LMICs, resulting in more than 80% mortality from the disease.[2] The 5-year survival for patients with esophageal cancer is low at 15% to 25%.[2]

The histology and incidence of esophageal cancer varies with geographic location and economic development.[2] In LMICs squamous cell cancer (SCC) is more common than adenocarcinoma; but the reverse is true for the developed world.[2] In the United States adenocarcinoma and SCC contribute 81% and 17% of the esophageal cancer, respectively. Black Africans are two to three times at higher risk for squamous esophageal cancer than Western populations.[2] Among Africans, the risk of SCC occurring at the middle third and distal third locations of the esophagus are similar.[2] Alcohol consumption is a primary risk factor and alcohol and tobacco use have synergistic effect with increased relative risk.[2] Smoking is a risk factor for SCC and adenocarcinoma, whereas alcohol is a significant factor for SCC.[2] Alcohol reduces metabolic activity of detoxification enzymes while promoting oxidation (ie, increased damage to DNA and increased sensitivity to other environmental toxins).[2] Other risk factors include age 45 to 70 years and regular and repeated consumption of hot beverages causing chronic esophagitis, environmental smoke (eg, cooking), human papilloma virus infection, diet (eg, maize [increased level of prostaglandin E_2], increased Wnt signaling and proliferation), Helicobacteraceae infection, wild herbs, and western diet (eg, fats and animal protein).[2] Obesity is a risk factor for adenocarcinoma, whereas fruits and vegetables reduce the risk of esophageal cancer (**Table 1**).[2]

Studies in LMICs have demonstrated specific risk factors for esophageal cancer and are summarized here. In Tanzania, risk factors are young age, lack of resource for treatment, and consumption of hot milky tea. Risk factors in Kenya are low socioeconomic condition, level of education, and general living conditions. In India, risk factors are drinking hot salted tea and human papilloma virus type infection.[2] China has half of the world's new cases of esophageal cancer, and it is the fourth most diagnosed cancer and fourth leading cause of cancer-related death in China.[2] Factors associated with esophageal cancer in China include rural residence, alcohol consumption, tobacco use, meat, salted and pickled vegetables, moldy food, hot green tea, passive smoking, *Helicobacter pylori* infection, low socioeconomic status, poor oral hygiene, and family history of cancer.[2] In Brazil, alcohol ingestion, smoking, and hot mate consumption are said to be associated with esophageal cancer.

CURRENT STATE OF HEALTH SERVICES?

In LMICs, late presentation and diagnosis, inefficient referral systems, and gaps in policy guideline compromise the efficacy of treatment of thoracic diseases, resulting in poorer outcomes.[4] Furthermore, economic hardship, patient circumstances, and poor health literacy further lead to delays in seeking care.[4] Cancer-related mortality is significantly higher in LMICs compared with high-income countries, despite the overall lower incidence of cancer in LMICs.[4] About 70% of global

Table 1
Esophageal cancer: demographics, risk factors, and histology type

	Demographics	Risk Factors	Histology Type
LMICs	M >/ = F 40–75 y	Alcohol Smoking HPV	Most SCC
High-income countries	M >> F 55–75 y	Alcohol Smoking Obesity GERD	Most adenocarcinoma

Abbreviations: GERD, gastroesophageal reflux disease; HPV, human papilloma virus.

lung cancer deaths occur in LMICs.[4] Pathology services were available only in 26% of LMICs and 90% of high-income countries in 2017.[4]

THE ROLE OF PATHOLOGY

One of pathology's urgent, needed contributions to thoracic disease in LMICs is confirmation and support through cancer registries of the true epidemiology of disease while also providing actionable diagnosis for patients. Pathology has helped in prevention, such as vaccine development by studying the clinical and subclinical inflammatory changes in the genital mucosa and by characterization of foreskin barrier functions and antibody transudation in HIV-positive patients.[13] It also helps in identifying other treatable diseases, such as tuberculosis and cryptococcal disease, which informs public health decisions.[13] Blind closed pleural biopsy has a role in the diagnosis of exudative pleural effusion in resource-limited settings, especially in patients suspected to have tuberculosis or malignancy.[14] Pathology helps in staging of esophageal cancer, which dictates the best mode of treatment of a specific patient, nonsurgical or surgical.[2] Pathology also helps to evaluate the response to treatment in nonsurgical situations (eg, neoadjuvant chemo radiotherapy) and recurrence following surgical treatments.[2]

Chest radiograph alone is inadequate for the diagnosis of asbestos-related diseases, because of similarity with diffuse interstitial fibrosis.[15] Mesothelioma and lung cancer require histologic and immunohistochemical confirmation because radiology is misleading.[15,16] Inaccuracies in pathology diagnosis impacting survival is difficult to study in the setting of limited resources, because of inadequate data capturing and high rates of loss to follow-up and treatment abandonment.[13] Other major challenge in LMIC pathology is the frequent reliance on routine and inexpensive hematoxylin and eosin staining rather than more definitive techniques to make cancer diagnoses.[13]

Fine-needle aspiration cytology contains disaggregated tissue, whereas Tru-Cut, operation room (incisional or excisional biopsy) retain the complex architecture.[13] It may be easier to differentiate malignant cells from normal cells in that a solid tumor's individual cancer cells look different from the normal cells, whereas in liquid tumors (eg, hematopoietic origin) the growth pattern needs to be seen.[13] Although hematoxylin and eosin histology is usually sufficient to distinguish benign from malignant cells in adequately fixed and processed tissue, it is often not sufficient to determine the exact tumor cell type among malignancies, particularly for metastatic cancers identified in secondary locations, such as lymph node, liver, lung, and brain.[13]

It is important to appreciate a potential increased risk of incorrect diagnosis in LMICs because the resources for appropriate tissue procurement, tissue processing, and pathologic interpretation are limited.[13] Challenges in tissue processing in routine sectioning and staining, absence of specialized equipment, trained staff, and access to consumables and reagents are poor in LMICs.[13] Many pathology laboratories in LMICs lack the resources to perform immunohistochemistry, and therefore run a much greater risk of misclassifying tumors compared with laboratories in which immunohistochemistry is performed.[13] To address these deficiencies, in general, a model of assessment, gap analysis, implementation planning, and execution is effective in pin-pointing internal laboratory needs and external preanalytical and postanalytical needs. The next sections detail two examples for consideration.

Rwanda

In 2012 through the Human Resources for Health Program, Rwanda embarked on increasing performance of thoracic surgical procedures and training of local specialists and increasing the pathology workforce.[17] In collaboration with 20 US-based medical institutions, three national referral hospitals (University Teaching Hospital of Butare [CHUB], University Teaching Hospital of Kigali, and King Faisal Hospital) participated.

In a period of 23 months, 33 thoracic surgical procedures were performed in 32 patients. Most procedures (85%) were in one hospital, CHUB. Seventy percent of the procedures were performed by surgery residents and junior faculty under supervision of a thoracic surgeon. A limited number of patients underwent preoperative CT scanning largely because of the fact there was no scanner at CHUB. A few of the CT scans were performed at another referral hospital. Preoperative bronchoscopy was done in two patients, one caused by massive hemoptysis and the other by a posttrauma tracheoesophageal fistula. Pulmonary function tests, cardiac stress tests, and arterial blood gas measurements were not available.

Of the 33 procedures, 10 (30%) were decortications to allow for lung expansion following parapneumonic effusions and suspected empyema, 5 were open thoracotomies caused by pyogenic empyema, 4 were anterior mediastinotomies caused by mediastinal masses suspected to be malignant, 2 were pericardial window operations caused by cardiac tamponade, 2 underwent thoracotomy and resection of lung neoplasms, and 1 was a pericardiectomy for acute constrictive pericarditis. There were no intraoperative complications, three postoperative complications, and two deaths. However, results of the histologic evaluations of the specimens are unknown.

The findings showed that amid challenges, specialized surgery can be performed in LMIC settings with satisfactory outcomes. Thoracic surgery has a role in the management of infectious diseases-related pathology and more emphasis is needed in the training of more thoracic surgeons and enhancement of support services.

In parallel, since 2013, a local pathology residency training program has been in place, which has graduated 15 new pathologists with five additional pathologists in training. The juxtaposition of training new surgeons in cardiothoracic procedures in parallel with pathology trainees results in a shared understanding of the needs for these patients and increases the diagnostic workflow efficiency for best outcomes.

South Africa

An upper middle income economy country, South Africa has a diverse population comprising different ethnicities.[18] This diversity reflects in the differences in genetic, ethnic, and epidemiologic risk factors of lung cancer. Lung cancer significantly contributes to the burden of thoracic pathology in the country. The state of thoracic pathology is discussed using lung cancer as a proxy. Patient diagnostic and management services vary across the nation depending on the availability of funding in the public and private health care sectors.

The public health care system suffers from understaffing and lack of resources in contrast to the modern state-of-the-art treatment and high population of oncologists in the private sector. Morphology-based histologic diagnosis and a full panel of biomarkers are routinely available in both sectors. Advanced testing, such as next-generation sequencing and targetable DNA mutations, is also available but efforts are futile in the public sector because of the lack of funding for treatment. Liquid biopsy and programmed death ligand-1 testing are available but limited to a few laboratories.

Staging is done using CT scanning but there are severe delays in the public sector in comparison with the private sector, where it is easily accessible. PET is available in the private sector for staging early disease and unclear cases on CT. Regarding management, patients are discussed in multidisciplinary team settings comprising cardiothoracic surgeons, radiologists, pathologists, medical and radiation oncologists, and nuclear medicine physicians.

Surgical diagnostic and staging procedures, such as flexible and rigid bronchoscopies, open surgical and video-assisted thoracic surgery, pleural and lymph node biopsy, mediastinoscopy, ultrasound-guided transbronchial needle aspirations, and interventional radiology, are available.

Medical and radiation oncology services are also available, varying across sectors of the health care system and rural versus urban settings. Thus, in the South African setting, although all tools are available, the dichotomy of outcomes for patient groups falls largely across the public versus private sector divide and requires special considerations for how to overcome fiscal obstacles to achieve equitable patient outcomes.

Capacity Building

With the extreme challenges of oncologic services in general in LMICs, the importance of pathology to a functioning cancer treatment system must be reiterated at all levels including government, funders, and clinical systems. To that end, engagement in activities that demonstrate/reiterate the importance of pathology services and help to create those services are key.

The most important first step is assessment, internal and external, of a proposed or existing cancer treatment location to determine what resources are and are not available, how they relate to treatment options, and goals for the population. The second step is gap analysis to determine what is missing that must be replaced immediately and what should be replaced over time. This is especially important in consideration of coevolution of the diagnostics and treatment so that resources are not mismatched, leading to untreated patients. The third step is implementation planning where a clear timeline, set of activities, stakeholders, and outcomes are determined formally with funding. This could be internal to a government agency or done by a donor; however, it is crucial to make sure the plan is clear and success can be measured. The final step (which leads back to the first step) is execution where the plan is implemented and measured with an assessment of the results to continue the cycle again.

Each assessment dictates an implementation plan based on the gaps; however, some common solutions are in person and virtual trainings for grossing, processing, embedding, microtomy, staining, immunohistochemistry, workflow, and laboratory management; virtual training and telepathology ongoing support for diagnosis; provisions of study materials for trainees including books, glass slides, and virtual slide sets; equipment procurement (donation, purchase, or sharing); policy support; and networking. As an example, in Rwanda, in parallel with the Human Resources for Health program described, an assessment was performed in 2012 of the Butaro District Hospital laboratory space, which had no anatomic pathology services. After site visit, candidate selection, training of two technicians, equipment purchase and install, facility retrofitting for environmental specifications, reagent supply chain establishment, and static image telepathology installation, a fully functioning histology laboratory was available on site within just a 6-month period. Immunohistochemistry was added within 2 years. By 2016, a fulltime pathologist was employed locally, supported by a telepathology team and including immunohistochemistry locally with a turnaround time of 3 days.

The caveats for the consideration in pulmonary pathology specifically must be stated. Surgical, interventional radiology, gastrointestinal, and pulmonology clinical services are required to obtain lung tissue safely and are too complex to be performed in rural settings without supportive care. Thus, a systematic approach to address thoracic cavity lesions for possible treatment requires a multidisciplinary team that includes the pathology services. Once obtained, treatments for specific cancers often rely on special testing including molecular tools, which should be included in budget and logistics planning of the equivalent treatments that are available. Lastly, follow-up for patients posttreatment for recovery of function may include ancillary support specific to pulmonary function. Building capacity for these services can still be achieved but it requires a multidisciplinary approach as with all cancers including the special considerations for most impactful outcomes for patients.

OPPORTUNITIES FOR RESEARCH

The reasons for decrease in research in thoracic pathology in LMICs are multiple and include loss of surgeons with interest in thoracic surgery from academic practice because of lack of opportunities for specialist training in thoracic surgery, lack of equipment and resources for specialized surgery, retirement, and private practice. The few thoracic surgeons available suffer burn out and are unable to fully participate in empirical research.[1] A study from the Republic of South Africa depicted that since the 1980s there is a decrease in publication and a shift to a nonindexed journal for publication.[1] Most of the publications were on inflammatory pleuropulmonary disease, whereas literature is limited on chronic empyema, tuberculosis and HIV, and lung and esophageal cancer.[1] Most are observational in design and there was no systematic reviews, meta-analysis, and randomized controlled trials.[1] For this reason the influence of the available literature on thoracic pathologies on clinical practice is weak based on grade of recommendations.[1]

Between 2015 and 2018 the International Cancer Research Partnership's member organizations funded more than 400 projects in Sub-Saharan Africa that were wholly or partially focused on lung cancer. This represents about 7% of the total projects supported in the region. More than 75% of projects had a co-principal investigator in Sub-Saharan Africa or directly funded principal investigators in the region. Prevention was the main focus of lung cancer research (44% of projects active in 2018), followed by etiology (18% in 2018), biology (12% in 2018), cancer control and survivorship (9%), diagnosis and detection (9%), and treatment (8%) (Lynne Davies, ICRP 2021 and personal communication). Although these data are promising, as one of the leading cancers in LMICs, increased research study and focus on lung cancer is warranted using proper tools, skilled clinical teams, and available treatments to further impact the disease.

Box 1
Future improvement of thoracic care in LMIC

- Public health: risk factor prevention through increasing awareness and patient education, introducing screening measures, and availing vaccination are critical.
- System based: improving access, diagnostic methods, investing on equipment, infrastructures, and training and up-skilling health care workers at all levels, and improving availability of treatment cannot be overemphasized.
- Academic: provision of funding and facilitating collaborations among researchers on common thoracic pathologies in LMICs and researchers in LMICs and high-income countries is essential.

FUTURE DIRECTIONS

Recognizing the magnitude of the chest pathologies/diseases is essential (**Box 1**).[4] Prevention strategies include screening, vaccination, and risk reduction.[2] Increased diagnostic awareness among health care providers is necessary for asbestos-related disease particularly in poorly resourced public health care facilities.[15]

There is a great need for a database of clinical experience, which emphasizes the importance of rekindling interest and a culture of research in thoracic surgery.[1] Creating ongoing collaboration among African countries can lead to much needed funding, specific study design, local ethical review and informed consent of patients, high-quality collection of samples, and processing of material for long-term studies.[13]

There is a great need for more investment into rapid and accurate diagnostics for respiratory tract infection, especially in HIV-infected children and adults.[5] Securing instruments for bronchoscopy, pulmonary function tests spirometry, and so forth is important.[9] Patients with exudative pleural effusion may need sputum microscopy, bronchoscopy, or cytology; closed pleural biopsy remains valuable in resource-constrained setup; and the high volume of inadequate biopsy specimens submitted suggests further training in sampling technique may improve the diagnostic/accuracy rate.[14]

There are many reasons why clinical outcomes are inferior in LMICs, such as lack of access to cancer treatment centers, inability to give appropriate intensive treatment because of lack of supportive care and unavailable drugs, and treatment abandonment.[13] Streamlining the pathways of lung cancer care is key to achieving early detection of lung cancer.[4] Improved access and quality of health care remain important and all health care professionals must accept that a multidisciplinary team is required.

SUMMARY

The current burden of thoracic disease in LMICs is not sufficiently supported by the tools and skills that are needed for effective management. Specifically, diagnostic resources are limited and, when expanded and directed, will lead to earlier diagnosis and treatment for improved outcomes of neoplastic and nonneoplastic lung disease. Awareness of lung cancer as a disease that is preventable, treatable, and curable is needed across the health care spectrum from patients to treating clinicians. The role of pathology in the diagnosis of cancerous and noncancerous lesions is crucial in LMICs because of the highly variable differential diagnosis across outcomes and treatment, including infections. Investment in resources to screen, diagnose, and treat lung diseases and relevant research projects will greatly benefit LMICs.

CLINICS CARE POINTS

- Lung cancer is a common disease in LMICs and should be considered in the differential diagnosis in the context of history, age, and risk factors so that early detection and appropriate treatment may be achieved.
- Efforts to expand diagnostic capabilities in LMICs are necessary to address the significant morbidity and mortality of thoracic disease in LMICs. This may be done through international collaboration, financial investment, and research initiatives.
- The pathologic confirmation of lung cancer requires a tissue biopsy or cytology sample, which may be challenging in many settings; however, the broad (often infectious) differential diagnosis requires it.
- Patients properly screened and diagnosed with lung cancer who receive directed therapies results in decreased mortality and downstaging of the population.
- Esophageal cancer is associated with a high mortality in LMICs mainly caused by absence of awareness and preventive measures; late presentations; and lack of screening tools, pathology services, and skilled staffs in preoperative and postoperative periods.

DISCLOSURE

The authors have no disclosures regarding this work, fiscal or otherwise.

REFERENCES

1. Linegar A, Smit F, Goldstraw P, et al. Fifty years of thoracic surgical research in South Africa. South Afr Med J 2009;99(8):592–5.
2. Hull R, Mbele M, Makhafola T, et al. A multinational review: oesophageal cancer in low to middle-income countries. Oncol Lett 2020;20(4):1.
3. Wang L, Li YM, Li L, et al. A systematic review and meta-analysis of the Chinese literature for the treatment of achalasia. World J Gastroenterol WJG 2008;14(38):5900.
4. Lubuzo B, Ginindza T, Hlongwana K. The barriers to initiating lung cancer care in low- and middle-income countries. Pan Afr Med J 2020;35:38.
5. Bates M, Mudenda V, Mwaba P, et al. Deaths due to respiratory tract infections in Africa: a review of autopsy studies. Curr Opin Pulm Med 2013;19(3): 229–37.
6. Van der Westhuizen G, Naude M, Nel M. The yield of pathological findings from routine screening chest X-rays in a military population. SA J Radiol 2017; 21(1):1.
7. Ouattara MA, Togo S, Kané B, et al. Compressive congenital giant segmental emphysema: diagnosis and treatment. Pan Afr Med J 2016;23(1).
8. Meghji J, Nadeau G, Davis KJ, et al. Noncommunicable lung disease in sub-Saharan Africa. a community-based cross-sectional study of adults in urban Malawi. Am J Respir Crit Care Med 2016; 194(1):67–76.
9. Kirenga BJ, Nakiyingi L, Worodria W, et al. Chronic respiratory diseases in a tertiary healthcare facility in Uganda. Afr J Respir Med 2013;8(2):21–3.
10. Pefura-Yone EW, Kengne AP, Balkissou AD, et al. Prevalence of obstructive lung disease in an African country using definitions from different international guidelines: a community based cross-sectional survey. BMC Res Notes 2016;9(1):1–10.
11. Bruce-Brand C, Allwood BW, Koegelenberg CF, et al. Postmortem lung biopsies from four patients with COVID-19 at a tertiary hospital in Cape Town, South Africa. S Afr Med J 2020;110(12):1195–200.
12. O'Neill OM, Johnston BT, Coleman HG. Achalasia: a review of clinical diagnosis, epidemiology, treatment and outcomes. World J Gastroenterol 2013;19(35): 5806–12.
13. Lemos MP, Taylor TE, McGoldrick SM, et al. Pathology-based research in Africa. Clin Lab Med 2018; 38(1):67–90.
14. Edgar JR, Wong ML, Hale M, et al. Histopathological diagnoses on pleural biopsy specimens over a 15-year period at Chris Hani Baragwanath Academic Hospital, Johannesburg, South Africa: a retrospective review. South Afr Med J 2019;109(1):53–7.
15. Ndlovu N, Rees D, Murray J, et al. Asbestos-related diseases in mineworkers: a clinicopathological study. ERJ open Res 2017;3(3):00022–2017.
16. Denning DW, Page ID, Chakaya J, et al. Case definition of chronic pulmonary aspergillosis in resource-constrained settings. Emerg Infect Dis 2018;24(8): e171312.
17. Sibomana I, Sinclair MC. A descriptive retrospective cohort study of thoracic surgery experiences from September 2015 to July 2017 at three referral hospitals in Rwanda. East Cent Afr J Surg 2018;23:5–10.
18. van Eeden R, Tuner M, Geldenhuys A, et al. Lung cancer in South Africa. J Thorac Oncol 2020; 15(Issue 1):22–8.

Anesthesia for Global General Thoracic Surgery

Janey R. Phelps, MD[a],
Henry Lizi, ACO, BSA, BAI (Bachelor of Science in Anesthesia and Intensive Care)[b],
Bryant A. Murphy, MD, MBA[a,*]

KEYWORDS

• LMIC • Global health • Anesthesia • Thoracic anesthesia

KEY POINTS

- There is a significant surgical and anesthesia workforce need in low-to-middle income countries (LMICs).
- Capacity building, as opposed to short-term mission trips, should be the goal when developing thoracic surgery programs in LMICs.
- Careful preoperative consideration of patient's baseline medical status and capabilities for postoperative care should be a part of the surgical planning for thoracic surgeries in LMICs.
- Intraoperative one-lung ventilation strategies need to be based on the resources available in LMIC and may differ significantly from strategies in high-resourced countries.

INTRODUCTION OF GLOBAL SURGICAL BURDEN AND WORKFORCE

The Lancet Commission of Global Health estimated that surgical conditions account for 28% to 31% of the overall global burden of disease.[1] The 2015 Bangkok Global Surgery Declaration states that 5 billion people, ~70% of the world's population, cannot access safe emergency and essential surgical care and anesthesia.[2] Holmer and colleagues reported in 2015 that only 12% of the surgical specialist workforce practice in Africa and Southeast Asia, although a third of the world's population lives there.[3] The Lancet Commission acknowledges that although 44% of the World's population lives in countries with a specialist surgical workforce density lower than 20 per 100,000 population, only 28% lives in countries with a specialist surgical density greater than 40 per 100,000, which is an optimum number. In 2015, the Lancet Commission estimated a worldwide shortage of more than 1 million specialist surgical, anesthesia and obstetric (SAO) providers. For example, in an effort to reach a 40 SOA per 100,000 by 2030, additional 2.28 million specialist SAO providers must be trained. The World Fedaration of Societies of Anesthesiologists (WFSA) is a federation of 135 member societies representing anesthesiologists in approximately 150 countries. Between 2015 and 2016, the WFSA conducted a survey and received data from 153 out of 197 countries, which represents 97.5% of the world's population. This survey revealed that 77 countries had less than 5 physician anesthesiologists per 100,000 population, which is the minimal recommendation for safe surgeries. In Sub-Saharan Africa, most of the countries have less than 1 anesthesiologist per 100,000. Many countries use nonphysician anesthetists and if they are included then 70 countries still had a total anesthesia provider density of less than 5 per 100,000[4] (**Fig. 1**).

In an effort to meet the surgical burden in low-to-middle income countries (LMICs), there needs to not only be more high-quality training programs but also a plan to retain the local providers. The country of Malawi in Sub-Saharan Africa has increased the enrollment of their Anesthesia

[a] Department of Anesthesiology, University of North Carolina School of Medicine, N2198 UNC Hospitals, CB#7010 Chapel Hill, NC 27599-7010 USA; [b] Kamuzu University of Health Sceinces Blantyre, Malawi Africa
* Corresponding authors.
E-mail addresses: Janey@unc.edu (J.R.P.); lizihenry@yahoo.com (H.L.); bryant_murphy@med.unc.edu (B.A.M.)

Thorac Surg Clin 32 (2022) 307–315
https://doi.org/10.1016/j.thorsurg.2022.04.001
1547-4127/22/

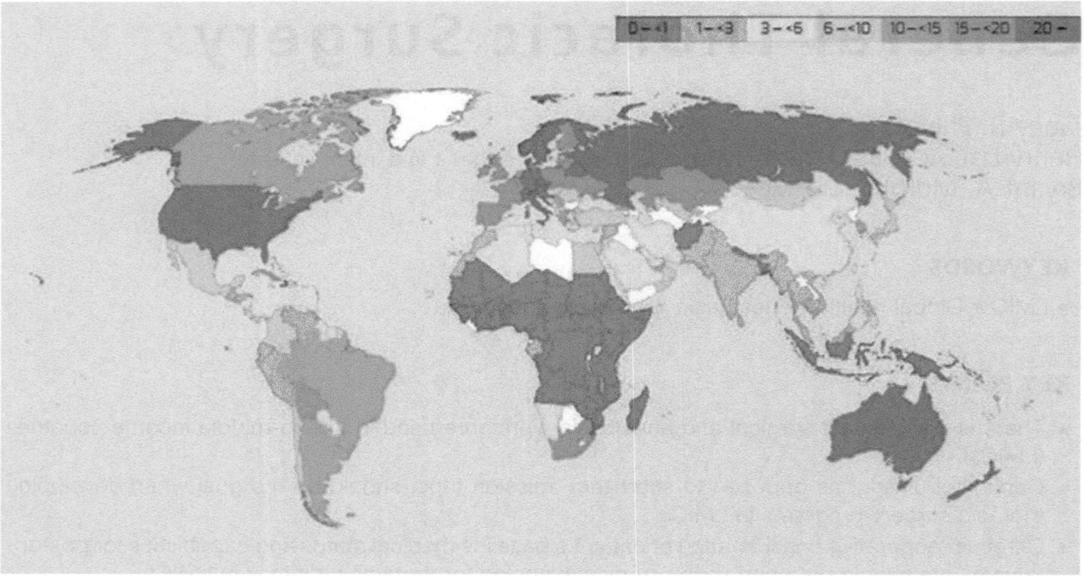

Fig. 1. WFSA survey delineating how many MD anesthesiologists there are per 100,000 people based on countries. (*From* Kempthorne P, Morriss WW, Mellin-Olsen J, Gore-Booth J. The WFSA Global Anesthesia Workforce Survey. Anesth Analg. 2017;125(3):981-990.)

Clinical Officer program from 16 students to 33 students over a 5-year period to meet the increased need of anesthesia providers. Malawi currently has 1.5/100,000 anesthesia clinical officers and 0.04/100,000 anesthesia medical doctors, so the need to increase providers and physicians is great. However, the students increased in number without a parallel increase in instructors, infrastructure, modification of the curriculum design to reach more students, or an increase access to theaters for clinical training. To produce high-quality anesthetist, both quantity and quality of the training programs must increase. Dr Mark Newton and his team in Kijabe Kenya created a nurse anesthetist problem with a robust consistent curriculum and a tool to access their impact throughout Kenya on surgical care.[5] His group also developed a program in which all surgical staff received training to address the surgical burden in remote locations.[6] These types of training programs and impact follow-up are needed throughout Sub-Saharan Africa.

"Brain Drain" is a term coined to define when local physicians from LMIC leave their home country to pursue professional opportunities in higher resourced countries. Up to 18% of all physicians in high-income countries are international medical graduates, and up to 66% of these may have come from low-income countries.[7] To be more specific to surgical specialties in 2015, it was reported that ~12% of all specialist surgeons, anesthesiologists, and obstetricians in high-income countries are foreign nationals that have graduated from medical schools in LMIC.[7] Some of the factors believed to lead to migration of local physicians away from LMICs include poorly equipped hospitals, unclear career pathways, better living conditions, and lack of role models. There must be an incentive program to retain these vital physicians in their home countries.

The 2015 Lancet report highlighted the surgical burden in LMICs and lack of trained surgical and anesthesia providers in those areas to meet the current and growing demand. At the opening meeting of the Lancet Commission on Global Surgery in January 2014, Jim Kim, President of the World Bank, stated that "surgery is an indivisible part of health care."[8] Along with this must come adequate support for anesthesia. The executive summary from the Lancet Commission states that the reduction of death and disability hinges on access to surgical and anesthesia care, which should be available, affordable, timely and safe to ensure good coverage, uptake, and outcomes.[1] The Lancet Commission noted that of the 313 million procedures undertaken worldwide each year, only 6% occur in the poorest countries where over a third of the world's population lives.[1] The Lancet report estimates that 93% of the population in Sub-Saharan Africa and 97% of the population in South Asia do not have access to safe, timely and affordable surgical and anesthesia care compared with 3.6% of the population in higher income regions (**Fig. 2**).

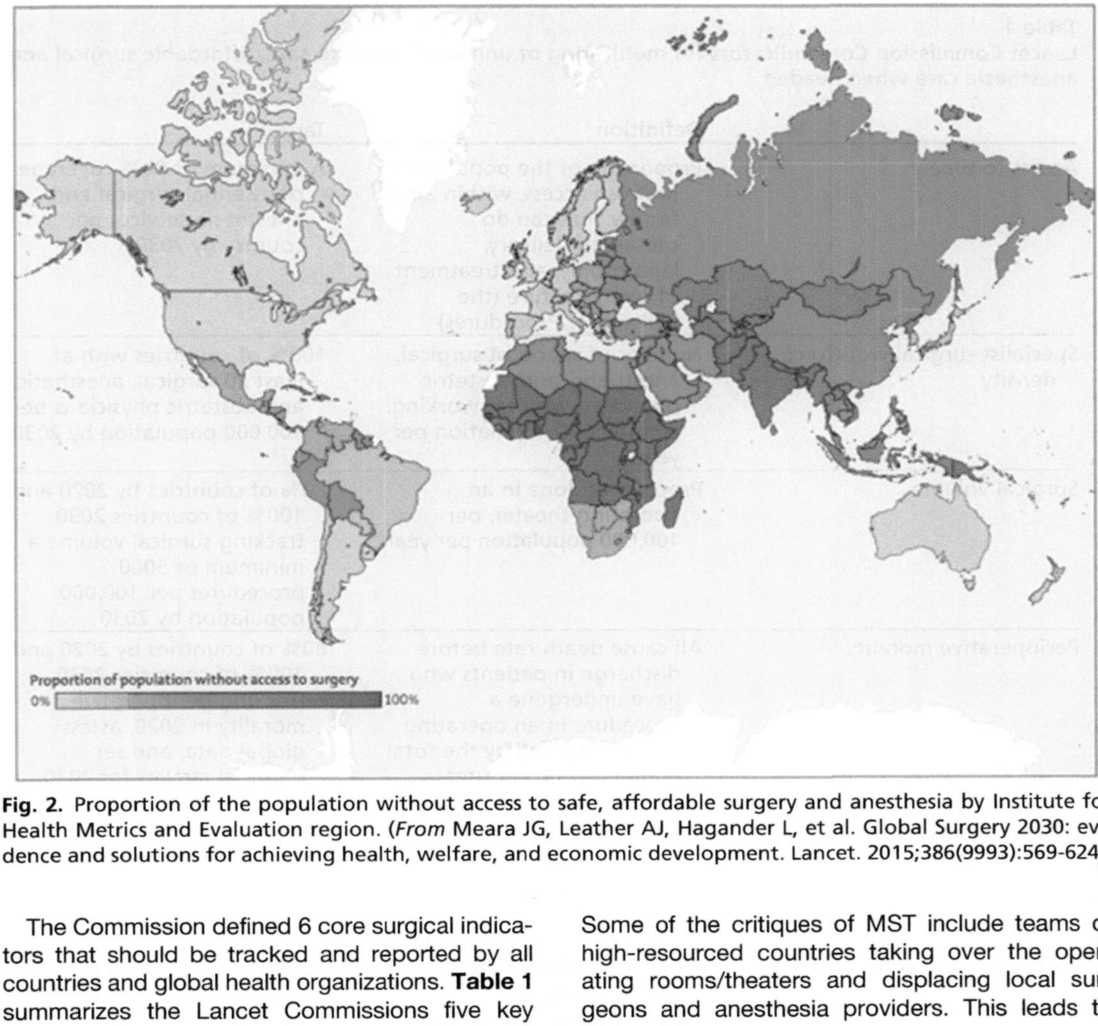

Fig. 2. Proportion of the population without access to safe, affordable surgery and anesthesia by Institute for Health Metrics and Evaluation region. (*From* Meara JG, Leather AJ, Hagander L, et al. Global Surgery 2030: evidence and solutions for achieving health, welfare, and economic development. Lancet. 2015;386(9993):569-624.)

The Commission defined 6 core surgical indicators that should be tracked and reported by all countries and global health organizations. **Table 1** summarizes the Lancet Commissions five key messages, and **Box 1** outlines the desired goals to be achieved by 2030.

CAPACITY BUILDING VERSUS MEDICAL SERVICE TRIPS

There has been a distinct shift over the past decades from medical service trips (MSTs) to capacity building trips. MSTs are well intended and meet many needs in host countries. There are a number of well-established organizations that sponsor MST, such as Operation Smile, Smile Train, and Interplast. These groups have a well-established safety record and provide surgical needs that would not otherwise be met in these areas. As these organizations have grown, they too have identified the need to provide "continual medical education" to the providers in the host country during the trips. This includes asking local anesthesia and surgical providers to work with them and offering lectures, mentoring, and proctoring. Some of the critiques of MST include teams of high-resourced countries taking over the operating rooms/theaters and displacing local surgeons and anesthesia providers. This leads to increasing the length of time for elective surgeries of the host country's citizens and delaying some emergency surgeries. In addition, many of these teams will bring all of their own equipment and medications. Although this seems generous on the surface, it is hard to teach and train the local providers on anesthetic equipment and drugs that they will not have further access to. It also highlights the discrepancy between the care that high-income countries can offer from what they can offer in their host countries. When medical teams from high-income countries come to LMIC for short-term mission trips, the local citizens may develop the perception that the care they receive from their local providers is inferior and this leads to an erosion of their trust of local providers.

Participants of MSTs must ensure that the procedures they are performing will have an appropriate postoperative long-term follow-up and

Table 1
Lancet Commission Core Indicators for monitoring of universal access to safe, affordable surgical and anesthesia care when needed

	Definition	Target
Access to timely	Proportion of the population that can access, within 2 h a facility that can do caesarean delivery, laparotomy, and treatment of open fracture (the Bellwether Procedures)	A minimum of 80% coverage of essential surgical and anesthesia services per country by 2030
Specialist surgical workforce density	Number of specialist surgical, anesthetic, and obstetric physicians who are working, per 100,000 population per year	100% of countries with at least 20 surgical, anesthetic, and obstetric physicians per 100,000 population by 2030
Surgical volume	Procedures done in an operating theater, per 100,000 population per year	80% of countries by 2020 and 100% of countries 2030 tracking surgical volume a minimum of 5000 procedures per 100,000 population by 2030
Perioperative morality	All cause death rate before discharge in patients who have undergone a procedure in an operating theater, divided by the total number of procedures, presented as a percentage	80% of countries by 2020 and 100% of countries 2030 tracking perioperative morality in 2020, assess global data, and set national targets for 2030
Protein against impoverishing expenditure	Proportion of households protected against impoverishment from direct out-of-pocket payments for surgical and anesthesia care	100% protection against impoverishment from out-of-pocket payments for surgical and anesthesia care by 2030
Protein against catastrophic	Proportion of households protected against catastrophic expenditure from direct out-of-packet payments for surgical and anesthesia care	100% protection against catastrophic expenditure from out-of-pocket payments for surgical and anesthesia care by 2030

These indicators provide the most information when used and interpreted together, no single indicator provides an adequate representation of surgical and anesthesia care when analyzed independently

From Meara JG, Leather AJ, Hagander L, et al. Global Surgery 2030: evidence and solutions for achieving health, welfare, and economic development. Lancet. 2015;386(9993):569 to 624.

support. For example, many countries cannot provide long-term anticoagulant therapy for artificial heart valves. Although an MST may have the ability to place these valves, there needs to be careful consideration of long-term care of these patients. MSTs are also very costly and some argue that the money spent on short-term mission trips could be used to support training, retention, equipment, and infrastructure in LMIC.

Capacity-building trips, on the other hand, engage in a long-term relationship with the LMIC host country to increase the local providers ability to care for surgical cases within their own infrastructure. The goal is to train the local surgical and anesthesia providers to become self-sufficient. It is said that an anesthesiologist working with an LMIC through capacity-building ultimate goal is to make his or her role obsolete due to the LMIC developing to a degree that outside support from high-income country physicians is not needed. Providing both clinical and classroom instruction is a key to achieving this. Developing long-term trusting relationships is a vital part of capacity building. This is especially true for complex

Box 1
Lancet Commission five key messages[1]

The Lancet Commissions Global Surgery 2030 Five Key Messages

Five billion people lack access to safe, affordable surgical and anesthesia care when needed.

One hundred forty-three million additional surgical procedures are needed each year to save lives and prevent disabilities.

Thirty-three million individuals face catastrophic health expenditure due to payment for surgery and anesthesia each year.

Investment in surgery and anesthesia services is affordable, saves lives, and promotes economic growth.

Surgery is an indivisible, indispensable part of health care.

Data from Meara JG, Leather AJ, Hagander L, et al. Global Surgery 2030: evidence and solutions for achieving health, welfare, and economic development. Lancet. 2015;386(9993):569-624.

specialized surgical interventions, such as thoracic surgeries. In addition to the surgical intervention, there must be careful consideration for the whole perioperative capacity to care for these surgical patients.

University of North Carolina, (UNC) Global Anesthesia is associated with UNC Project Malawi, and was established to improve the care of all surgical patients, and was composed of several components (**Table 2**). These items are an important part of capacity building which helps to improve the foundation for the development of more complex surgical procedures (eg,. thoracic procedures).

Table 2
UNC Global Anesthesia partnership with Kamuzu Central Hospital

Visiting Anesthesiologist Role	Host Anesthesiologist Role
Participated in clinical care in the operating rooms	Conducted clinical examinations for the Training Anesthesia Clinical Officers
Introduced a "flipped classroom" approach to teaching and problem-based learning discussions	Developed written examinations for the Training Anesthesia Clinical Officers
Conducted ultrasound guided regional anesthesia workshops	Developed a code box for emergencies
Introduced the use of intralipids for local anesthetic toxicity	Developed a sustainable simulation program
Introduced evidence-based protocols	Identified and prioritized quality improvement projects
Provided prepared and on-the-fly didactic lectures to both students and clinical officers	

INFRASTRUCTURE ASSESSMENT

The World Health Organization (WHO) Surgical Assessment Tool database surveyed almost 800 facilities in LMICs to discover what proportion of them did not have reliable electricity (31%), running water (22%), oxygen (24%), a dedicated area for emergency care (31%), and provisions for postoperative care (47%).[1] Internet is scarce at many LMIC hospitals, so that the ability for remote continual medical education resources is limited. In addition, the availability of advanced airway equipment for thoracic surgeries must be evaluated before starting a thoracic surgery program, such as fiber-optic scopes, double-lumen tubes, and ability to provide postoperative ventilation, if needed. In addition, the ability to provide consistent cardiovascular monitoring (eg, oxygenation and invasive blood pressure monitoring) is essential to patient safety and the success of the thoracic surgery program. Advanced training of operative and postoperative staff must also be considered. The ability to provide blood products for high-risk surgeries should be explored. The Lancet commission reported that only 27% of hospitals in LMIC reported an on-site blood bank.[1]

Anesthesia for Thoracic Surgery in Resource-variable Settings

The surgical burden for basic general, orthopedic, and obstetric operations comprises the most of the literature on surgical capacity building in LMIC. Very few articles are written on more complex procedures, such as thoracic surgeries in LMIC. These procedures are very specialized and provide unique challenges for the surgeon and anesthesia providers. The WHO lists death associated with trachea, bronchus, or lung cancer as the sixth leading cause of death worldwide, suggesting the need to expand access to thoracic surgeries in LMICs.[9] Tracheal, bronchus, and lung (TBL) cancer was the leading cause of cancer in high–middle sociodemographic index (SDI) countries, and it was the most common cause of cancer deaths by absolute cases globally as well as in all SDI quintiles. For men, TBL cancer was the most common incident cancer in 48 countries and the most common cause for cancer deaths in 110 countries based on data reported in 2017.[10] In addition, the ability to diagnose and treat these cancers is especially limited, which can lead to a disproportionate rate of morbidity and mortality.

When thoracic surgeries are discussed in LMIC, the mantra of "first do no harm" must be remembered. Many LMICs do not have the resources needed to safely provide thoracic surgery and the required anesthesia, which is why blunt chest trauma in LMIC has such a high mortality. Many poorly resourced rural hospitals in LMIC cannot operate on blunt chest trauma so the patients must be sent to larger district hospitals for surgical repair. This also introduces the risks associated with the transport of a critically ill patient with thoracic disease.

When a hospital in a low reourced setting is ready to start a thoracic surgery program is advised to start small and increase the complexity of surgical cases, once both experience and equipment are acquired. The LMIC hospital is encouraged to partner with experts from either regional sites with thoracic surgery programs or high-income country hospitals to gain the training and identify vital resource needs. Preoperative planning, intraoperative, and postoperative care must all be considered when starting thoracic surgery programs in LMICs. Special consideration also has to be given to hospital infrastructure and staffing when considering thoracic surgical procedures. It has been noted that many hospitals lack basic anesthetic equipment, such as machines, oxygen, pulse oximeters, and airway management equipment. These are essential to care of the thoracic surgical patient.

Kamuzu Central Hospital (KCH) is the central referral hospital in the capital city of Lilongwe, serving the middle region of Malawi. It is an 800-bed hospital that will flex to over 1000 beds during the busy season. KCH is overseen by the Ministry of Health and is affiliated with the Malawi College of Medicine and Malawi College of Health Sciences with on-site facilities for the third-year Malawian medical students.

In the author's experience at KCH, the surgical suite was frequently limited with regards to basic monitors and lacks specialized airway equipment, such as double-lumen tubes and fiber-optic scopes, which are needed for the safe care of thoracic surgical patients. Establishing supply chains will be as important as developing training models for these highly specialized anesthetic techniques to support thoracic surgical care. In addition, many LMICs do not have adequate number of staff who are properly trained in the delivery of specialized thoracic care, and this has a direct impact on patient safety and outcomes.

PREOPERATIVE EVALUATION

Selecting appropriate patients for thoracic surgery in LMIC is of the utmost importance. Careful consideration of the patient's fitness, as well as the limitations of perioperative care, should be weighed together with the acuity of the condition and long-term benefit of the operation.

The preoperative evaluation for thoracic surgery starts with the basic considerations of any anesthetic. A full history and physical must be obtained including previous anesthesia history, airway examination, allergies, nil per os, NPO status, functional capacity, American Society of Anesthesiology (ASA) score, baseline vital signs, and physical examination. In addition to this, careful evaluation of both pulmonary, cardiovascular, and renal status must be obtained.

In high-income countries, pulmonary function test, echocardiograms, and sleep studies are all readily available. This is not true in LMICs. Many LMICs do not have consistent access to radiographs or computed tomography, CT scans to evaluate lung status. In these settings, extra attention must be paid to the patient's functional status and physical examination findings. **Table 3** lists the important preoperative questions to determine a patient's metabolic equivalent (METS)of oxygen consumption. MET scores are the best

Table 3
Metabolic equivalent score to determine cardiovascular health

1–4 METs (poor)	Standard light home activities Walking short distances Walk 1–2 blocks on level ground at 3–5 km/h
5–9 METs (moderate)	Climb a flight of stairs Walk on level ground at >6 km/h Run a short distance Moderate exercise (dance, hiking, bicycle around town)
>10 METs (excellent)	Strenuous sports (swimming, tennis, basketball) Heavy professional work

noninvasive measures of cardiovascular health. Scores of less than 4 are an indicator of poor cardiovascular status, where 4 to 9 indicates moderate cardiac status and greater than 10 delineates excellent cardiovascular status.

Patients who are greater than 70 years old, ASA greater than 3 (**Table 4**), obese, obstructive sleep apnea, smokers, or alcoholics have an increased risk of complications.[11] The patient's chest X-ray and CT scan, if available, should be reviewed. If the LMIC has the ability to obtain arterial blood gas analysis, the results on room air can be useful in the perioperative setting. If not, baseline oxygen saturations sitting, standing and with exertion, such as walking, will be helpful as a surrogate for PFTs. Laboratory test should include complete blood count and creatinine at a minimum.[11]

Table 4
American Society of Anesthesiology, physical status classification scale

1	Normal Healthy patient
2	Patient with mild systemic disease
3	Patient with severe systemic disease that limits activity, but is not incapacitating
4	Patient with incapacitating systemic disease that is a constant threat to life
5	Moribund patient not expected to survive 24 h with or without the operation

If a patient is a smoker then cessation should be highly encouraged for at least 2 to 3 weeks before surgery, ideally 4 weeks. This is also true for daily consumption of alcohol. Increasing physical activity, as tolerated, before elective thoracic surgery will improve pulmonary outcomes. Patients should be encouraged to use incentive spirometers, if available, both before and after surgery.

INTRAOPERATIVE CONSIDERATIONS

Thoracic surgery requires careful monitoring of oxygenation and cardiovascular function, which is frequently done via invasive monitoring modalities (intra-arterial cannulas). Lung isolation is frequently required for surgical exposure but may also be required for broncho-pleural fistulas or infectious processes involving one lung.

Lung isolation is commonly performed using a double-lumen endotracheal tube (DLETT) (**Fig. 3**); however, there are methods that can be used if a DLETT is unavailable including mainstem endobronchial intubation. There are several potential problems with endobronchial intubation that should be anticipated including tube movement during the procedure, inability to provide complete isolation to the dependent lung, and inability to ventilate the upper lung. Bronchial blockers and Fogarty embolectomy catheters can also be used; however, they lack the ability to provide suction to the dependent lung and will require a fiberoptic scope to place.[12,13] The availability of fiberoptic bronchoscopy to confirm proper positioning of the double lumen tube, DLT or other endobronchial device may be limited in LMIC, necessitating careful auscultation and physical examination. In addition, surgical rigid bronchoscopy may be used for placement of the single-lumen tube in the mainstem position or placement of an endobronchial device.

Positioning of the surgical patient is also an important consideration as most thoracic surgery is performed with the patient in a lateral decubitus position with the exception of procedures that require a median sternotomy.[12] After positioning, it is imperative that the endotracheal tube or other endobronchial device remains in the optimal position and confirmation may be necessary.

POSTOPERATIVE CARE

Postoperative care of the thoracic surgical patient is challenging, and special attention must be paid to the cardiovascular and respiratory system, the potential for postoperative hemorrhage, and

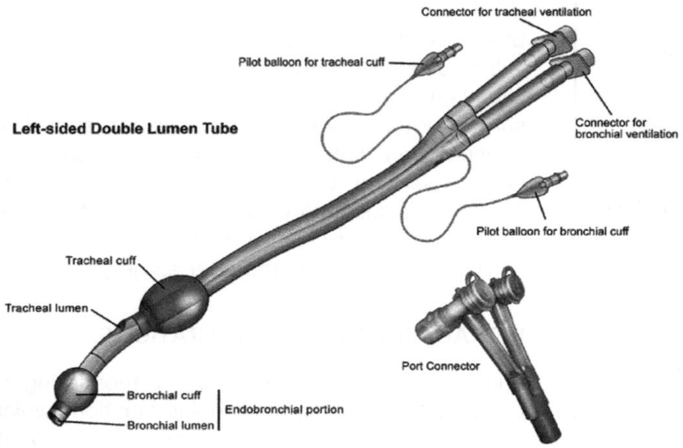

Fig. 3. Left-sided double lumen endotracheal tube. (*From* Bonavia A, Barbeito A. Double Lumen Tube for Single-Lung Ventilation. In: Doyle DJ, Abdelmalak B, eds. Clinical Airway Management: An Illustrated Case-Based Approach. Cambridge: Cambridge University Press; 2000:265-270.)

postoperative pain control.[14] Arrhythmias can be common in the postoperative period and must be anticipated. Common causes, such as respiratory failure and electrolyte abnormalities, should be corrected initially. Medications such as beta blockers, calcium channel blockers, and other antiarrhythmics should be considered for unstable patients, if available.[15]

Neuraxial pain control via intrathecal morphine or epidural analgesia is an option but may be limited by equipment availability. Postoperative pain relief using intrapleural blockade (IPB) should also be considered. IPB involves infusing local anesthetic into the paravertebral gutter where it can diffuse through the parietal pleura and intercostal muscles to provide pain relief. Most commonly Bupivacaine is used for IPB in the 0.5% or 0.25% concentration.[15] In addition, multimodal pain relief with non-opioid medications including anti-inflammatory and neuropathic drugs may be used, if available.[12] With any regimen, careful attention must be paid to potential complications such as postoperative respiratory depression.

SUMMARY

Anesthetic care for patients in LMIC is complex and frequently limited by access to equipment, staff, and other resources. When considering more complicated surgical procedures, such as thoracic surgery, it is recommended that the LMIC develops a partnership with other institutions that can provide education, training, and assess resource needs. At a minimum, there must be the capacity for the preoperative evaluation of the patients with chest-radiography, complete pulmonary assessment, and baseline bloodwork. Intraoperative anesthetic management, including the ability to perform one-lung ventilation, is also important. Finally, considerations for postoperative monitoring with pulse oximetry and pain control must be a part of any thoracic surgical program.

CLINICS CARE POINTS

- Capacity building should be a part of all short-term mission trips and global health endeavors with the goal of enhancing education and resources of low-to-middle income countries (LMICs).
- Preoperative assessment of pulmonary and cardiovascular status in LMICs is based on a thorough history and physical.
- Assigning a patient a metabolic equivalent (MET) score is a good surrogate for cardiovascular status and should be used when advance testing is not available to assess patient's fitness for thoracic surgery.
- Less than five METs is poor, 5 to 9 METs is moderate, greater than 10 METs is excellent.
- If a patient is a smoker then cessation should be highly encouraged for at least 2 to 3 weeks before surgery, ideally 4 weeks.
- The ability to provide lung isolation is key and traditional techniques used in high-resourced countries may not be available.

DISCLOSURE

The authors have nothing to disclose.

REFERENCES

1. Meara JG, Leather AJM, Hagander L, et al. 2030:evidence and solutions for achieving health, welfare, and economic development. The Lancet 2015;386: 569–624.
2. McQueen KA, Coonan T, Derbew M, et al. The 2015 Bangkok Global Surgery Declaration: A Call to the Global Health Community to Promote Implementation of the World Health Assembly Resolution for Surgery and Anesthesia Care. World J Surg 2017;41: 7–9.
3. Holmer H, Lantz A, Kunjumen T, et al. Global Distribution of surgeons, anaesthesiologists, and obstetricians. Lancet Glob Health 2015;3:S9–11.
4. Kempthorne P, Morris WW, Mellin-Olsen J. *etal.* WFSA Global Anesthesia Workforce Survey. Anesth Analg 2017;125(3):981–90.
5. Umutesi G, McEvoy MD, Starnes JR, et al. Safe Anesthesia Care in Western Kenya: a preliminary assessment of the impact of nurse anesthetists at multiple levels of government hospitals. Anesth Analg 2019;129(5):1387–93.
6. Newton M, Bird P. Impact of parallel anesthesia and surgical provider training in sub-Saharan Africa: a model for a resource-poor setting. World J Surg 2010;34(3):445–52.
7. Lantz AH, Holmer H, Finlayson S, et al. International migration of surgeons, anaesthesiologists, and obstetricians. Lancet Glob Health 2015;3:S11–2.
8. Kim JY. Opening address to the inaugural “The Lancet Commission on Global Surgery” meeting. The World Bank. Jan 17, 2014. Boston, MA, USA.
9. Available at: https://www.who.int/data/gho/data/themes/mortality-and-global-health-estimates
10. Fitzmaurice C. Global, regional and national cancer incidence, mortality, years of life lost, years lived with disability, and disability-adjusted life-years for 29 cancer groups, 1990 to 2017. JAMA Oncol 2019; 5(10):1749–68.
11. Jacob R. Challenges in the practice of thoracic anesthesia in developing countries. In: Slinger P, editor. Progress in thoracic anesthesia. Baltimore (MD): Lippincott Williams and Wilkins; 2004. p. pp267–85.
12. Jacob R. Anesthesia for thoracic surgery in children in developing countries. Pediatr Anesth 2009;19: 19–22.
13. Available at: https://www.cambridge.org/core/books/abs/clinical-airway-management/double-lumen-tube-for-singlelung-ventilation/FC0D1EF7312DE7E2B6C31C0EF45A0D38
14. Piccioni F, Droghetti A, Bertani A, et al. Recommendations from the Italian intersociety consensus on Perioperative Anesthesia Care in Thoracic Surgery (PACTS) part 2: intraoperative and postoperative care. Periop Med (Lond) 2020;9:31.
15. Amar D. Post thoracotomy arrhythmias. In: Slinger P, editor. Progress in thoracic anesthesia. Baltimore (MD): Lippincott Williams and Wilkins; 2004. p. pp267–85.

Development of an Endoscopy Training Partnership in a Developing Country

Eileen S. Natuzzi, MD, MPH[a,*], Chris Hair, FRACP, MBBS, BSc, AMICDA[b,c,d,e], Elizabeth Ha'upala Wore, MD, MBBS/MMED[f], Virginia Litle, MD[g]

KEYWORDS

• Endoscopy • Sustainability • Capacity building

KEY POINTS

- Developing an endoscopy training partnership in a developing country can be challenging.
- A team approach that includes local and international team members must commit to excellence
- Endoscopy equipment and supply procurement can be challenging
- Availability for maintenance of endoscopy equipment can be the linchpin of any program and must be built in from the program's inception.

Cancers of the esophagus, stomach, colon and rectum, and liver are ranked among the top 10 cancers killers worldwide.[1] In many developing countries the burden from gastrointestinal diseases, including cancers, is not known. This is particularly true in Sub-Saharan Africa and the southwestern Pacific whereby disease prevalence is often underestimated due to limited screening and early diagnoses.

This article describes the components of and challenges in developing a multinational training partnership to establish local, sustainable endoscopic services. The program highlighted as an example in this article is one that has been established in the Solomon Islands and Fiji. The overarching goal of this type of program should be to define the epidemiology of gastrointestinal disease in the country while providing quality care for its citizens.

BACKGROUND

Many developing countries have high rates of both infectious and chronic diseases. This includes infectious diseases that contribute to the development of gastrointestinal cancers including *Helicobacter pylori*, Hepatitis B, and Hepatitis C. *H pylori* infection rates in Asia are 35% to 58%.[2] In the Pacific Islands, the rates seem to be as high as 94% although limited population-based data are available.[3] Infection with Helicobacter pylori is the strongest recognized risk factor for gastric adenocarcinoma.[4] More than 240 million people worldwide have chronic Hepatitis liver infections and 780,000 die annually from Hepatitis. The highest incidences of Hepatitis B are in Southeast Asia and the Pacific Region whereby transmission is largely vertical from mother to child. In Solomon Islands, an estimated 19.6% of the population is seropositive for Hepatitis B antigen.[5] When acquired in childhood, Hepatitis B progresses to cirrhosis, portal hypertension varices, and in some cases cancer in 15% to 25% of individuals, and therefore represents a major cause of mortality in endemic settings.[6]

A robust screening, diagnostic and therapeutic endoscopy program is the cornerstone of

[a] ANZGITA, San Diego, CA USA; [b] University Hospital, Geelong, Australia; [c] Epworth Private Hospital, Geelong, Australia; [d] Deakin University, Waurn Ponds, Australia; [e] ANZGITA, Melbourne, Australia; [f] National Referral Hospital, Honiara, Solomon Islands; [g] Intermountain Healthcare
* Corresponding author.
E-mail address: esnmd@mac.com

Thorac Surg Clin 32 (2022) 317–327
https://doi.org/10.1016/j.thorsurg.2022.03.002

addressing a wide range of gastrointestinal cancers. In 2008 an endoscopy training partnership was formed between Fiji National University (FNU), Australian and New Zealand Gastroenterology International Training Association (ANZGITA), and the World Gastroenterology Organization. Before the establishment of this training scheme, endoscopy services were lacking in most Pacific Island countries. This partnership established comprehensive centralized gastroenterology and endoscopic training program at Fiji National University's Colonial War Memorial Hospital in Suva, Fiji. The centralized training "hub" meant that clinicians and nurses from other regions in Fiji and the Pacific Island nations could meet, train and upskill in an environment that was similar to their own health care systems. The FNU-ANZGITA program has trained doctors and nurses from throughout the Pacific Island nations over the last decade. A few years after this program was established endoscopy training was extended to include a regional-based "in-country" training partnerships model. The first site for this training model was established in Solomon Islands in 2012.

Both programs have demonstrated the ability to develop endoscopy services that provide valuable epidemiologic and clinical information on the incidence, prevalence, and risk factors for a wide range of gastrointestinal diseases, especially cancers. Pairing centralized training in Fiji along with in-country training in Solomon Islands has allowed training to incorporate local medical conditions as well as challenges in setting up an endoscopy service while establishing a university-based training hub. The information gleaned from both partnerships is vital to allowing health providers and local Ministries of Health to design medical as well as public health interventions that address treatment as well as prevention (**Box 1**, **Fig. 1**).

ESTABLISHING THE PROGRAM

Local Buy in

The most important consideration when establishing a training partnership is to understand local health care needs and priorities. This includes understanding what the local health care system can support. There are 3 key goals to consider when establishing this type of capacity-building partnership: [11]

1. Ensure the program is responsive to local needs, with adequate buy-in from local health care providers
2. Ensure the program is of high quality and must take into account the local context.
3. Establish an overarching commitment to long-term sustainability

Having a local champion who knows what is needed and how to negotiate within the health system is key during the initial phase of the program. This local champion can motivate fellow participating physicians, registrars, and nursing staff who contribute to making a tremendous difference in the success of the program. The local champion serves as the contact person for planned visits, tele-consults, and digital meetings. That person also communicates what is working and what is not. Programs should include registrars as well as nurses-in-training as the training of the future generation helps to build a robust.

To ensure the program is of high-quality minimum standards for training should be established. This includes endoscopy procedure competencies. This is discussed further in the Certification and Credentialing of Training section of this article.

Committing to long-term sustainability is a major challenge, which can be addressed by forming partnerships with industry, professional organizations, and the Ministry of Health.

Additional considerations in establishing a training partnership includes language barriers, cultural differences and ease of travel to the site whereby training will take place. How is health care paid for? Is it government funded, private pay, third-party payment, or a combination of all of the above? Economic roadblocks can hinder patients from accessing the program.

Centralized Versus Regional Training

Beginning a training partnership should first consider whether a centralized, regional, or hybrid training program will be the best strategy. A centralized program is efficient and cost-effective. It brings together trainees for collective education while it serves as professional training center in the future. It also establishes protocols, minimal training criteria and can foster widespread involvement in a community-based cancer registry. A regional program has the advantage of solving problems on a local level, such as electricity outages and water availability. It also allows the trainers to learn about the endemic gastrointestinal diseases the endoscopists will be treating.

The endoscopy training partnership program in the Pacific started as a centralized training at Colonial War Memorial Hospital (CWMH) in Suva, Fiji. CWMH offers an ideal location for training as it is close to the Fiji National University, the major clinical training hospital for medicine and nursing in Fiji, and can be accessed by postgraduate

Box 1
Region information

The Pacific Islands are comprised of hundreds of remote islands and coral atolls distributed over an area equivalent to 15% of the earth's surface. Three ethno-geographic groups define the collective population of 2.3 million people spread across those islands; Melanesia, Micronesia, and Polynesia. Health care challenges in the Pacific Islands suffer from similar problems identified in other developing countries such as: under-resourcing of manpower, training, and supplies.

The Solomon Islands is an independent nation located in the Melanesian portion of the western Pacific. The country is an archipelago made up of 999 islands scattered across a 450,000 square miles area of ocean. The Solomon Islands is one of the least developed countries in the Pacific Region with a 2020 United Nations Development Program Human Development Index ranking of 151 of 189 countries.[7,8] The population is just more than 600,000. 80% of the population lives in outer islands, however, the highest population density is in urban areas such as Honiara, the capital city.

The health system in Solomon Islands is largely a public system accounting for 5.5% of the GDP or roughly $75 US per capita.[9] The government funds 65% of health care costs while external development sources provide an additional 29%. The remaining 6% comes from out-of-pocket payments and fees.[10] The National Referral Hospital (NRH), located in Honiara on Guadalcanal delivers complex and acute care. Patients are referred to the NRH from 7 provincial and 4 private hospitals. There is no CT scanner in the country and until the initiation of this in-country endoscopy training partnership program doctors did not have access to video endoscopic equipment.

medical and surgical trainees from across the Pacific. Through the program local Fijian physician endoscopists were given intensive skills training as well as training in teaching. This included short intense training fellowships in Australia and New Zealand. This allowed the physicians in Fiji to rapidly upskill over a short time period and become part of the teaching team alongside visiting ANZGITA volunteers. It also created local consultants who can offer clinical and technical advice to new programs starting out. Our initial approach of providing training to the nurses and doctors at CWMH has evolved into their becoming the Pacific region's resource for endoscopy. CWMH endoscopy teams now performed outreach training visits to other Pacific Islands whereby endoscopy programs are under development. These have included Pohnpei, Marshall Islands, Kiribati, Tonga, Vanuatu, and Samoa.

Since the central training scheme's inception in 2008, 45 gastroenterologists and 30 nurse trainers from Australia and New Zealand have visited the training center in Suva and participated in the program with 68 visits. Several have participated in multiple training visits. We have found commitment from the trainees to the program is the key to their success.

There have been 104 Pacific Island doctor attendees to the Fiji program which includes physicians, surgeons, and registrars from Fiji and other Pacific Island Countries. Pacific Island Nurse Trainees have totaled 96 attendances over the past 10 years. Some have attended on more than one occasion. The nurses are an integral part of the program, accompanying their physician colleagues, so that they can both learn together as a team. Many of these teams have returned to their Pacific Island community and established their own gastroenterology and endoscopy services. The impact of the centralized program can be demonstrated by the expanded regional service provision in nations including Timor Leste, Solomon Islands, Vanuatu, Tonga, Samoa, American Samoa, Cook Islands, Marshall Islands, Kiriabti, Micronesia, and Palau. Based on our experience we encourage the development of a hybrid model with a central knowledge and training hub in addition to regional outreach training.

General Structure

A training partnership agreement should be clearly defined by the medical staff and trainees. The goals of the program, who will be involved in the team and what requirements are essential for certification need to be identified and described. The Ministry of Health (MOH) should be included in these discussions to ensure implementation is aligned with national goals. If there are other capacity-building partners working within the same country, collaborative discussions with them are important. Partnering with other stakeholders could offer the expansion of the program and enhance knowledge of the new endoscopy services available for patients. Planning should include frequency of in-country training visits, connectivity for remote consultations, and specifics about equipment supply and maintenance. A Memorandum of Understanding (MOU) between the training partners and the MOH can serve to

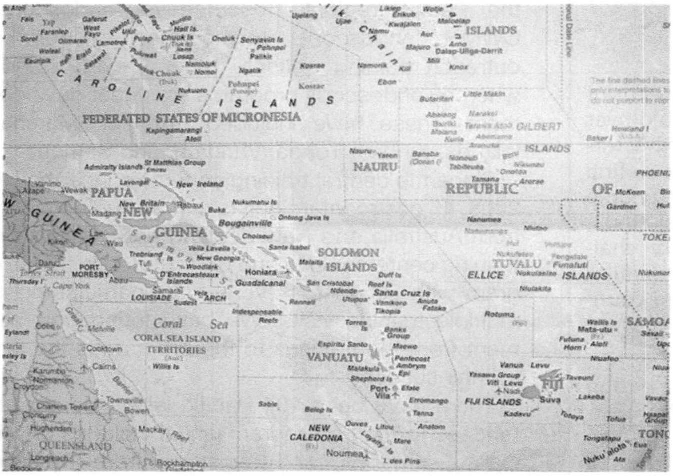

Fig. 1. Map of the western Pacific region and Solomon Islands. (*From* Hema Maps.)

solidify the commitment in writing. Our training visits in the Solomon Islands included:

1. Lectures on gastrointestinal diseases pertinent to the region.
2. Hands-on dry laboratory training on care and use of endoscopic equipment.
3. Instruction on endoscopic record-keeping.
4. Supervised endoscopic procedures.
5. Audit of current endoscopy cases (**Fig. 2**).

Build a Core Team

The core partnership team includes physician endoscopists, endoscopy nurses or technicians, and registrars. Endoscopic nurse training is an essential part of building a strong program. Nurses should be encouraged to attend all of the training and receive additional education in assisting with endoscopic procedures, cleaning and disinfecting and care of equipment. During our training partnership visits, local endoscopy nurses were paired with a visiting partner nurse. This allowed one-to-one knowledge sharing and peer-to-peer problem-solving.

Additional team members should include supply chain experts, radiologists, pathologists and, if available, oncologists. Clearly defined roles and expectations for each team member should be available in the partnership agreement and reviewed with the team as needed.

Additional team members should be included to meet local and regional needs. For example, moving goods in and out of a foreign country can be challenging, especially when there are custom fees and clearance issues; therefore, we included a shipping company as part of our team to facilitate the acquisition and delivery of supplies from Australia and the US. In addition, partnership with local government officials as well as embassy representatives may be beneficial in keeping them appraised of the partnership's progress.

The gastroenterologist teaching team should be broad and include doctors, nurses, and a country coordinator. It is important to establish a core group of nurses and doctors who become familiar with the country, any local challenges in doing endoscopy, and the diseases that are endemic to it. In our programs, we pair nurse and physician instructors who are familiar with the country and the endoscopy training program with those visiting for the first time. This allows for smoother integration of new volunteers.

Funding for volunteer travel and lodging can be challenging. We were fortunate early on to receive funding from endoscopic industry and support from the American Society for Gastrointestinal Endoscopy's Ambassador Program. As the program developed it folded into ANZGITA. ANZGITA has a large number of Australian and New Zealand gastroenterologist and nurse volunteers who are involved in the training programs in Fiji as well as Solomon Islands.

Endoscopy Equipment

Procurement of endoscopy equipment is *the* lynchpin of any new program. At the inception of our partnership video, endoscopic equipment was obtained through donations from the endoscopic industry including Olympus and Pentax. One very important consideration when acquiring endoscopy equipment is knowing whether its electrical voltage is compatible with the local infrastructure. If a donation does not match, a step-up or step-down converter may be needed. As

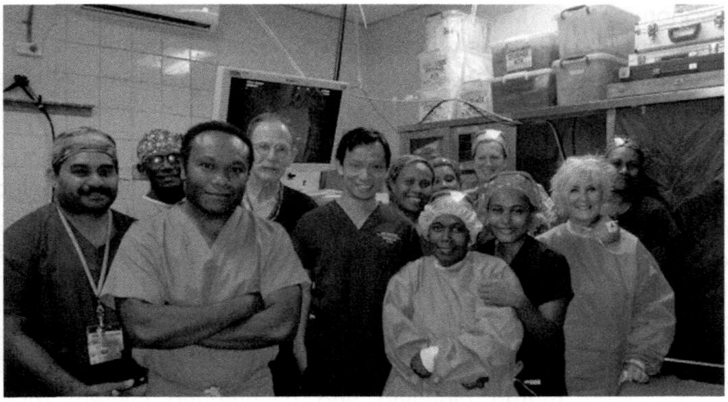

Fig. 2. Solomon Islands Endoscopy Partnership team made up of members of the NRH hospital staff and the ANZGITA team. (*Courtesy of* Eileen Natuzzi, MD, MPH, San Diego, CA.)

equipment is obtained over time emphasis should be placed on voltage-compatible equipment to enhance shelf life.

The basic endoscopy starter equipment for any new or developing program should include:

1. A pair of gastroscopes, if possible, one should have a large biopsy channel
2. A pair of colonoscopes, if possible one should have a large biopsy channel
3. Biopsy forceps
4. Biopsy Brushes
5. Endo needles for tattooing
6. Savory Gilliard over wire dilators
7. A video processor
8. At least one monitor and, if possible, a second slave monitor
9. A USB image capture system if not built into the video processor
10. A leak tester

Over time additional equipment can be added and should include endoscopic intervention equipment such as diathermy, and C-arm fluoroscopy.

After establishing the program, it is ideal to move toward the standardization of the equipment used. In the Solomon Islands, we formed an MOU with Pentax to allow for interchangeability of scopes and parts while creating a reliable mechanism for equipment maintenance and replacement. A major factor in determining sustainability is to have a dedicated maintenance support program for the facility and its equipment. Endoscopic equipment is fragile and requires advanced technical skills for repair. It is not possible to simply repair the equipment in a Pacific Island nation at this stage, so the equipment must be sent overseas for repair. Establishment of a regular, timely maintenance and repair program and a way to ship equipment to that site is necessary to sustain the life of the equipment. One big decision in the establishment of any new facility or training site is whether to incorporate new endoscopes and maintenance agreements or to rely on older equipment that would be expected to degrade quickly.

Considerations for Setting up the Endoscopy Suite

The in-country team members should identify whereby the endoscopy procedures will take place, whereby patients will be interviewed, prepped, and recovered and whereby the equipment will be cleaned and stored. This can be challenging in a space-limited hospital or clinic. If possible, a space designated for equipment set up would be preferred. Early on in our programs in Fiji and Solomon Islands endoscopy was performed in the minor operating theater. The equipment was installed on a rolling endoscopy cart. The hospital carpenters made a wooden scope hanging system that assisted with "drip drying" equipment. Because many developing countries are tropical, especially those in the Pacific region, an air conditioning unit should be installed in the procedure and scope storage area. This can reduce some of the effects of heat and humidity on equipment and supply degradation. As the program matures finding funding for renovating or building a designated endoscopy suite, cleaning, and storage area should be emphasized. In the Solomon Islands, the doctors converted a large storage space into a state-of-the-art endoscopy suite thanks to our partners (ANZGITA, Australia DFAT, the US WWII veterans, Taiwan AID and the MOH) and industry support. Not every program can do this but presenting program outcomes to the MOH, government representatives and other stakeholders can be helpful to garner financial support.

Disposable Versus reusable equipment

While donated reusable and disposable supplies are a reasonable way to prime the program, access to a reliable supply chain and economic considerations need to be put in place as the program achieves success. Whether to use disposable or reusable supplies will depend on availability, quality, and cost. The partnership should include environmental considerations on how disposable equipment such as biopsy forceps, cleaning solutions, and disinfectants will be handled. Will disposables be incinerated, end up in a landfill, or possibly be discarded in the ocean or other body of water? The discussion should include the possibility that some supplies will be reused. This is a matter of practicality in a resource-limited environment, so it should be addressed up front. In the Solomon Islands, the endoscopists perform variceal banding, at times repeatedly on the same patient. They designate and label the variceal banding kit per patient reusing it on the same person until all the bands have been deployed. In Fiji, a patient receiving repeat endoscopic dilation of luminal strictures using a balloon device will commonly receive the same, cleaned balloon marked and tagged for individual reuse at their follow-up.

If disposables are going to be reused decisions should be made on how to best clean and disinfect them. Single-use biopsy forceps can be manually washed and then placed in an ultrasonic cleaner with 2% glutaraldehyde solution; however, manufacturer practices of coating disposable forceps with plastic can interfere with ultrasonic cleaning. For this reason, it is recommended that the reusable biopsy forceps be used when possible rather than disposable ones.

Emphasize Infection Control

Cleaning and disinfection of endoscopic equipment is key to preventing the transmission of diseases that may be endemic to the region such as H. pylori, Hepatitis B or C. The nursing staff should be trained in infection control measures and when and how to order cleaning supplies and disinfectants. Training should include disinfecting the endo unit as well. The World Gastroenterology Organization (WGO) has provided an excellent cascade of care for endoscopic disinfection in developing countries, reflecting the gold standard of care against the economic capacity of the nation.[12]

Training on the handling of scopes postprocedure should include:

1. Precleaning or wiping down the scopes at the bedside
2. Leak testing to prevent cross-contamination and scope leak damage
3. Manual cleaning using biofilm and microorganism active solutions (eg: Matrix)
4. High-level disinfection with 2% glutaraldehyde
5. Proper drying and storage

Early in our experience, we used a 3 tub manual cleaning system that included enzymatic cleaning and disinfecting. One key consideration is doing cleaning in a well-ventilated room, if possible, as all of these products can be toxic. As our program expanded, we were able to install cleaning systems, such as the Cantrel system. Any program that moves toward an automated or semiautomated cleaning and disinfecting system must include comprehensive nursing training on its uses as well as troubleshooting the system and a mechanism to maintain and repair the system, similar to the challenges of maintaining endoscopes.

Peripheral Services

Pathology services are important to define types of tumors and to best direct care. Not every region will have on-site pathology due to manpower, supply, and infrastructure problems. The use of remote telepathology and/or sending pathology specimens to another countries for processing and reading is a good alternative to on-site processing.[13,14]

If send out services are used the request should contain pertinent clinical information that can assist the pathologist in making an accurate gross as well as microscopic diagnosis. This can also decrease delays in processing. Overseas specimen processing will incur delays in receiving results and so these issues should be anticipated and streamlined, wherever possible. Pathology reports that diagnose cancer should be added to the regional cancer registry.

If Helicobacter pylori is endemic to the region testing for it should be routine. If test kits are not available consider asking the pathologist to stain for the organism during the biopsy specimen processing.

Laboratory services on site are important for diagnosis and for assessing treatment response. If the laboratory does not have a comprehensive list of assays that are needed, such as CEA or CA19 to 9 tumor markers, creating a partnership with another country to provide send out analysis can be helpful.

Radiology services can help in diagnosis as well as during endoscopy procedures such as esophageal stent placements and foreign body retrievals. We have used flat plate and fluoroscopy imaging to check the placement of over-the-scope esophageal stents. A CT scanner is an important imaging modality but due to cost may not be readily available. Ultrasound and barium studies can be used for diagnostics when a CT scanner is unavailable.

Work with What Works in the Country

Not all assays and supplies will be readily available in a developing country. These include rapid H. pylori tests and bowel preps. We found less expensive solutions to some supply problems without compromising quality.

The capacity of local infrastructure is important to consider as well. In some locations, a consistent supply of reliable clean water could be an issue. In the Pacific Islands, most communities use captured rainwater as well as public water. Knowing whereby the water is sourced at the site whereby endoscopic services will be provided can reduce interruptions of services and assure the source is clean. Reliability of the electrical supply either as a part of the local grid or through the use of generators is another important consideration. Above all the program needs flexibility in the event of a power outage or contamination of the city or public water supply.

Plan for the Evolution of the Program

Members of the team should be aware of additional services, needs, and skill sets that come up as the training program progresses. The additional training in interventions should be led by the prevalence of gastrointestinal disease as defined by diagnostic endoscopy. This could include interventional endoscopy such as esophageal stents, variceal banding, and Percutaneous Endoscopic G-tube (PEG) placement. Training in advanced endoscopic interventions should focus on physicians with the most experience with diagnostic endoscopy first. The program in Fiji has trained the senior endoscopists in Endoscopic retrograde cholangiopancreatography. (ERCP) procedures. With the establishment of these higher-level services, local referrals can save time and money in repatriating patients following treatment provided internationally.

Establish Durable and Reliable Consultation and Virtual Education Linkages

As mentioned earlier our program provides ongoing consultations as a bridge between in-country visits through the use of email, Viber, and WhatsApp. This allows the team to share new and pertinent information and knowledge. It also solidifies the partnership as readily available consultations prevent local providers from feeling isolated. During the SARsCoV2 pandemic, while Pacific Islands were locked down, we found digital communication particularly helpful in maintaining the program. We added Zoom conferences covering pertinent topics and as a means to analyze data and plan future programs. This approach has also served the program well during recent geopolitical unrest in Solomon Islands. We were able to discuss safety, and other issues posed by the rioting with our in-country peers. Any program should consider local challenges such as political unrest, adverse economic impacts as well as natural disasters that can adversely impact the working partnership.

Data and Record-Keeping

Records of endoscopic procedures, including analysis of procedure findings, are key to defining the incidence and prevalence of diseases as well as treatments and outcomes. There are internet-based endoscopy reporting systems. Some interface with electronic health records. The local broadband capability and reliability need to be taken into consideration when choosing this type of recording system. A computer-based system that is uploadable is an ideal method of record keeping. Every member of the endoscopy team should be trained on and have access to whichever record-keeping program is selected. It is important to stress that the case data are used in the credentialing process and in determining individual competency. Where possible the addition of images taken at the time of endoscopy is a plus. The reports from each endoscopist should be collated together into a monthly department report. This data defines productivity and outlines the type and pattern of cases the program is seeing. A monthly audit should be held and shared with the local medical community with deidentified case discussions on the most interesting cases.

The partnership should encourage local team members to present this data to MOH, Public Health and other stakeholders to garner support for the program.

Encourage and Support Analysis, Sharing and Publication of Data

Include training and support on collecting, collating, and synthesizing information collected from endoscopic services. This should include incidences of diseases, relative risks, and odds ratios of diseases found. Encourage regular presentations of the data to the MOH and any funders or partners. Inviting political representatives and stakeholders to visit the endoscopy suite can go a long way to garner support. Include an economic assessment of the monies saved by providing endoscopic services locally as opposed

Box 2
Summary of the Solomon Islands program

Established in 2012 the program has evolved into a multinational training partnership when merged with the ANZGITA program in 2016.

Total staff trained: 13 doctors (9 surgeons, 4 medical), 7 Nurses, 8 Registrars

Total endoscopies performed: 2956 cases

- Upper: 2349
- Lower: 607
- Interventions: 75 esophageal dilations, 28 esophageal stents, 83 variceal banding

Bronchoscopy: 41

Source of funding: Solomon Islands MOH, ANZGITA funding through DFAT and donations, Funding by the Solomon Islands Living Memorial Project, Olympus America and Taiwan AID.

to people traveling internationally to receive care. The goal should be to share information and use that information for establishing support programs for sustainability as well as adding oncological services or public health prevention measures. Encourage the publication of findings and data by members of the endoscopy partnership with active participation by local team members.

Data should be shared locally as well as regionally during professional conferences and meetings as well as during monthly audits. In the case of cancers, participation in the regional cancer registry should be encouraged. The Global Initiative for Cancer Registry Development (GICR) has established six regional hubs that serve as catchments for the countries within the hub region.[15] Identifying which hub the program functions within and creating linkages with it is important in sharing cancer data. GICR provides training and guidance for establishing a health information specialist who inputs data into the cancer registry.

Certification and Credentialing of Training

As the program becomes more proficient training certification should be established to define the minimum number of cases to determine competency. This is whereby good individual procedure record-keeping is important (see above).

In our program, we use the Gastroenterological Society of Australia (GESA) definition of minimal standards for the endoscopists[16] and the nurses follow the Gastroenterological Nurses College of Australia (GENCA) standards.[17]

Box 3
What our partnership learned in the Solomon Islands

Malignancies made up a significant portion of the endoscopic diagnoses. We found significant numbers of advanced left-sided colon and anorectal cancers. The higher left-sided distribution might reflect difficulty in reaching the cecum. As experience increases rates of reaching the cecum during colonoscopy we may see more right-sided tumors.[24]

Esophageal cancers found on endoscopy were largely squamous cell carcinomas and tended to involve the middle portion of the esophagus. This is in contrast to the more distal distribution of adenocarcinomas of the esophagus seen in Australia and the United States and is in keeping with findings in East Africa and China. Our finding may reflect lower rates of reflux and Barrett's metaplasia and the carcinogenic impacts of betel nut chewing and tobacco use which are reported in 60% and 40% of individuals, respectively, in the Solomon Islands.[25] Betel nut is classified as a Group 1 carcinogen by the International Agency for Cancer Research (IARC).[26] A number of studies have linked esophageal cancer with betel nut use and its synergistic combination with tobacco use.[27]

One significant but often overlooked cobenefit of this program is a doctor's ability to diagnose advanced disease in a patient, to communicate that with the patient as well as their family and allow them to return to their village or community knowing their fate. Many of the patients treated at the National Referral Hospital are referred in from rural outer islands. The ability to diagnose an incurable disease process, explain what that process is, and what to expect from the patient as well as their accompanying family member allows them to accept their diagnosis, return to the care of their relatives and friends and address it as is culturally appropriate within their own surroundings.

These competencies can be modified for the region but should be made available to everyone doing endoscopy. If the program has a central training facility, this facility should define what the region's competencies will be. Our centralized program at FNU in Fiji oversees this process along with partnership assistance. Housing the competency and certification can be within regional medical organizations or as a de novo new association.

Encourage a Commitment to Learning

All team members should be encouraged to participate in centralized training as well as local training. Attending clinical education conferences should also be encouraged. This allows team members to share their own experiences and difficulties while getting information from their regional as well as international peers. Participation by registrars and nurses in training is very important as it builds depth to the program. One point our program stresses is "all of us are learning all of the time, even the most seasoned trainers."

Shift the Program Toward Being a Regional Training Site

As members of the team gain experience, the program should encourage those members with competent endoscopic skills to become trainers themselves. New trainers can be involved locally as well as in assisting in training regionally. With competency a program can invite regional peers to visit to develop their skills or go to other regional sites to assist them in getting programs off the ground. Senior endoscopists should be encouraged to participate in a Train the Trainer program sponsored by The World Gastroenterology Organization (WGO). A number of programs are offered by the WGO per year and in some cases, WGO can assist in offsetting the cost of attending. The program includes education on publications, clinical trial design as well as credentialing guidelines.[18]

Addressing Challenges

Affordable endoscopy equipment and reliable supply chains in developing countries are a universal issue for any health capacity-building program. A program can initially be built on donated supplies but consideration and planning for a slow transition to a sustainable locally directed purchasing program should be part of the plan. Tiered pricing for endoscopic equipment purchases is very much needed and in many cases is negotiable with endoscopy suppliers. Where possible the use of reusable supplies should be encouraged to keep costs down and avoid contributing to environmental degradation. Biomedical equipment repairs can be problematic. An MOU with the industry for repairs should be established but as the program progresses the establishment of a regional repair and servicing center should be considered (**Box 2**).

Final thoughts

Global health data sources documenting mortality, such as Globocan, provide only estimates of the prevalence of cancers in some resource-limited parts of the world, including many Pacific Island countries. Until recently gastrointestinal diseases in the Pacific Region have been underdiagnosed. This has resulted in inaccurate accounting for disease prevention and treatment needs. Establishment of endoscopy training in Fiji and a local program in the Solomon Islands has allowed health providers to begin to define cancers and diseases at a time when they are potentially curable. This type of burden of disease data can help policymakers better shape health policy within the country and in the region.

Video endoscopy programs have been established in a number of developing countries.[19–22] Many of these programs have consisted of distant training symposiums. In-country endoscopy programs have been slow to be adopted in the Pacific Region despite the active Fiji centralized regional training programs. Our partnership paired in-country endoscopy training with a comprehensive centralized endoscopy training provided by FNU, ANZGITA, and the World Gastrointestinal Organizations Regional Training Program at Fiji National University School of Medicine. This approach was undertaken to accelerate the adoption of safe and accurate endoscopic services at the

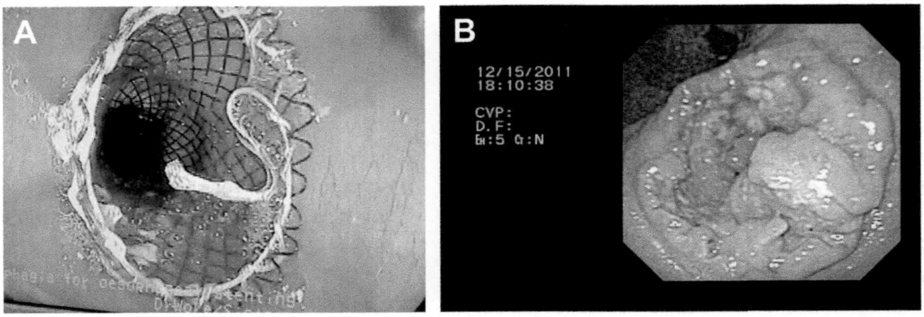

Fig. 3. (*A*) Gastric cancer. (*B*): Esophageal cancer poststent placement. (*Courtesy of* [*A*] Elizabeth Wore, Honaria, SB; [*B*] Scott Siota, Honaria, SB.)

National Referral Hospital in Honiara, Solomon Islands.

Many arguments have been put forth against establishing video endoscopic programs in resource-limited environments and these arguments have included challenges with training, cost and availability, and upkeep of equipment.[23] Our multinational training partnership has addressed many of these challenges and in doing so developed a locally owned video endoscopy program that has begun to deliver valuable local burden of gastrointestinal disease information (**Box 3**, **Fig. 3**).

The collection and analysis of data representing the burden of disease, along with epidemiologic investigation, can empower local health care providers and influence the effectiveness of limited health resources. Educational training partnerships with local providers can increase job satisfaction, reduce brain drain and contribute valuable, accurate information on disease prevalence and risk factors which can be used by MOH, public health services and add valuable information to regional cancer registries.

REFERENCES

1. Globocan 2012 Estimated cancer incidence, mortality and prevalence worldwide. Available at: http://globocan.iarc.fr/Pages/fact_sheets_population.aspx.
2. Fock KM, Ang TL. Epidemiology of Helicobacter pylori infection and gastric cancer in Asia. J Gastroenterol Hepatol 2010;25:479–86.
3. Isaac BA. Helicobacter pylori infections at a family practice in Pohnpei, Federated States of Micronesia. Health in Palau and Micronesia 2005;12(1):47–51.
4. Correa P, Piazuelo. Helicobacter pylori Infection and Gastric Cancer. US Gastroenterol Hepatol Rev 2011; 7(1):59–64.
5. Furusyo N, Hayashi J, Kakuda K, et al. Markedly high seroprevalence of hepatitis B virus infection in comparison to hepatitis C virus and human T lymphotropic virus type-1 infections in selected Solomon Islands populations. Am J Trop Med Hyg 1999;61:85–91.
6. WHO Hepatitis B fact sheets. Available at: http://www.who.int/mediacentre/factsheets/fs204/en/. Accessed November 15 2021.
7. UNDP human development Index. Available at: http://hdr.undp.org/en/content/latest-human-development-index-ranking. Accessed November 15 2021.
8. Solomon Island National Census Report. Solomon Island Government and National Statistic Office, SPC website. 2009. Available at: http://www.spc.int/prism/solomons/. Accessed November 15 2021.
9. The Kaiser Family Foundation. Total Expenditure on Health (as Percent of Gross Domestic Product). Available at: http://kff.org/global-indicator/total-expenditure-on-health/. Accessed November 15 2021.
10. WHO and Ministry of Health Health Delivery Profile: Solomon Islands 2012. Available at: http://www.wpro.who.int/health_services/service_delivery_profile_solomon_islands.pdf. Accessed November 15 2021.
11. Macpherson L, Collins M. Training responsibly to improve global surgical and anaesthesia capacity through institutional health partnerships: a case study. Trop Doct 2017;47(1):73–7.
12. Endoscopic Disinfection: A resource-sensitive approach. Available at: https://www.worldgastroenterology.org/UserFiles/file/guidelines/endoscope-disinfection-english-2011.pdf. Accessed November 15 2021.
13. Shashidhar VM, Brauchli K, Oberholzer M, et al. Pacific Telepathlogy Service at Fiji School of Medicine. Pac Health Dialog 2003;10(2):178–81.
14. Brauchli K, Jagilly R, Oberli H, et al. Telepathology on the Solomon Islands–two years' experience with a hybrid Web- and email-based telepathology system. J Telemed Telecare 2004;10(Suppl 1):14–7.
15. IARC Regional Hubs. Available at: https://gicr.iarc.fr/iarc-regional-hubs-for-cancer-registration/. Accessed November 15 2021.
16. Credentialling in endoscopy training. Available at: https://www.gesa.org.au/education/credentialing. Accessed November 15 2021.
17. Credentialing of Gastroenterology Nurses. Available at: https://www.genca.org/credentialling/cogen. Accessed November 9 2021.
18. WGO Train the Trainers Course. Available at: https://www.worldgastroenterology.org/education-and-training/train-the-trainers. Accessed November 9 2021.
19. Mothes H, Chagaluka G, Chiwewe D, et al. Do patients in rural Malawi benefit from upper gastrointestinal endoscopy? Trop Doctor 2009;39:73–6.
20. Asombang A, Turner-Moss E, Seetharam A, et al. Gastroenterology training in a resource-limited setting: Zambia, Southern Africa. World J Gastroenterol 2013;19(25):3996–4000.
21. Ismaila B, Misauno M. Gastrointestinal endoscopy in Nigeria: a prospective two year audit Pan African. Med J 2013;14:22. https://doi.org/10.11604/pamj.2013.14.22.1865. Available at: http://www.panafrican-med-journal.com/content/article/14/22/full/.
22. Makmun D. Present status of endoscopy, therapeutic endoscopy and the endoscopy training system in Indonesia. Dig Endosc 2014;26(Suppl. 2):2–9.
23. Chuks N. Challenges of gastrointestinal endoscopy in resource-Poor countries. 2011. Available at: intechopen.com/pdfs-wm/24152.pdf.

24. Rabeneck L, Davila J, El-Serag H. Is There a True "Shift" to the Right Colon in the Incidence of Colorectal Cancer? Am J Gastroenterol 2003;98(6): 1400–9.

25. Solomon Islands 2010 NCD Risk Factor STEPS Report. Available at: https://www.who.int/ncds/surveillance/steps/2006_Solomon_Islands_STEPS_Report.pdf. Accessed November 9 2021.

26. WHO Review of areca (betel) nut and tobacco use in the Pacific: a technical report. Available at: https://iris.wpro.who.int/bitstream/handle/10665.1/5281/9789290615699_eng.pdf. Accessed November 15 2021.

27. Akhtar S. Areca nut chewing and esophageal squamous-cell carcinoma risk in Asians: A meta-analysis of case–control studies. Cancer Causes Control 2013;24:257–65.

Chest Trauma Management in Low- and Middle-Income Countries

Brittney M. Williams, MD, MPH[a], Gift Mulima, MBBS, FCS(ecsa)[b], Anthony Charles, MD, MPH[a,b,*]

KEYWORDS

• Chest trauma • Thoracic injury • Global surgery

KEY POINTS

- The burden of thoracic trauma in low- and middle-income countries (LMIC) is high and is associated with significant morbidity and mortality.
- Efforts to increase access to basic airway supplies, tube thoracostomy, regional analgesia, and radiology services are needed to improve chest trauma care in LMICs.
- The healthcare workforce skilled in managing chest trauma is also severely limited in LMICs. Collaboration with established organizations and the creation of local training programs have been shown to help close this gap in care.
- Trauma registries can help define the local chest trauma burden, quality improvement, and priority setting.

Trauma is a leading cause of death and disability worldwide. Over 1.5 billion injuries occur each year, including 4.4 million injury-related deaths.[1] This global burden of traumatic injury disproportionately affects low- and middle-income countries (LMICs), where approximately 90% of all trauma-related mortality occurs.[2] In addition to high mortality, non-fatal injuries result in significant disability. In 2017, the age-standardized disability-adjusted life year (DALY) rates from injury were estimated at over 3000 per 100,000 persons in LMICs and over 4000 per 100,000 persons in parts of sub-Saharan Africa.[1] There is a preponderance of traumatic injury for a relatively younger population. The reduced functional outcomes associated with injury-related morbidity can have a profound societal and economic impact on developing countries. Many long-term sequelae would be preventable given access to essential trauma services and safe, affordable surgical and anesthesia care.[3,4]

CHEST TRAUMA IN LMICs

An estimated two-thirds of trauma patients sustain an injury to the thoracic cavity.[5] Chest injuries are associated with high morbidity and mortality, contributing to an estimated 25% to 50% of trauma-related mortality worldwide.[6] Mortality rates of patients with chest trauma vary depending on the mechanism, anatomic location and injured structure, presence or absence of pre-hospital care, and available resources. Still, some studies in LMIC have cited mortality as high as 60%.[7] Attributing mortality solely to chest trauma is problematic given that most patients will have multisystem trauma and the exact cause of prehospital death is unknown.

MECHANISM OF INJURY

The mechanism of injury in trauma is largely categorized as either blunt or penetrating. The most

[a] Department of Surgery, University of North Carolina-Chapel Hill; [b] Kamuzu Central Hospital, Lilongwe, Malawi

* Corresponding author. UNC School of Medicine, 4008 Burnett Womack Building, CB 7228.
E-mail address: anthchar@med.unc.edu

Thorac Surg Clin 32 (2022) 329–336
https://doi.org/10.1016/j.thorsurg.2022.04.008
1547-4127/22/

common cause of chest injury in civilian settings is blunt trauma following motor vehicular collisions (MVC). LMICs are particularly susceptible to MVCs due to ill-enforced traffic laws, unsafe road infrastructure, and limited resources for safety equipment.[8] Secondary causes of blunt chest trauma in LMICs are falls, occupational injuries, and assault.[9–11] While penetrating chest injuries are far more common in conflict zones, the use of firearms, knives, arrows and other weapons has become commonplace in urban areas with increased rates of crime and violence.[10,12,13]

ANATOMIC CONSIDERATIONS AND MANAGEMENT CHALLENGES

Chest wall injuries, particularly rib fractures, are among the most commonly injured structure and are associated with a high degree of injury severity and underlying pulmonary or abdominal injuries.[14,15] Flail chest, defined as three or more consecutive ribs fractured in 2 or more places, is the most severe form of chest wall injury as the resultant paradoxic chest wall movement, alteration of pulmonary mechanics, and underlying pulmonary contusion can yield significant pulmonary complications, long-term morbidity, and increased mortality.[16] The primary treatment strategy of chest wall injuries is managing pain and pulmonary dysfunction.[14,17] While management of chest wall injuries is predominantly non-surgical, patients in LMICs still face challenges due to limited access to mechanical ventilatory support and pain control, including locoregional analgesia such as epidural catheters and intercostal nerve blocks.

Pneumothorax, hemothorax, and hemopneumothorax are common complications of chest wall trauma, present in approximately 20% to 50% of patients in chest trauma series from LMICs.[10,11,18,19] Tube thoracostomy is indicated for clinically significant hemothorax due to the risk of fibrothorax and empyema with retained hemothorax[20] and for all large or symptomatic pneumothoraces.[14] Due to the rapidly fatal nature of tension pneumothoraces, patients in LMICs that lack robust pre-hospital care systems are at risk of high mortality without prompt recognition and treatment. Similarly, injuries to the great vessels are highly lethal, with aortic disruption identified in up to a quarter of blunt trauma patients in autopsy series from the U.S.[21] While blunt cardiac injuries, such as myocardial contusion, have better prognoses, other types of blunt cardiac injury like pericardial rupture and, rarely, coronary artery injuries can also lead to devastating injuries.[22]

Injuries caused by stab and puncture wounds depend on tissue disruption and trajectory identified on imaging. Ballistic trauma such as a gunshot wound is often more unpredictable and complex due to variation in energy transfer and tissue effect. As most penetrating injuries involve the chest wall and lung tissue, initial CXR completed with a radiopaque marking of entry and exit wounds helps gauge the injury trajectory. Injury to the chest that does not involve the mediastinum is typically treated with a chest tube and follow-up imaging.[23,24] An immediate output of more than 1000 mL blood or a continuous output of 200 mL/h or greater for 4 hours is an indication of a thoracotomy.

Penetrating cardiac injuries are often fatal, with only 10% to 20% of patients presenting to the hospital alive even in developed countries.[25,26] In addition to limitations of the pre-hospital care system, management of cardiac and great vessel injuries in LMICs is also limited by the surgical anesthesia, critical care, and blood bank resources at first-level and even many tertiary care hospitals in LMICs. Interventions ranging from pericardiocentesis to sternotomy and thoracotomy are often necessary, requiring equipment, infrastructure, and trained personnel to safely and effectively provide these services. Across sub-Saharan Africa, retrospective series from South Africa are the only available literature on operative management of these injuries, with mortality rates ranging from 8% to 35% for stab wounds to the heart to 80% following firearm injuries.[25,27]

Diaphragmatic injuries are under-recognized in both low- and high-income countries. There is limited data on traumatic diaphragm injuries in LMICs. However, an incidence of between 1.6% to 12.8% has been cited in hospital-based series from South Africa, India, and Nigeria.[13,28,29] Diaphragm injuries can result in early mortality secondary to the cardiopulmonary effects of intra-abdominal organ displacement of the lung and mediastinum. Diaphragmatic injuries more commonly present with the long-term morbidity related to late herniation, such as gastric or intestinal obstruction and ischemia.[30,31] These injuries can be difficult to diagnose during the initial trauma evaluation in LMICs as the sensitivity of chest radiography for identifying diaphragm injuries is low. In left-sided diaphragmatic injury, seeing the gastric bubble in the chest with or without the coiling of a nasogastric tube in the chest is pathognomonic.[32,33] Many occult injuries to the diaphragm are only identified at the time of laparotomy for other injuries. Those diagnosed radiographically at the presentation, particularly left-sided injuries, should be repaired immediately via laparotomy. Those detected remotely from the injury should be electively repaired via laparotomy or a thoracotomy.[28]

Traumatic esophageal injuries are similarly rare. Penetrating injuries to the esophagus commonly occur in the cervical esophagus from a weapon to the neck. Esophageal firearm injuries often have pre-hospital death from concomitant cardiovascular injuries. Due to deceleration injury, blunt trauma to the esophagus usually occurs at the thoracic outlet.[34] While esophageal perforation can be evaluated using plain radiographs, the standard for diagnosis is a contrast esophagram. Management has evolved over the years with increasing use of endoscopic stenting[35]; however, these advanced endoscopic techniques and supplies are limited in LMIC.

STRENGTHENING CHEST TRAUMA CARE IN LMICs

In response to significant disparities in trauma outcomes among LMICs, the World Health Organization (WHO) published a series of guidelines from 2004 to 2009 on essential trauma care, pre-hospital trauma systems, and trauma quality improvement programs.[4,36,37] Within these guidelines is a framework for suggested physical and human resources, designated by priority level (essential, desired, possibly required, or irrelevant). These resources are then further stratified by the priority level appropriate for each type of healthcare facility (community facilities, first-level hospitals staffed by general practitioners, specialty hospitals, and tertiary care centers). Priority levels may vary based on local needs assessment.

ESSENTIAL SKILLS, SUPPLIES, AND EQUIPMENT

The WHO includes basic airway and ventilatory techniques and low-risk, high-value procedures like needle decompression as essential components of trauma care that should be available at either community facilities or first-level hospitals (**Box 1**). Advanced airway supplies are desired but not necessary in the community or first-level hospital setting (**Box 2**).[4] For specialty and tertiary care hospitals, an algorithmic approach is helpful for the management of chest trauma. We have adapted an algorithm used in South Africa for a generalized approach to managing chest trauma across LMICs (**Fig. 1**).[38]

RADIOLOGIC SERVICES

Radiologic imaging is essential to ensure timely diagnosis and appropriate treatment of chest diseases. Diagnostic imaging services are critical components in safe and effective chest trauma care and as an adjunct following therapeutic procedures. However, approximately two-thirds of the global population whose imaging needs can be fulfilled by plain radiography and ultrasound lack access to adequate radiologic resources.[39]

Where available, a chest radiograph is an essential first step in the diagnostic evaluation of a trauma patient. CT may help identify the missed injuries on the initial chest X-ray (CXR). Despite CT's superior diagnostic capabilities in identifying pulmonary, pleural, and bony abnormalities, its routine use in the initial assessment of blunt thoracic injury has been controversial. Many LMICs in sub-Saharan Africa have less than one computed tomography scanner per million

Box 1
Essential skills, supplies, and equipment needed for chest trauma management at a basic facility or first-level hospital

Airway and breathing assessment

Basic maneuvers to relieve airway obstruction that is, manual, oral or nasal airway, suction device, bag-valve-mask

Supplemental oxygen

Needle or tube thoracostomy, underwater seal device

Adequate analgesia

Respiratory therapy

Intravenous fluids

Data from Mock C, Lormand J, Goosen J, et al. Guidelines for essential trauma care. Geneva: World Health Organization; 2004.

Box 2
Desired skills, supplies, and equipment for chest trauma management at a basic facility or first-level hospital

Endotracheal intubation

Cricothyroidotomy

Advanced airway equipment (laryngoscope, capnography)

Pulse oximetry

Autotransfusion from chest tubes

Data from Mock C, Lormand J, Goosen J, et al. Guidelines for essential trauma care. Geneva: World Health Organization; 2004.

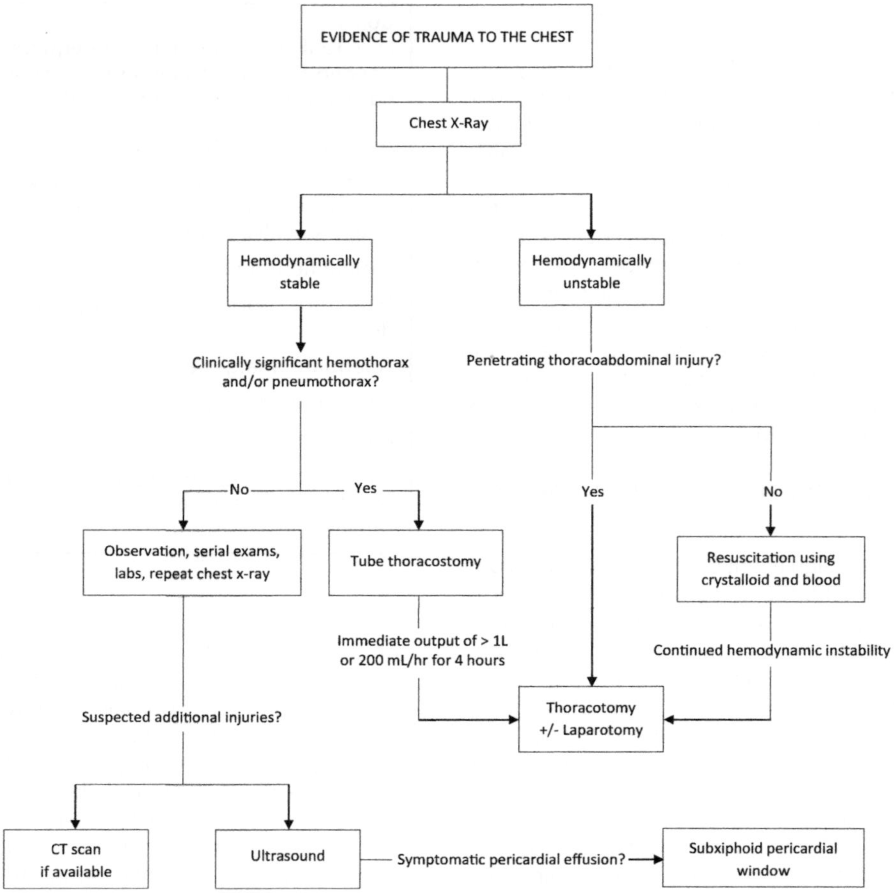

Fig. 1. Proposed algorithm for management of chest trauma in LMICs. (*Adapted from* Willett JK. Imaging in trauma in limited-resource settings: A literature review. Afr J Emerg Med. 2019;9(Suppl):S21-S27).

population.[40] In the absence of a CT scan in a stable patient, close observation with serial clinical examinations can help recognize chest injury severity, particularly traumatic parenchymal injuries. Operator-dependent, ultrasound is an effective, low-cost technique for evaluating thoracic trauma.[41] Because of its ease of use and feasibility, ultrasound has become an increasing focus of trauma care in LMICs, particularly among organizations such as RAD-AID. They seek to develop sustainable radiology capacity through education and training efforts.[39]

ANESTHESIA TECHNIQUES

Anesthesia is uniquely embedded into thoracic trauma care as adequate analgesia is essential to preventing pulmonary complications, and advanced airway techniques such as single lung ventilation are often desirable for surgical management. As access to basic anesthesia care is severely limited in low-resource settings, equipment such as bronchial blockers, double-lumen endotracheal tubes, and bronchoscopes are of even more limited capacity.[42,43] Although adequate analgesia is imperative to post-chest trauma care, only an estimated 6.7% of the global supply of medical opioids is available in LMICs.[44] Regional anesthesia techniques, such as epidurals and intercostal nerve blocks, can provide an opportunity to fill this gap; however, prioritization of the necessary supplies, such as local anesthesia and spinal needles, is needed.[45,46]

CRITICAL CARE NEEDS

The cardiopulmonary derangements associated with severe chest injuries require critical care monitoring. The appropriate infrastructure to care for these patients, including intensive care units

(ICUs) equipped with mechanical ventilators and hemodynamic monitoring systems and staffed with trained critical care providers and nurses, is necessary for chest trauma management. ICU capacity is low in many LMICs, often limited to referral centers within major cities with a median of only 8 available beds and 1/4 of reporting ICUs without access to a mechanical ventilator.[47] Additionally, effective critical care in the management of chest trauma requires access to a blood bank. Transfusion services are limited in LMICs due to lack of infrastructure for donation, limited public awareness of transfusion needs, and stigma surrounding disease transmission.[48] Many sub-Saharan African countries utilize a government-sponsored centralized blood bank system to overcome these challenges. While this strategy was developed by the WHO to improve access to blood bank services, in some LMICs it has unintentionally decreased the amount of safe, available blood products due to decreased ability for directed family donation and overreliance on healthy volunteers.[49]

HEALTH CARE WORKFORCE IN LMIC

The World Health Organization (WHO) defines a health workforce crisis as less than 22.8 skilled health professionals per 10,000 population, a threshold for which 83 countries fell below in 2016.[50] In certain LMICs, the density of medical doctors is estimated as low as 0.4 per 10,000 in Malawi (2018) and Niger (2016), and the density of nursing staff is as low as 0.7 per 10,000 population. Further, critical shortages exist in subspecialty surgeons.[51] Increasing the health care workforce capacity in LMICs is challenging due to socioeconomic factors, training access, and internal or external brain drain of skilled health care providers. Therefore, chest trauma is often managed by untrained or unsupervised health care providers resulting in variable outcomes, such as this malpositioned chest tube which is placed in too anterior of a location to provide adequate drainage of hemothorax (**Fig. 2**). Successful models for addressing these limitations include training community health workers and general practitioners to perform essential procedures, creating local surgical training programs, partnerships with institutions and non-governmental organizations (ie, "twinning" programs), and humanitarian efforts.[52] While several criticisms of surgical volunteerism have been well-established, transfer of knowledge and creation of training programs can be more effective long-term solutions to surgical workforce capacity building in LMICs. These strategies, however, require significant investment and buy-in from multiple stakeholders from the medical facility level to the ministry of health and local government.

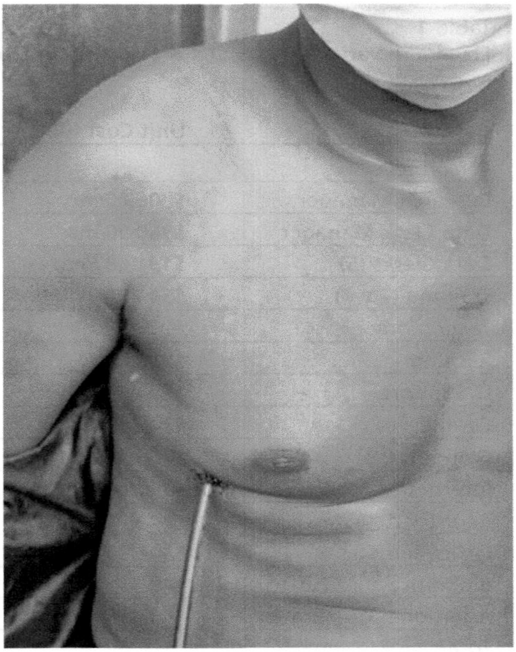

Fig. 2. Malpositioned intercostal chest drain. (*Courtesy of* Natasha Ngwira, MD, Lilongwe, MW).

BETTER RESEARCH TO INFORM HEALTH CARE PRIORITIES

Further data collection is needed to define the gaps in chest trauma care in each LMIC. Hospital-based trauma registries have become increasingly useful for gathering the epidemiologic and outcome data necessary to assess the local trauma burden and provide a means for public health priority setting. The trauma registry-based at Kamuzu Central Hospital (KCH) in Lilongwe, Malawi is one example of how this data collection can yield successful capacity-building efforts through academic partnerships. A robust trauma registry was developed to establish the local trauma burden through collaboration with the Malawi Surgical Initiative at the University of North Carolina in Chapel Hill. **Table 1** outlines the features including the personnel, materials, and data sources/elements of the KCH trauma registry, which has been in place since 2008. This trauma registry has since been utilized to develop quality improvement strategies, promote prioritization of trauma care at the Ministry of Health level, and has helped lead to the development of a surgical

Table 1
Fixed and variable costs of start-up and annual maintenance of the Trauma Surveillance Registry in Malawi

	Unit Cost (USD)	Start-up Cost (USD)	Annual Cost (USD)
Personnel			
Research Manager	$806.00/mo	$806.00	$9672.00
Data Clerk Manager	$350.90/mo	$350.90	$4210.80
Data Clerks (5)	$1317.87/mo	$658.94	$15,814.44
Training (2 wk)	$34.25/d	$342.50	-
Technology			
REDCap	$200	$200	-
IT Support	$50/edit	$50	$600
Facility	$14.25 sqft/y	-	$852.60
Computers	$300	$600	-
Internet	$390/device/year	-	$780
Registry Activities			
Office supplies	$107.90/mo	$107.90	$1294.80
Blood pressure cuff	$40	$80	-
Additional training	$34.25/d	-	$137.00
Total		$3196.24	$33,361,64

Modfied from Purcell LN, Nip E, Gallaher J, Varela C, et al. Design and Implementation of a Hospital-based Trauma Surveillance Registry in a Resource-Poor Setting: A Cost Analysis Study. Injury 2020;51(7):1548 to 1553.

residency program that has improved outcomes with the increasing workforce.[53,54]

SUMMARY

Chest trauma which disproportionately affects LMICs is associated with high morbidity and mortality. As many LMIC lack pre-hospital care systems and have limited access to basic anesthesia, and surgical care, management of chest trauma can prove challenging. As outlined by the WHO, increasing access to the services and supplies needed for basic airway maneuvers and low-risk procedures are essential to improving chest trauma outcomes in resource-limited settings. At the specialty and tertiary care hospital level, we have provided a proposed algorithm for a chest trauma management approach. Further data collection and capacity building in human and physical resources is needed to improve access to safe and effective chest trauma care.

DISCLOSURE

No conflicts of interest.

FUNDING

NIH Fogarty International Center Grant #D43TW009340.

REFERENCES

1. James SL, Castle CD, Dingels ZV, et al. Global injury morbidity and mortality from 1990 to 2017: results from the Global Burden of Disease Study 2017. Inj Prev 2020;26:i96–114.
2. Gosselin R. Injuries: the neglected burden in developing countries. Bull World Health Organ 2009; 87(4):246.
3. Meara JG, M Leather AJ, Hagander L, et al. The lancet commissions Global Surgery 2030: evidence and solutions for achieving health, welfare, and economic development the lancet commissions. Lancet 2015;386(9993):569–624.
4. Mock C, Lormand J, Goosen J, et al. Guidelines for essential trauma care. Geneva: World Health Organization; 2004.
5. Ludwig C, Koryllos A. Management of chest trauma. J Thorac Dis 2017;9(Suppl 3):S172–7.
6. Okonta KE, Ocheli EO. Blunt Chest Injury: epidemiological profile and determinant of mortality. Int Surg J 2018;5(5):1622–7.
7. Veysi VT, Nikolaou VS, Paliobeis C, et al. Prevalence of chest trauma, associated injuries and mortality: a level I trauma centre experience. Int Orthop 2009; 33(5):1425–33.
8. Global status report on road safety 2018. Geneva: World Health Organization; 2018.
9. Demirhan R, Onan B, Oz K, et al. Comprehensive analysis of 4205 patients with chest trauma: a 10-

year experience. Interact Cardiovasc Thorac Surg 2009;9(3):450–3.
10. Al-Koudmani I, Darwish B, Al-Kateb K, et al. Chest trauma experience over eleven-year period at al-mouassat university teaching hospital-Damascus: a retrospective review of 888 cases. J Cardiothorac Surg 2012;7:35.
11. Mefire AC, Jean JP, Fokou M, et al. Analysis of epidemiology, lesions, treatment and outcome of 354 consecutive cases of blunt and penetrating trauma to the chest in an african setting. S Afr J Surg 2010;48(3):90–3.
12. Thomas MO, Ogunleye EO. Penetrating chest trauma in Nigeria. Asian Cardiovasc Thorac Ann 2005;13(2):103–6.
13. Ali N, Gali BM. Pattern and management of chest injuries in maiduguri, nigeria. Ann Afr Med 2004;3(4): 181–4.
14. Majercik S, Pieracci FM. Chest wall trauma. Thorac Surg Clin 2017;27(2):113–21.
15. Dennis BM, Bellister SA, Guillamondegui OD. Thoracic Trauma. Surg Clin North Am 2017;97(5): 1047–64.
16. Dehghan N, de Mestral C, McKee MD, et al. Flail chest injuries. J Trauma Acute Care Surg 2014; 76(2):462–8.
17. Simon B, Ebert J, Bokhari F, et al. Management of pulmonary contusion and flail chest. J Trauma Acute Care Surg 2012;73(5):S351–61.
18. Lema MK, Chalya PL, Mabula JB, et al. Pattern and outcome of chest injuries at Bugando Medical Centre in Northwestern Tanzania. J Cardiothorac Surg 2011;6:7.
19. Atri M, Shlgh G, Ch M, et al. Chest trauma in Jammu region an institutional study. Indian J Thorac Cardiovasc Surg 2006;22:219–22.
20. Zeiler J, Idell S, Norwood S, et al. Hemothorax: a review of the literature. Clin Pulm Med 2020;27(1): 1–12.
21. Brinkman WT, Szeto WY, Bavaria JE. Overview of great vessel trauma. Thorac Surg Clin 2007;17(1): 95–108.
22. Embrey R. Cardiac trauma. Thorac Surg Clin 2007; 17(1):87–93, vii.
23. Restrepo CS, Gutierrez FR, Marmol-Velez JA, et al. Imaging patients with cardiac trauma. Radiographics 2012;32(3):633–49.
24. Shanmuganathan K, Matsumoto J. Imaging of penetrating chest trauma. Radiol Clin North Am 2005;44: 225–38.
25. Kong VY, Oosthuizen G, Sartorius B, et al. Penetrating cardiac injuries and the evolving management algorithm in the current era. J Surg Res 2015;193(2):926–32.
26. Nicol AJ, Navsaria PH, Hommes M, et al. Sternotomy or drainage for a hemopericardium after penetrating trauma. Ann Surg 2014;259(3):438–42.
27. Degiannis E, Loogna P, Doll D, et al. Penetrating cardiac injuries: recent experience in south africa. World J Surg 2006;30(7):1258–64.
28. D'Souza N, Clarke D, Laing G. Prevalence, management and outcome of traumatic diaphragm injuries managed by the Pietermaritzburg Metropolitan Trauma Service. Ann R Coll Surg Engl 2017;99(5): 394–401.
29. Narayanan R, Kumar S, Gupta A, et al. An analysis of presentation, pattern and outcome of chest trauma patients at an urban level 1 trauma center. Indian J Surg 2018;80(1):36–41.
30. Fair KA, Gordon NT, Barbosa RR, et al. Traumatic diaphragmatic injury in the American College of Surgeons National Trauma Data Bank: a new examination of a rare diagnosis. Am J Surg 2015;209:864–9.
31. Hanna C, Ferri LE. Acute traumatic diaphragmatic injury. Thorac Surg Clin 2009;19:485–9.
32. Hammer MM, Raptis DA, Mellnick VM, et al. Traumatic injuries of the diaphragm: overview of imaging findings and diagnosis. Abdom Radiol 2017;42(4): 1020–7.
33. Sangster G, Ventura VP, Carbo A, et al. Diaphragmatic rupture: a frequently missed injury in blunt thoracoabdominal trauma patients. Emerg Radiol 2007;13(5):225–30.
34. Bryant AS, Cerfolio RJ. Esophageal Trauma. Thorac Surg Clin 2007;17:63–72.
35. Kumar Kuppusamy M, Hubka M, Felisky CD, et al. Evolving Management Strategies in Esophageal Perforation: Surgeons Using Nonoperative Techniques to Improve Outcomes. J Am Coll Surg 2011;213:164–72.
36. Sasser S, Varghese M, Kellermann A, et al. Prehospital trauma care systems. Geneva: World Health Organization; 2005.
37. Mock C, Juillard C, Brundage S, et al. Guidelines for trauma quality improvement programmes. Geneva: World Health Organization; 2009.
38. Willett JK. Imaging in trauma in limited-resource settings: a literature review. Afr J Emerg Med 2019;9: S21–7.
39. Mollura DJ, Azene EM, Starikovsky A, et al. White paper report of the RAD-AID conference on international radiology for developing countries: identifying challenges, opportunities, and strategies for imaging services in the developing world. J Am Coll Radiol 2010;7(7):495–500.
40. World Health Organization. Total density per million population: Computed tomography units. Available at: https://www.who.int/data/gho/data/indicators/indicator-details/GHO/total-density-per-million-population-computed-tomography-units. Accessed November 15, 2020.
41. Chan KK, Joo DA, McRae AD, et al. Chest ultrasonography versus supine chest radiography for diagnosis of pneumothorax in trauma patients in the

emergency department. Cochrane Database Syst Rev 2020;7(7):CD013031.
42. Hadler RA, Chawla S, Stewart BT, et al. Anesthesia care capacity at health facilities in 22 low- and middle-income countries. World J Surg 2016;40(5): 1025–33.
43. Ramirez AG, Nuradin N, Byiringiro F, et al. General thoracic surgery in rwanda: an assessment of surgical volume and of workforce and material resource deficits. World J Surg 2019;43(1):36–43.
44. Goucke CR, Chaudakshetrin P. Pain: a neglected problem in the low-resource setting. Anesth Analg 2018;126(4):1283–6.
45. Schnittger T. Regional anaesthesia in developing countries. Anaesthesia 2007;62(Suppl 1):44–7.
46. Rukewe A, Fatiregun A. The use of regional anesthesia by anesthesiologists in Nigeria. Anesth Analg 2010;110(1):243–4.
47. Murthy S, Leligdowicz A, Adhikari NKJ. Intensive care unit capacity in low-income countries: a systematic review. PLoS One 2015;10(1):e0116949.
48. Kralievits KE, Raykar NP, Greenberg SLM, et al. The global blood supply: a literature review. Lancet 2015;385(S2):S28.
49. Gallaher JR, Mulima G, Kopp D, et al. Consequences of centralised blood bank policies in sub-Saharan Africa. Lancet Glob Heal 2017;5(2):e131–2.
50. Campbell J, Dussault G, Buchan J, et al. A universal truth: no health without a workforce. Forum report. Third global forum on human resources for health. Brazil: Recife; 2013.
51. World Health Organization. Global health workforce statistics. Geneva: World Health Organization; 2018.
52. Dearani JA, Jacobs JP, Bolman RM, et al. Humanitarian outreach in cardiothoracic surgery: from setup to sustainability. Ann Thorac Surg 2016;102: 1004–15.
53. Tyson AF, Varela C, Cairns BA, et al. Hospital mortality following trauma: an analysis of a hospital-based injury surveillance registry in sub-Saharan Africa. J Surg Educ 2015;72(4):e66–72.
54. Grudziak J, Gallaher J, Banza L, et al. The Effect of a Surgery Residency Program and Enhanced Educational Activities on Trauma Mortality in Sub-Saharan Africa. World J Surg 2017;41(12):3031–7.

Surgical Management of Mycobacterial Infections and Related Complex Pleural Space Problems

From History to Modern Day

Miyako Hiramatsu, MD, PhD*, Jun Atsumi, MD, PhD, Yuji Shiraishi, MD, PhD

KEYWORDS

• Tuberculosis • Surgery • Thoracoplasty • Destroyed lung • Chronic empyema

KEY POINTS

- Thoracic surgical procedures evolved for control of tuberculosis before the advent of effective drugs are still useful for management of complex refractory thoracic pathology owing to chronic infectious conditions in the present day.
- Patients with sequelae of tuberculosis (eg, hemoptysis, destroyed lung) are both surgically and medically challenging to manage.
- Thoracoplasty as a primary procedure or staged after open window thoracoplasty may be used in an adjuvant setting for refractory mycobacterial disease related complex pleural space trouble.

CURRENT STATUS OF SURGERY FOR TUBERCULOSIS

Since the latter half of the twentieth century, the incidence of tuberculosis (TB) has decreased worldwide,[1] which was more evident in high income countries owing to both improvement of socioeconomic conditions and the introduction of the first anti-TB drugs. Thus, the days when surgery once played the leading role in TB treatment are being forgotten. In the end of the twentieth century when multidrug-resistant TB and extended drug-resistant TB emerged as the predominant issues,[2,3] there was a resurgence of the need for lung resection as an adjuvant therapy for active pulmonary TB also in Japan.[4,5] Recently, in addition to better medical control of resistant strains through newly developed antimicrobial agents such as delamanid and bedaquiline, shifting immigration patterns during the global coronavirus disease 2019 pandemic have led to a further decreases in the incidence of TB in Japan (10.1 per 100,000 population in 2020). Most recently, the number of lung resections for TB in Japan performed was only 46 (including diagnostic resection) and the registered cases of TB empyema decreased to only 30 cases annually; therefore, surgery for active TB is literally disappearing in our country.[6,7]

However, lung resection (lobectomy, segmentectomy, or wedge resection) for active TB may still be needed in regions with moderate to high endemicity, low- to middle-income countries (eg, the Russian federation, South Africa, and China), and where multidrug-resistant strains are prevalent. In these regions, the indication for lung resection for TB may also be driven by local socioeconomic issues, because the completion of long-term and expensive medication regimens for multidrug-resistant TB with substantial side effects is very challenging and may far be a greater burden on the local health care system.[8,9]

Section of Chest Surgery, Fukujuji Hospital, Japan Anti Tuberculosis Association, 3-1-24, Matsuyama, Kiyose, Tokyo, 204-0052, Japan
* Corresponding author.
E-mail address: mykhrmt@a07.itscom.net

Thorac Surg Clin 32 (2022) 337–348
https://doi.org/10.1016/j.thorsurg.2022.04.009
1547-4127/22/© 2022 Published by Elsevier Inc.

Finally, the steady global increase of the incidence and number of deaths from nontuberculous mycobacterial lung disease, which is more indolent but more insistent lung disease than TB owing to a lack of definitive medical therapies, gave rise to another need of adjuvant resectional surgery for mycobacterial lung disease[10,11]

Therefore, this article focuses on a historical review of the role of surgery for TB, starting with the rationale for resectional surgery for mycobacterial lung disease and moving to the history of thoracic surgery itself, which is rooted in treatment for TB. Next, detailed descriptions of the techniques of "thoracoplasty," including "open window thoracostomy (OWT)," are provided. These historical techniques and concepts are not just the basis of present thoracic surgery, but also practically reliable in dealing with refractory infectious thoracic disease in the present day. Finally, the surgical management of recent sequelae of TB are described.

RATIONALE FOR RESECTIONAL SURGERY FOR MYCOBACTERIAL LUNG DISEASE

For mycobacterial lung disease, the rationale for resectional surgery is to decrease the amount of lung tissue with intractable pathology as a reservoir of infection and to decrease the bacterial load. As an adjuvant means, the role of surgery needs to be flexible according to the efficacy, costs, and merits of drug treatment. After adequate optimal chemotherapy for at least 2 to 3 months, surgery for localized cavitary lesions or destroyed lobes amenable to anatomic resection was considered for those patients who had persistently positive sputum. Further, even patients who achieve sputum conversion but are deemed at high risk of relapse based on drug resistance patterns, radiographic findings, or immune-compromising conditions owing to diabetes and others should be considered for elective partial lung resection. However, owing to lack of adequate data, further research is needed to clarify the type and the timing of surgery, postsurgical chemotherapy, and long-term survival.[8–11]

Lung resection for mycobacterial lung disease can achieve a favorable treatment outcome; however, this type of surgery is associated with a relatively high morbidity and should be performed at centers with substantial experience with surgery for the treatment of infectious lung diseases.

HISTORY OF THORACIC SURGERY WITH ROOTS IN SURGERY FOR TUBERCULOSIS

The history of surgery for pulmonary and pleural TB has long predated the introduction of antibiotics (streptomycin) in 1944.[12,13] The fundamental components of surgical procedures, at any place at any time, have always been to cut, to remove or drain the lesion, and to close. Although many of the archival surgical procedures currently performed outside of the chest had been introduced by the end of the nineteenth century,[14] it was not until 1935 that the first successful pulmonary lobectomy for TB treatment was performed by Samuel Freedlander.[15] The major principles in performance of this resectional procedure included (I) "stable respiratory management under adequate anesthesia," (II) a "profound understanding and control of postoperative intrathoracic negative pressure," (III) the "control or prevention of bleeding and air leak when cutting into lung tissue," and (IV) most of all, an "understanding and control of tubercle bacilli." Before that, Thoracoplasty had been the main strategy, which was developed and refined through the long fight against pulmonary and pleural TB.

Rationale of Collapse Therapy

Before discussing thoracoplasty, collapse therapy for pulmonary TB should be understood. The general concept of "rest" to allow the healing of damaged tissue was applied to the diseased lung by Carson in 1819.[16] At that time, TB was rampant, especially in industrializing Europe, and without any effective drugs. Based on autopsy series, pulmonary cavities were believed to play the leading role in the pathogenesis of TB.[17,18] According to Carson, consolidations or nodules generated within the lung by tubercular process contain fragile infiltrating necrotic tissues with less elasticity compared with the surrounding healthy lung. By continuous exposure to the repeated traction from labored respirations in infected patients, these lesions would occasionally result in internal lacerations and cavitations from the adjacent (leading) bronchus owing to mechanical dynamics, particularly in the apical and dorsal parts of the lung. Recent reports have proved this theory by taking a sequence of computed tomography scans in animal models.[19,20] Once the leading bronchus is created, this nodular–bronchial fistula becomes a gateway to the vicious cycle of refractory infection within the pathologic space owing to constant motion during respiration.

Stockes and colleagues described the positive effect of pleural effusion and pneumothorax on healing and arresting pulmonary TB in 1838.[21] After this, the concept of putting the lung at rest and immobilization of patients came to be regarded as not only the prevention of cavities, but also a treatment, by collapsing the lung and decreasing mechanical stress to the lesion.

To summarize, the rationale of collapse therapy are as below[22]:

- Cavitary closure by external compression
- To stop aerogenous spread of the disease by bending and closing of leading bronchus to the cavity
- To decrease the oxygen supply to the aerobic tuberculous bacilli within the cavity
- To induce lymphoedema to collapse of the cavity

After the introduction of artificial pneumothorax by Forlanini in 1882[23] (**Fig. 1**), this procedure became very popular all over the world and played the main role in the treatment of TB until the introduction of effective drugs.[24] Among the recipients of this procedure, there developed a growing need for an additional surgical approach to manage refractory open cavities after artificial pneumothorax, which was mainly due to apical adhesions, as well as a need to manage artificial pneumothorax–induced empyema and chronic tuberculous empyema.

THORACOPLASTY

Thoracoplasty is to remove a series of ribs (decostalization) overlying the pathologically altered lung parenchyma (refractory cavity) or the infectious pleural space (empyema). The aim of this procedure is to decrease or adjust the size of the chest wall to fit to the diseased lung inside to heal and to function well. Then, the thoracic wall that lost its skeletal support was expected to slump toward the mediastinum naturally by intrathoracic negative pressure, compressing and obliterating an infected pleural space or pulmonary cavity and promoting a definite internal self-healing process.

It should be noted that thoracoplasty in the nineteenth century was actually derived from 2 major streams, one as the second choice of treatment for a refractory tuberculous cavity that had not been collapsed and healed despite repeated artificial pneumothorax (extrapleural thoracoplasty) and the other for managing pyogenic or tuberculous empyema (intrapleural thoracoplasty).

Extrapleural Thoracoplasty (without opening of parietal pleura)

Based on its rationale, extrapleural thoracoplasty was developed as an additional treatment for refractory TB cavities after the creation of an artificial pneumothorax. Direct approaches to drainage or to remove the TB cavity were known to have failed so repeatedly that entering the pleural space for lung resection was considered to be taboo at that time. Therefore, only the ribs from the subperiosteal plane were removed in this procedure (**Fig. 2**). In 1885, de Cerenville removed only the second and the third ribs in the aim of arresting pulmonary TB, which is known to be the first extrapleural thoracoplasty,[12] followed by many others as described later in this article (**Table 1**). This process of refining versions of extrapleural thoracoplasty continued until effective drugs for TB were available worldwide. Tuffier, who is also known for the first successful removal of apical portion of a lung, had introduced a very selective procedure (extrapleural apicolysis and extrapleural plombage) in 1893.[25] Plombage is one of the forms of thoracoplasty and was used for patients too ill for invasive surgery. Plombage endeavors to compress the underlying lung by inserting a variety of materials in the extraperiosteal plane to seal the space. As an alternative for patients who were able to tolerate the procedure, to achieve a better sputum conversion rate, more and more ribs (II–IX) were removed subosteally by Friedlich, Sauerbruch, and others; however, mortality and morbidity were high with these nonselective procedures.[12,26] The procedure was ultimately regarded as too morbid and resulted in only lateral gross collapse and was inefficient in the apex with the apical cavity remaining open. Alexander made successful modifications by separating these processes into 3 staged procedures every 3 weeks to decrease morbidity. He also insisted on the importance of selectively removing I through III ribs from transverse process until costochondral junction to achieve good results, while leaving the anterior and lateral part of ribs to avoid deformity and a loss of pulmonary function.[27] The most selective approach was Jacobeu's thoracoscopic cauterization of the adhesive apex intrapleurally, which achieved closure of the cavity without removing ribs. However, intraoperative instability was severe owing to uncontrollable bleeding from subclavian vessels.[28] Finally, the highest collapse rate with the least invasive approach was achieved by Semb's thoracoplasty (ribs I–IV, V) with extrafascial apicolysis, which is the blunt separation of the ribs in the most external plane.[29] Through the long list of surgeons and procedures, 2 main trends have emerged:

- To improve the success rate of cavity collapse and eventually the sputum conversion rate, remove selected ribs cranially and posteriorly.
- To decrease mortality and morbidity, including later deformity and respiratory dysfunction,

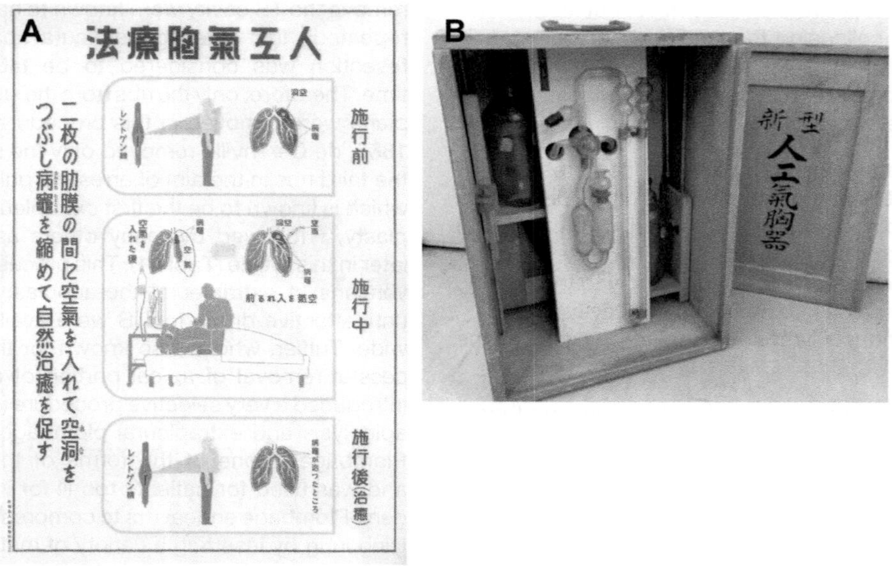

Fig. 1. (*A*) An advertising poster of artificial pneumothorax therapy. (*B*) An old device for artificial pneumothorax therapy used in the mid-twentieth century in Japan. ([*A*] *Courtesy of* Japan Anti-Tuberculosis Association, Tokyo, JP.)

separate the ribs at the external plane in step-by-step manner.

Intrapleural Thoracoplasty to Manage Empyema Space (with opening of parietal pleura)

Finnish surgeon Jacob August Estlander and German surgeon Max Schede are famous for their introduction of another type of thoracoplasty for chronic empyema.[30] This type of thoracoplasty became known as intrapleural thoracoplasty, which was aiming to open and enter the infectious intrapleural space (see **Fig. 2**). According to Schede's procedure, from the intrapleural space the musculoskeletal thoracic wall and thickened parietal pleura is widely taken off, which is notorious for its disfiguring big U-shaped incision. The mortality and blood loss (known as Schede's clot) used to be considerably high and morbidities such as paradoxic chest wall motion, paresis of the abdominal wall, and deformity were outstanding. Moreover, it took quite a long time for the musculocutaneous flaps that were left open to be healed and closed after.

Open Window Thoracostomy

To improve this treatment result and to decrease the burden of an already debilitated patient, this procedure was modified to allow efficient drainage of the empyema with minimal invasion.

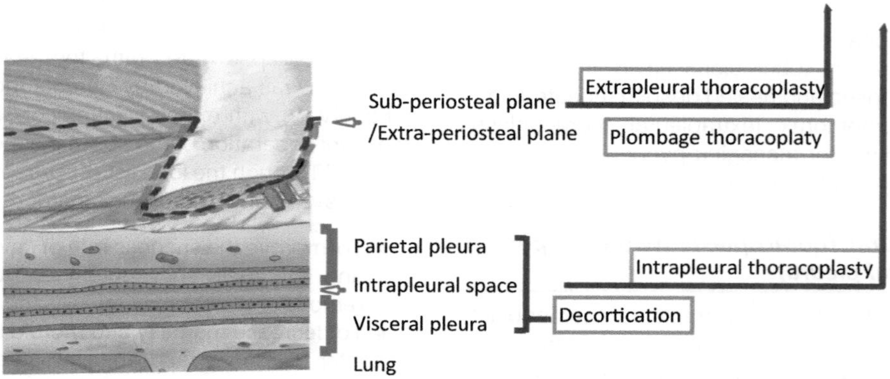

Fig. 2. The chest wall and thoracoplasty: layers to separate from the rib to be excised.

The procedure of OWT was established and handed down with many attempts and modifications.

Among them, 2 types of OWT named after 2 famous surgeons work are well-known.

- The Eloesser flap: This flap was originally designed to act as a tubeless 1-way valve to drain chronic pleural effusion.[31] It is small U-shaped skin flap that was folded inward and sutured to the upper edge of the opened parietal pleura, which was plastied as a one-half labial fistula promoting stable drainage with the remnant outer skin edge of the U-shaped flap being sewn together as a valve. This original design was later modified and introduced as a type of OWT.[32]
- The Clagett procedure: Clagett and Geraci described a 2-stage procedure for the treatment of postpneumonectomy empyema.[33] Their window was created by removing a rib (VII) originally aiming to promote active and thorough drainage of the pleural infection through gauze packing. Then, patients were asked to return to the hospital in approximately 6 to 8 weeks to close the window using antiseptic solutions. The skin flap was designed to cover the orifice of the window circumferentially and it should be adequately large to achieve sufficient temporal drainage.

Various skin incisions for an OWT including U-shape,[34] H-shaped,[35] and triradiate incisions[36] have been described so far. We prefer a single linear incision, which minimizes the ischemia of the wound edge and yet allows adequate drainage with its wide spindle shaped stoma (**Fig. 3**).[37]

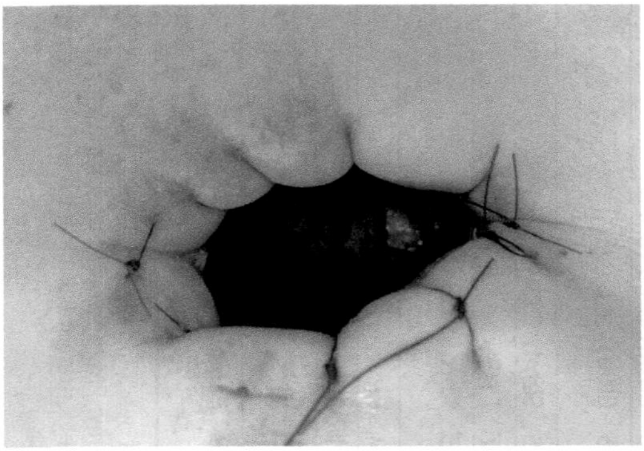

Fig. 3. Open window thoracostomy designed and plastied from a single linear incision.

Technique#1: OWT

- A single long skin incision of about 10 cm or more is laid along the costal bone just at the middle level of the empyema cavity (see **Fig. 3**).
- We prefer an anterolateral incision ventral to the edge of latissimus dorsi muscle to preserve an generous muscle flap for closure.
- A too dorsal or too caudal incision will sometimes be inconvenient because of the later elevation of hemidiaphragm. Also the window, which is out of the patient's reach, often tends to soil linens and clothes.
- After muscle dissection to the thoracic wall, a rib just under the incision is removed as 8 to 10 cm long, and the empyema cavity is entered and explored.
- From there, cranially and caudally 2 to 3 more bones are removed.
- Thickened parietal empyema wall will be resected leaving an outer wall edge of about 1.0 to 1.5 cm to affix and pull the skin inward firmly.
- A need for additional rib resection should be considered to adjust the length of the ribs so that its stump does not stick to or out from the subcutaneous tissue and skin.
- Skin edges, starting from the middle point of the incision, are folded inward and are adjusted to match the edge of parietal pleura with mattress sutures using #2 nylon.
- If necessary, we add additional stiches to both ends of the wound with mattress suture.

This technique can also be applied to refractory cavities with uncontrollable infection with medication, such as *Aspergillus fumigatus* and nontuberculous mycobacteria. If the cavity is located close to the chest wall and the relevant pleural layers are fused, a cavernostomy, a technique to open the cavity by removing the outer cavity wall together with chest wall and fused visceral/parietal pleura, can be a lifesaving drainage technique in selected cases.

Closure

To obliterate and close the space safely, countless attempts were followed by another list of surgeons. What should be emphasized here is the introduction and establishment of pedicled extrathoracic muscle flap transposition gave a great step forward in improving the result of window closure with little functional or cosmetic defect.[36] As time went by, the indication of thoracoplasty has changed from TB related and

Table 1
Evolution of indications for thoracoplasty

year	Surgeon	Indication: Pulmonary TB	Indication: Pyogenic Empyema	Indication: Postresectional Empyema	Opening of Parietal Pleura	Resected ribs[a]	Steps	Comment
1879	Estlander (Finland)[30]		✔		✔	Multiple	1	Subperiosteal rib resection
1885	de Cerenville E (Switzerland)[12]	✔				II III	1	
1890	Schede M (Germany)[30]		✔		✔	I–X	1	Thorax-resection, OWT
1893	Tuffier T (France)[25]	✔				NA	1	First successful removal of apical lung extrapleural apicolysis and plombage
1908	Friedrich PL (Germany)[26]	✔				II–X	1	Thoracoplastic pleuropneumolysis
1913	Sauerbruch F (Germany)[12]	✔				II–VII	1	Extrapleural paravertebral thoracoplasty
1913	Jacobeus HC (Sweden)[28]	✔			✔	0	1	Thoracoscopic intrapleural apicolysis
1916	Robinson S (USA)[38]		✔		✔	ND※	1	Muscle flap (LD), OWT
1935	Eloesser L (USA)[31]	✔			✔	VII?	1	One-way valve drainage skin flap
1935	Semb C (Sweden)[29]	✔				I–IV, V	1	Extrafascial apicolysis
1937	J Alexander (USA)[27]	✔				I–IX	3	Paravertebral thoracoplasty
1953	Kergin FG (Canada)[39]		✔	✔	✔	ND※	1	Muscle flap (IC), parietal pleural resection
1954	Bjork VO (Sweden)[40]	✔	✔	✔	✔	I–VII	1	Osteoplastic technique
1961	Andrews NC (USA)[41]		✔	✔	✔	ND※	1	Thoracomediastinal plication
1963	Clagett and Galaci (USA)[33]			✔	✔	VII	2	Primary closure of BPF, OWT antiseptic solution
1983	Pairolero PC (USA)[37]		✔	✔	✔	ND (II)	1–7	Muscle flap (LD, PM, SA, Pm, RA)

※, ribs overlying the empyema cavity; BPF, bronchopleural fistula; IC, intercostal muscle; LD, latissimus dorsi muscle; NA, not available; ND, not described; OWT, open window thoracostomy; PM, pectoralis major muscle; Pm, pectoralis minor muscle; RA, rectus abdominis muscle; SA, serratus anterior muscle.

[a] Greek numerals indicate the ribs resected. Mean number of resected ribs were 7.5 for pneumonectomy, 3.6 for lobectomy, 4.8 for others.

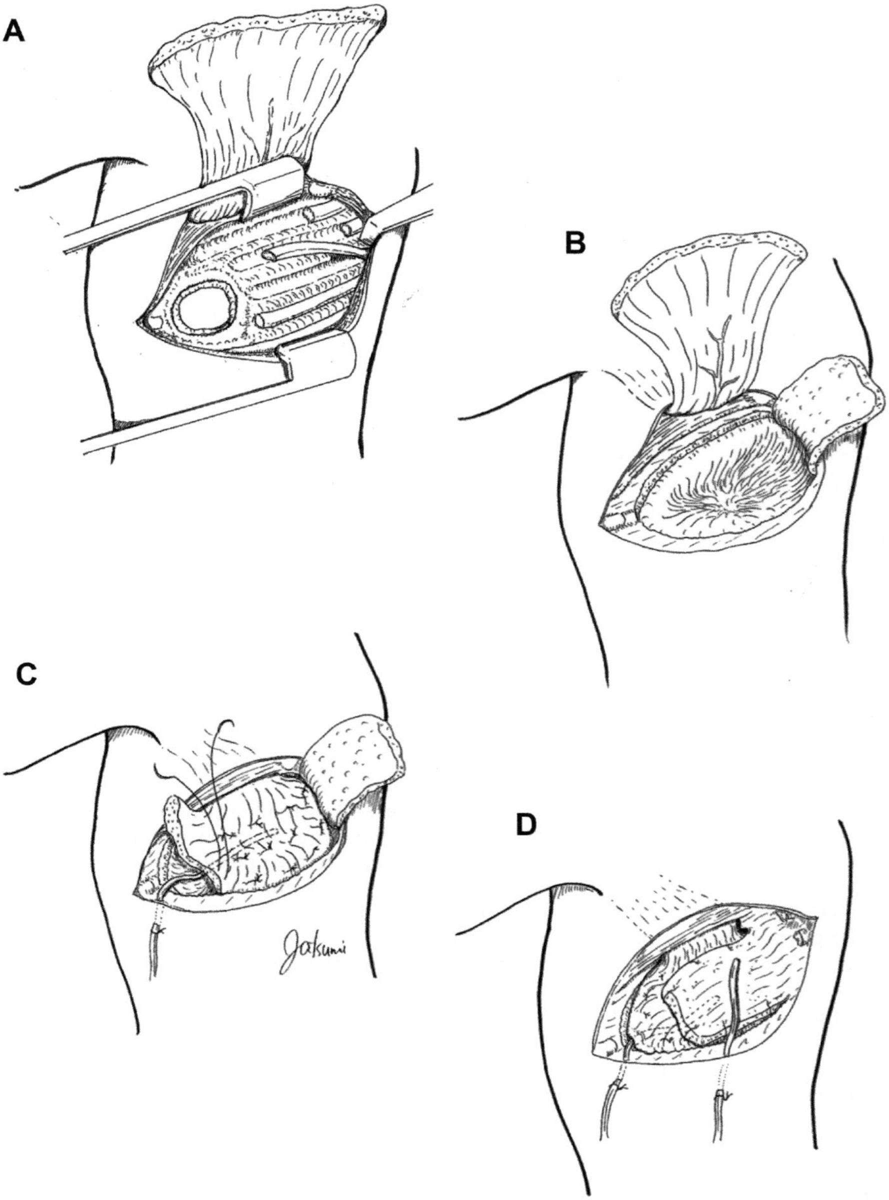

Fig. 4. The diagrams illustrate the reoperation to close a chronic empyema cavity with a latissimus flap. (*Courtesy of* Jun Atsumi, MD, PhD, Tokyo, JP.)

pyogenic empyema to postresection empyema (**Table 1**).

The 2 main questions to address were:

- How to handle the grossly thickened infected pleura, and
- The use of integral autologous tissue (muscle flap or omental flap) to close bronchopleural fistula and to fill the space.

A detailed description of techniques is as follows.

Technique#2: Closing an OWT with Muscle Flap

Closure of the OWT is planned after adequate wound drainage and sufficient improvement of the patient's general condition (**Fig. 4**). By this time, the size of the cavity has decreased considerably.

- Make sure there is no malignant disease (including pyothorax associated malignant lymphoma, pleural angiosarcoma) in the empyema cavity.

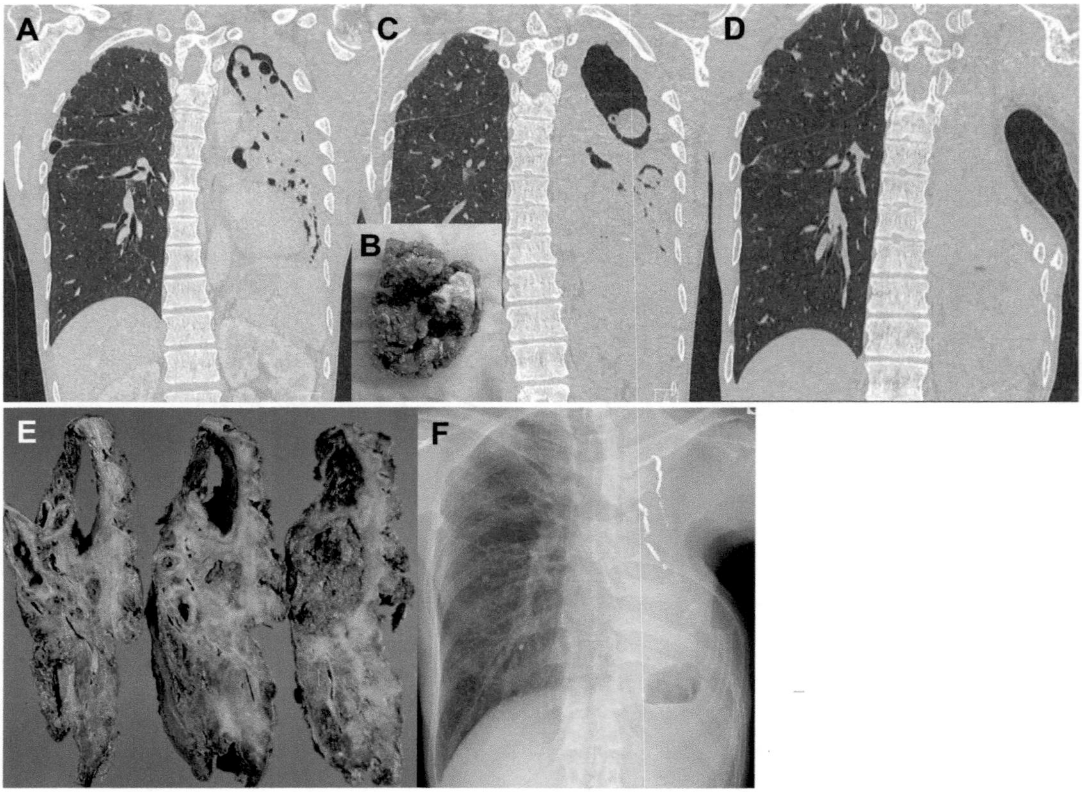

Fig. 5. (*A*) A 40-year-old man, who had a history of pulmonary TB, was admitted with recurrent hemoptysis and daily high fever. His left lung was totally destroyed, containing large cavities with fungus balls each inside. (*B*) (inset) As a primary drainage, the fungus ball of the largest cavity in the apex was removed under general anesthesia. (*C*) A balloon catheter was in situ to drain the cavity. The more inferior cavity was still filled with a fungus ball. Bronchial arterial embolization and antimicrobial/antifungal agents were administered to stabilize his condition. Intensive physical therapy, nutritional supply, dental and parasinus cleaning were thoroughly done during his hospitalization. (*D*) After rehabilitation at home, he was admitted to hospital again for surgery. Extrapleural pneumonectomy was conducted together with posterior II to VI rib resections in advance. About one-third of the inferior left scapula was cut to prevent its dislocation. Pedicled latissimus dorsi muscle flap was harvested to cover the stump of left main bronchus and mediastinum. (*E*) Excised specimen. The parietal and visceral pleura were prominently thickened and fused, especially around the cavities with fungus balls inside. The specimen shows that the extrapleural dissection was conducted at the extraperiostal plane with electrocautery, resulting in cauterized intercostal muscle bundles attached to the resected pleura. This practice helped to decrease blood loss and improve visualization during surgery. (*F*) The patient returned to regular activities with a capacity for light work. Note that the ipsilateral lung and mediastinum are free from malretraction to the left side owing to the effect of a thoracoplasty.

- A posterolateral incision is made, which excises the pleurocutaneous fistula.
- Harvest the pedicled latissimus dorsi muscle flap (preserving the proximal vascular blood supply) (see **Fig. 4**A).
- Resect all the ribs overlying the space (extrapleural approach) (see **Fig. 4**A).
- An incision is made in the parietal pleura to turn it open and fully expose the empyema cavity (Intrapleural approach).
- The empyema wall should be curetted until only clean fibrous tissue remains (see **Fig. 4**B).
- The empyema cavity is thoroughly irrigated with sterile water and povidone-iodine.
- Spread the muscle flap to cover the visceral pleura and add mattress sutures persistently to anchor and obliterate the space (see **Fig. 4**C).
- A bronchopleural fistula, if present, is closed by direct suturing or by using muscle flap, which is sutured into the bronchopleural fistula with reasonable interrupted stiches.
- Close the parietal layer together with any remaining intercostal muscle bundles over the muscle flap and add anchoring interrupted sutures as well (see **Fig. 4**C).

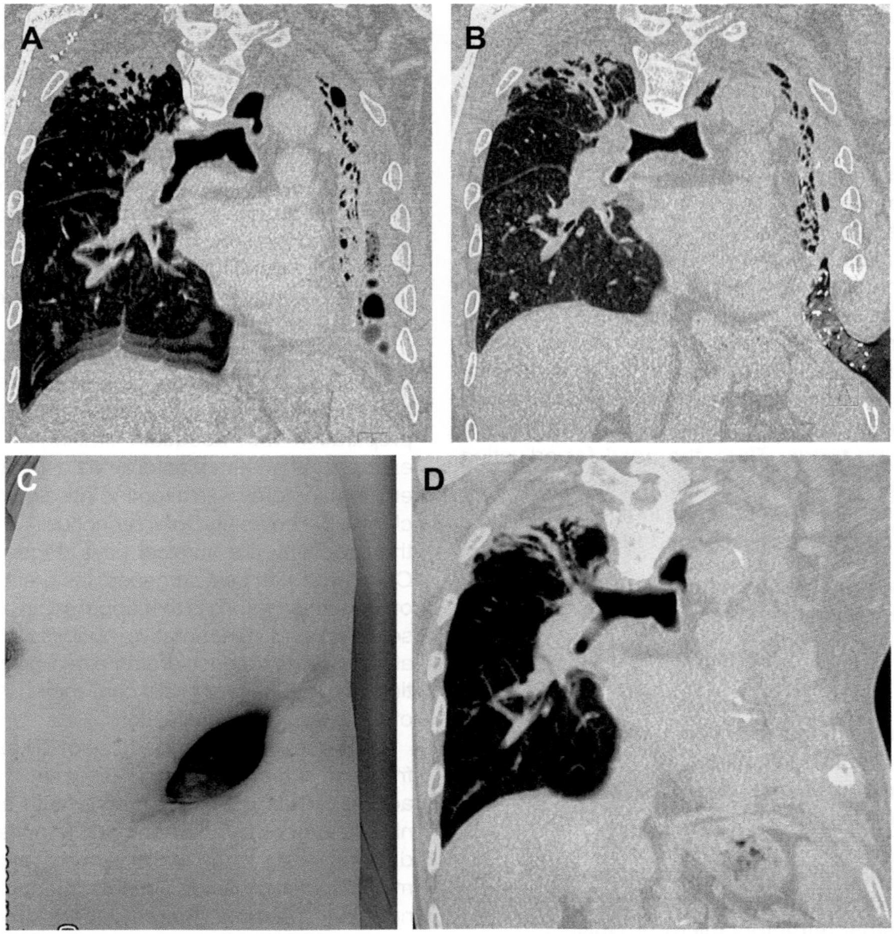

Fig. 6. (*A*) A 65-year-old man who had a history of pulmonary TB, was admitted with cough, massive airway secretions, weight loss and fever. Underlying destroyed lung causing empyema with bronchopleural fistula was apparent. He was prescribed amoxicillin/clavulanate (CVA/AMPC) for 2 years with reference to drug sensitivity. (*B*) He came back to hospital owing to an uncontrollable infection. By resecting the seventh through the ninth ribs, an OWT was created. (*C*) A small window was created anterior to the latissimus dorsi muscle. He needed to visit the clinic every morning to change the dressings for 2 years. This practice was continued until his weight returned to normal. (*D*) Extrapleural pneumonectomy was conducted together with posterior second through ninth rib resections and in advance with excision of the pleurocutaneous fistula. A pedicled latissimus dorsi muscle flap was made to cover the main bronchial stump and mediastinum, including the defect of pericardium, and to obliterate the space. Note that his mediastinum and trachea are also in the middle, proving that the size of his chest wall fits well to his residual lung.

- At least 2 tubes are laid beneath the muscle flap and subcutaneous tissue, which are connected to closed suction drainage reservoirs (see **Fig. 4**D).
- The chest incision is closed by approximation of the muscles and subcutaneous tissues in layers with interrupted sutures.

It is essential to select sensitive antimicrobial agents by referring to culture results before surgery and administer them during the perioperative period. The culture results from intraoperative lavage fluid and drainage fluid are also important information in determining the timing of tube removal and selecting postoperative antimicrobial agents.

Decortication

Apart from thoracoplasty, another historical procedure—decortication—was also developed for cases whose underlying lung (trapped lung) was healthy and reexpandable.[42] By removing the empyema cavity with both pleural and visceral pleura (see **Fig. 2**), the released lung is expected to fill the infectious space.

THORACOPLASTY FROM NOW ON

Now a days, thoracic surgical techniques are increasingly used for the treatment of malignancy. Improved general anesthesia, effective targeted antimicrobial agents, sophisticated techniques, modern stapling devices, and uniformly guided perioperative management ensures the safety of lung resection. In addition to pervasive general public health and vaccination reducing the chance of bronchiectasis and deformity to the underlying lung, most lung lesions are recognized in earlier stages and can be removed with minimal loss of lung parenchyma. These are favorable factors for safe lung resection because the residual space is not a major issues if there remains sufficient healthy lung tissue. Thus, the need for adjusting the size of hemithorax has become less important.

As described previously, the indication of thoracoplasty has gradually changed from:

- Chronic pyogenic and tuberculous empyema
- Tuberculous pulmonary cavity

to

- Chronic pyogenic empyema
- Postresectional empyema with or without a bronchopleural fistula
- Destroyed lung (extensive bronchiectasis, fibrocicatoricias lung, mostly as a sequela of TB)
- A cavity with uncontrollable infection with nontuberculous mycobacterial, *Aspergillus*, and other refractory micro-organisms

Although the incidence of severe pulmonary infections resulting in destroyed lung are dramatically decreased, the need to manage these issues will never be completely obsolete. In the modern day, surgery for benign thoracic diseases (such as sequala of TB as described as follows in this article, aspergilloma) is known to be fraught with danger, with quite high morbidity and mortality because patients with these issues are often severely debilitated from the underlying conditions, which resulted in their infectious problems.[43,44] Looking to the future, we will be interested to know if severe coronavirus disease 2019, which occasionally results in empyema, bronchiectasis, and distortions of the lung parenchyma, may increase the need for these procedures.

SEQUELAE OF TUBERCULOSIS

Pulmonary TB may still lead to severe thoracic sequelae, including a so-called destroyed lung. The architectural distortion reaches its maximal degree with severe fibrocicatricis. Broncholith or bronchostenosis as a result of endobronchial TB, hemoptysis, chronic empyema, pulmonary hypertension, and refractory pneumothorax are other sequalae of TB. These issues are known to affect the left side more commonly. When host immunity is weakened, the lesion becomes a reservoir for intractable pathogens like fungus (aspergillus) and nontuberculous mycobacteria, and others. Owing to repeated respiratory symptoms, such as bronchopneumonia and hemoptysis, affected patients are usually debilitated and exhausted when they visit the hospital, making the management of these sequelae difficult.

Unfortunately, to manage such advanced situations surgically, pneumonectomy is often unavoidable. We prefer to consider preoperative preparation with adequate drainage at first, then extrapleural pneumonectomy via a wide posterolateral thoracotomy with a routine latissimus dorsi muscle flap covering of bronchus and tailored thoracoplasty are surgical keys (**Figs. 5** and **6**).[45] Compared with past surgeons, the greatest strength of modern surgeons is that appropriate antimicrobial selection and perioperative optimization are available; achieving bronchial stump healing and obliteration of spaces are critically challenging in the setting of preexisting active infection.

Destroyed lungs as sequelae of TB and other refractory infectious lung diseases should be addressed as described above with all the techniques, modern equipment, and knowledge. Coordinating all the skills and expertise of multidisciplinary fields such as infectious disease, nutrition, physical therapy, and other medical fields are indispensable requirements for success.

SUMMARY

It should be remembered that a thoracoplasty is a gift from the courage and passion of so many surgical predecessors who aimed to cure the patients presenting to them. They persevered with no access to modern equipment nor drug therapies and at the expense of their own risk of TB infection. Precise understanding and application of these techniques for care of our own patients and to pass them on to our successors is an important task with which we have been charged.

CLINICS CARE POINTS

- The initial surgical approach should ensure maximal drainage with the least invasive procedures possible.

- Divide the procedure into multiple steps after evaluating the patient's functional and nutritional status.
- Decortication can be attempted for cases with healthy underlying lung; on the other hand extrapleural pneumonectomy may be needed for empyema cases with fibrotic or destroyed underlying lung.
- Consider a pedicled muscle or omental flap for closing a bronchopleural fistula and obliterating the space.
- Selective thoracoplasty can be applied entailing resection of the posterior portion of the apical ribs from the costovertebral joint (leaving the 1st rib and anterolateral portions to avoid deformity) and the inferior one-third of the scapula to avoid impingement.
- Good clinical outcomes require coordination of multidisciplinary expertise.

DISCLOSURE

The authors have nothing to disclose.

REFERENCES

1. Hermans S, Horsburgh CR Jr, Wood R. A century of tuberculosis epidemiology in the northern and southern hemisphere: the differential impact of control interventions. PLoS One 2015;19: e0135179.
2. Galai N, Graham N, Chaisson R, et al. Multidrug-resistant tuberculosis. N Engl J Med 1992;327(16): 1172–3.
3. Dye C, Espinal MA, Watt CJ, et al. Worldwide incidence of multidrug-resistant tuberculosis. J Infect Dis 2002;185:1197–202.
4. Shiraishi Y, Nakajima Y, Katsuragi N, et al. Resectional surgery combined with chemotherapy remains the treatment of choice for multidrug-resistant tuberculosis. J Thorac Cardiovasc Surg 2004;128:523–8.
5. Statistics of TB in Japan 1999. Tokyo: Japan Anti-Tuberculosis Association.
6. Committee for Scientific Affairs, The Japanese Association for Thoracic Surgery. Thoracic and cardiovascular surgery in Japan during 2017: annual report by The Japanese Association for Thoracic Surgery. Gen Thorac Cardiovasc Surg 2020;68: 414–49.
7. Statistics of TB in Japan 2020. Tokyo: Japan Anti-Tuberculosis Association.
8. WHO consolidated guidelines on tuberculosis. Module 4: treatment - drug-resistant tuberculosis treatment. Geneva (Switzerland): World Health Organization; 2020. p. 60–1. License: CC BY-NC-SA 3.0 IGO.
9. Fox GJ, Mitnick CD, Benedetti A, et al. Surgery as an adjunctive treatment for multidrug-resistant tuberculosis: an individual patient data metaanalysis. Clin Infect Dis 2016;62:887–95.
10. Ratnatunga CN, Lutzky VP, Kupz A, et al. The rise of non-tuberculosis mycobacterial lung disease. Front Immunol 2020;11:303.
11. Daley CL, Iaccarino JM, Lange C, et al. Treatment of nontuberculous mycobacterial pulmonary disease: an official ATS/ERS/ESCMID/IDSA clinical practice guideline. Eur Respir J 2020;56:2000535.
12. Rosenblatt MB. Pulmonary tuberculosis: evolution of modern therapy. Bull N Y Acad Med 1973;49:163–96.
13. Walcott S, Sukumar M. The history of pulmonary lobectomy: two phases of innovation CTS net 2016. Available at: https://www.ctsnet.org/print/article/history-pulmonary-lobectomy-two-phases-innovation. Accessed June 30, 2022.
14. Raven WR. Principles of surgical oncology. 1st edition. New York: Plenum Book Company; 1977. p. 8.
15. Freedlander SO. Lobectomy in pulmonary tuberculosis. J Thorac Surg 1935;12:132–42.
16. Carson J. On the elasticity of the lungs. Phiols Trans Roy Soc Lond 1820;1:29–45.
17. Dubos R, Dubos J. The white plague: tuberculosis, man, and society. 2nd edition. New Brunswick (NJ): Rutgers University Press; 1987. originally published 1952.
18. Virchow R. Cellular pathology as based upon physiological and pathological histology. London: John Churchill; 1860. p. 511.
19. Ihms EA, Urbanowski ME, Bishai WR. Diverse cavity types and evidence that mechanical action on the necrotic granuloma drives tuberculous cavitation. Am J Pathol 2018;188:1666–75.
20. Chen RY, Yu Xy, Smith B, et al. Radiological and functional evidence of the bronchial spread of tuberculosis: an observational analysis. Lancet Microbe 2021;2:e510–26.
21. Davidson L, Fuhrman M, Rella J. Precursors of Forlanini and Murphy. Am Rev Tuberc 1939;40:292–305.
22. Arai T. Surgery. Kekkaku 2011;86:627–31.
23. Kurause AK. First attempts at artificial pneumothorax in pulmonary phthisis. By Carlo Forlaninni. Tubercle 1934;16:121–5.
24. Sakula A. Carlo Forlanini, inventor of artificial pneumothorax for treatment of pulmonary tuberculosis. Thorax 1983;38:326–32.
25. Tuffier T. De la résection du sommet du poumon. Sem Med Paris 1891;2:202.
26. Friedlich PL. The operative treatment of unilateral lung tuberculosis by total mobilization of the chest wall by means of thoracoplastic pleuropneumolisis. Surg Gynecol Obstet 1908;7:632–8.
27. Alexander J. Some advances in the technique of thoracoplasty. Ann Surg 1936;104:545–51.
28. Jacobaeus HC. The cauterization of adhesions in artificial pneumothorax. Treatment of pulmonary

tuberculosis under thoracoscopic control. At a Joint Meeting of the Section of electro-therapeutics with the Roentgen Society at Manchester, Nov 17. Available at: https://journals.sagepub.com/doi/pdf/10.1177/003591572301600506.
29. Semb C. Thoracoplasty with extrafascial apicolysis. Br Med J 1937;2:650–66.
30. Paget S. The surgery of the chest. Bristol: John Wright &Co. London: Simpkin, Marshall, Hamilton, Kent & Co., Ltd; 1896. p. 270–85.
31. Eloesser L. An operation for tuberculous empyema. Surg Gynecol Obstet 1935;60:1096–7.
32. Symbas PN, Nugent JT, Abbott OA, et al. Nontuberculous pleural empyema in adults. The role of a modified Eloesser procedure in its management. Ann Thorac Surg 1971;12:69–78.
33. Clagett OT, Graci JE. A procedure for the management of postpneumonectomy empyema. J Thorac Cardiovasc Surg 1963;45:141–5.
34. Samson PC. Empyema thoracis. Essentials of present-day management. Ann Thorac Surg 1971; 11:210–21.
35. Hurvitz RJ, Tucker BL. The Eloesser flap: past and present. J Thorac Cardiovasc Surg 1986;92:958–61.
36. Galvin IF, Gibbons JR, Maghout MH. Bronchopleural fistula. A novel type of window thoracostomy. J Thorac Cardiovasc Surg 1988;96:433–5.
37. Pairolero PC, Arnold PG, Piehler JM. Intrathoracic transposition of extrathoracic skeletal muscle. J Thorac Cardiovasc Surg 1983;86:809–17.
38. Robinson S. The treatment of chronic non-tuberculous empyema. Surg Gynecol Obstet 1916; 22:557–93.
39. Kergin FG. An operation for chronic pleural empyema. J Thorac Surg 1953;25:430, 1953;26:430-4.
40. Bjork VO. A new osteoplastic technique. J Thorac Surg 1954;28:194–211.
41. Andrew NC. A surgical technique for chronic empyema. J Thorac Surg 1961;41:809–16.
42. Fowler GR. A case of thoracoplasty for the removal of a large cicatricial fibrous growth from the interior of the chest, the result of an old empyema. Med Rec (1866-1922) 1893;44:838.
43. Reed CE. Pneumonectomy for chronic infection: fraught with danger? Ann Thorac Surg 1995;59: 408–11.
44. Massard G, Dabbagh A, Wihlm JM, et al. Pneumonectomy for chronic infection is a high-risk procedure. Ann Thorac Surg 1996;62:1033–8.
45. Shiraishi Y, Nakajima Y, Koyama A, et al. Morbidity and mortality after 94 extrapleural pneumonectomies for empyema. Ann Thorac Surg 2000;70: 1202–6.

Management of Pulmonary Hydatidosis and Lung Abscess in Low-Resource Settings

Alfredo Sotomayor, MD[a,*], Silvia Portilla, MD[b], Gita N. Mody, MD, MPH[c]

KEYWORDS

- Pulmonary hydatid cyst • Pulmonary hydatidosis • Echinococcosis • Pulmonary abscess
- Cystectomy • Zoonosis • Benign lung conditions

KEY POINTS

- Antimicrobial therapies have reduced the need for surgery for lung cysts and abscesses.
- Surgery is the treatment of choice in pulmonary hydatidosis and large lung abscesses (>5 cm) in low-resource settings because it is curative and has low morbidity and mortality.
- The clinical presentation and high level of suspicion in endemic areas are fundamental for the diagnosis in pulmonary hydatidosis and lung abscesses.
- Cystectomy is the most commonly used surgery for pulmonary hydatidosis, and the smallest volume of lung parenchyma should be resected when more resection is needed. Similarly, the smallest resection of the liquefactive and consolidative components of a lung abscess should be done.
- Public health prevention measures focused on reducing transmission and controlling risk factors are essential to reduce the incidence of benign lung conditions owing to infectious diseases.

SURGICAL MANAGEMENT OF PULMONARY HYDATIDOSIS *PATHOGENESIS*

Causative Organism

Pulmonary hydatidosis is a zoonosis of global public health importance, caused by the cestode *Echinococcus*.[1–3] Humans may become infested through oral contact and develop one or more hydatid cysts in the lung or liver.[1] There are 3 other species causing alveolar echinococcosis: (*Echinococcus multilocularis*), polycystic echinococcosis (*Echinococcus vogueli*), and unicystic echinococcosis (*Echinococcus oligarthrus*).[4,5]

This article focuses on *Echinococcus granulosus*, given its worldwide distribution. *E. granulosus* includes a complex of 10 strains (G1 to G10), of which G1 affects humans most often.[4,6] The tapeworm *Echinococcus* (adult form) lives in the small intestine of the dog (definitive host) and measures 3 to 7 mm in length and can contain 100 to 1500 eggs, 30 to 40 μm in diameter.[7,8]

Biologic Cycle

The eggs are expelled from the intestine with the dog's feces, adheres to their hair, and then infests the soil, grass, and water. If the intermediate hosts (sheep, cattle, pigs, horses, rabbits, rats, and so forth) or the casual host (human) ingests the eggs, they acquire the disease (**Fig. 1**).[1,4,6,8,9] Human beings unknowingly contribute to the cycle when they slaughter livestock for consumption without sanitary control, and also if they feed canines with infested viscera.[10]

Humans can develop disease when they ingest food contaminated with the parasite's eggs with

[a] Department of Thoracic and Cardiovascular Surgery, Hipólito Unanue National Hospital, Lima, Peru; [b] Department of Anesthesia, María Auxiliadora Hospital, Lima, Peru; [c] Division of Cardiothoracic Surgery, Department of Surgery, University of North Carolina Burnett-Womack Building, Suite 3041, Campus Box 7065, Chapel Hill, NC 27599, USA
* Corresponding author. Jr. La Floresta 319, Dpto. 505, Urbanización Camacho, Santiago de Surco, Lima, Peru.
E-mail address: alfredosotomayor19@gmail.com

Thorac Surg Clin 32 (2022) 349–360
https://doi.org/10.1016/j.thorsurg.2022.04.002

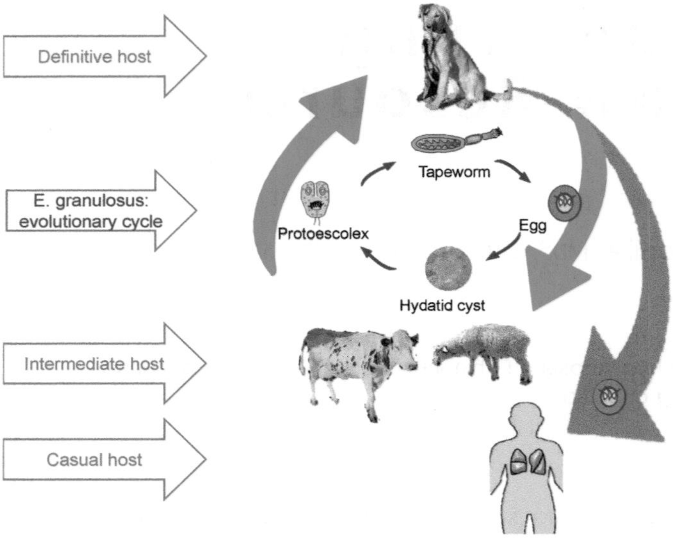

Fig. 1. Biological cycle: the adult tapeworm lives in the definitive host (the dog's intestine) and emits dozens of eggs that are excreted in the dog's feces. The egg is ingested by intermediate hosts (cattle, sheep, and pigs) and by the casual host (human), and they acquire hydatid disease. The cyst (metacestode) develops in the liver or lungs. When cattle, sheep, or pigs are slaughtered for human consumption, if the infested viscera (with cysts containing protoscolices) are ingested by a dog, then the biological cycle is closed, and the adult tapeworm will develop in its intestine.

improper hand hygiene. Once ingested, gastric and intestinal juices destroy the layers of the egg and release the exacanthus embryo into the duodenal lumen. It then enters the portal system and implants in the liver, lungs, or both.[4,8,11] In the lungs, these cysts develop in the lower lobes, predominantly on the right. They can develop in other organs if they pass through arteriovenous shunts.

Cyst Structure

Hydatid cysts measure from a few millimeters to 30 cm, and as they grow, they collapse the lung parenchyma. The cyst membranes are composed of the adventitial, cuticular, and germinative layers, as shown in **Fig. 2**[4,11,12,13]:

1. The adventitial membrane, formed by the host, is made up of fibroblasts, fibrous tissue, and cells as an immune response to prevent the spread of the parasite.
2. The cuticular membrane is acellular, laminar, and chitinous, measures 200 μm to 1 cm thick, protects the parasite, reduces the immune stimulus, allows the passage of nutrients from the host, rarely calcifies in the lung, and takes the spherical or ovoid shape.
3. The germinative membrane is unicellular and very thin, contains glycogen, produces scolices and hydatid fluid, and proliferous vesicles (rare in the lung). The hydatid liquid is clear and transparent, "rock crystal," is composed of water, sodium chloride, glucose, urea, and proteins with antigenic capacity, and has a pressure of 60 to 80 cm H_2O.

Epidemiology

E. granulosus is mainly distributed in countries with agricultural and livestock areas and temperate climates; it produces high morbidity and high health care costs despite being a preventable disease.[1,4,14] The incidence is high in South America, the Mediterranean coast, the Middle East, south and central Russia, central Asia, India, Nepal, China, Australia, Africa, and the United States.[1,4,6,15] The incidence reaches 50/100,000 people per year in endemic regions,[1] and the prevalence is between 5% and 10%, mainly in rural areas of Argentina, Peru, East Africa, central Asia, and China. In South America, the highest prevalence occurs in Argentina, Chile, Peru, Uruguay, Brazil (Rio Grande do Sul province), and to a lesser extent, Bolivia, Colombia, and Paraguay.[1,15,16,17] Peru has the highest incidence and prevalence in the Americas.[15,16,17] The risk factors for acquisition are as follows[13,18]:

- Poor hand washing before eating food
- Feeding dogs with livestock viscera infested with cysts
- Ineffective national echinococcosis control programs

Seventy percent of the people who fall ill are young adults of active working age. The World Health Organization reports that echinococcosis causes 19,300 deaths each year and the loss of 871,000 disability-adjusted life-years. Annual treatment costs and losses to the livestock industry amount to US $3 billion.[5,13]

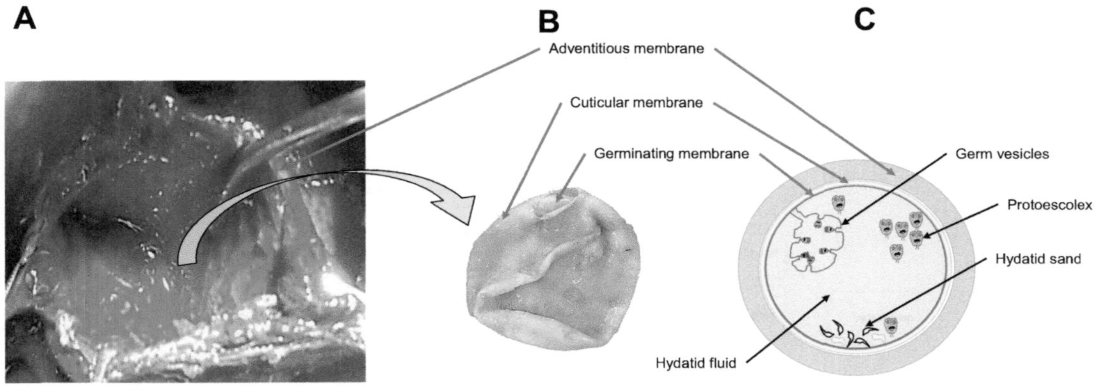

Fig. 2. Hydatid cyst membranes: the first photograph exposes the wall of the cystic bed formed by the adventitial membrane after having removed the cuticular membrane (*arrow*). This photograph corresponds to a cystectomy in a patient with a ruptured, complicated hydatid cyst, with hemoptysis (*A*). In the photograph in the center, the whitish cuticular membrane is observed, somewhat thickened, with a rupture at the level of its upper pole that allows us to see its interior where the transparent germinative membrane is adhered to the cuticular membrane (*B*) is found. The diagram explains the conformation of the 3 layers described and the presence of transparent hydatid fluid, germinative vesicles, protoscolices, and hydatid sand composed of membrane remains, hooks, and protoscolices remains (*C*).

Clinical presentation and diagnosis

Patients have 2 forms of presentation:

- *Asymptomatic* are those who generally have uncomplicated cysts and are frequently diagnosed incidentally by routine radiographic control for another cause.[11,18,19]
- *Symptomatic* are those patients who have large cysts, greater than 5 cm in diameter. Large cysts can cause chest pain if they are in contact with the pleura or dyspnea of varying degrees, depending on atelectasis they may cause. One of the most frequent symptoms is a forceful cough followed by hydatid vomica (expectoration of a transparent liquid with a salty taste with remnants of a whitish membrane and sometimes vesicles) for 1 or 2 weeks, after which the expectoration becomes mucopurulent or purulent owing to the rupture of the cuticular membrane and its subsequent infection of the cystic bed with colonizing bacteria from the airway. Symptoms of aspiration, pericystic pneumonitis, or atelectasis with or without fever may occur if the contents of the vomitus enter other bronchi. Hemoptysis sometimes occurs owing to rupture of blood vessels present in the adventitia.[3,7,11,18,19,20] Spontaneous anaphylaxis or hydropneumothorax (if the cyst ruptures into the pleural cavity) rarely occurs.[11,20]

The diagnosis is primarily clinical. The frequency of presentation of symptoms varies according to the different publications. Imaging examinations confirm the diagnosis, but do not replace the clinical impression.

Simple frontal and lateral chest x-ray (CXR) allows the following:

- Locating and estimating the size of the cyst.
- Determining if the cyst is complicated or not.
- Specifying pulmonary complications.
- Signs that guide the diagnosis and the evolutionary stage of the disease, as summarized in **Fig. 3**.

Features of an *uncomplicated* cyst on CXR (**Fig. 4**) are as follows[11,21]:

- Homogeneous, rounded, or oval radiopacities, with thin, defined borders
- Healthy surrounding lung parenchyma
- Rarely, calcifications and daughter cysts

The most important findings on a *complicated* cyst on CXR are as follows[11,21]:

- Pneumopericyst: The presence of air between the adventitial and cuticular membranes, rarely observed (**Fig. 5**)
- Double-arch sign: Similar to the pneumopericyst, but with the presence of air within the cuticular membrane, rarely observed
- Camalot sign: The cuticular membrane floats on the hydatid fluid after hydatid vomica, commonly seen (**Fig. 6**)
- Retained membrane, uncommon
- Empty cyst, very rare
- Thickening of the cystic wall presents in complicated cysts
- Pleuroparenchymal complications, for example, cysts ruptured into the pleural cavity causing hydropneumothorax

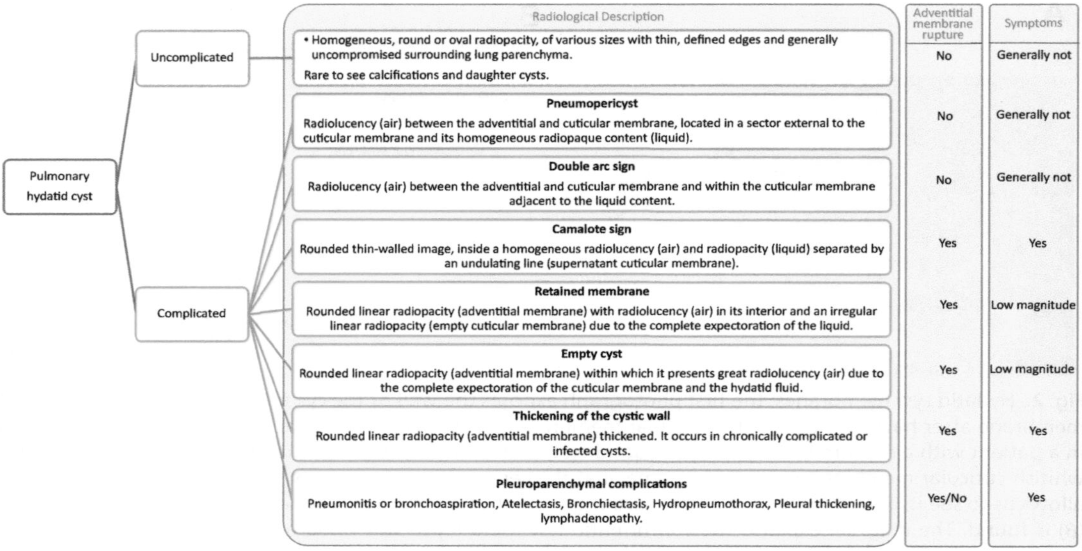
Pulmonary hydatid cyst
Uncomplicated
Complicated
Radiological Description
Adventitial membrane rupture
Symptoms
• Homogeneous, round or oval radiopacity, of various sizes with thin, defined edges and generally uncompromised surrounding lung parenchyma.
Rare to see calcifications and daughter cysts.
No
Generally not
Pneumopericyst
Radiolucency (air) between the adventitial and cuticular membrane, located in a sector external to the cuticular membrane and its homogeneous radiopaque content (liquid).
No
Generally not
Double arc sign
Radiolucency (air) between the adventitial and cuticular membrane and within the cuticular membrane adjacent to the liquid content.
No
Generally not
Camalote sign
Rounded thin-walled image, inside a homogeneous radiolucency (air) and radiopacity (liquid) separated by an undulating line (supernatant cuticular membrane).
Yes
Yes
Retained membrane
Rounded linear radiopacity (adventitial membrane) with radiolucency (air) in its interior and an irregular linear radiopacity (empty cuticular membrane) due to the complete expectoration of the liquid.
Yes
Low magnitude
Empty cyst
Rounded linear radiopacity (adventitial membrane) within which it presents great radiolucency (air) due to the complete expectoration of the cuticular membrane and the hydatid fluid.
Yes
Low magnitude
Thickening of the cystic wall
Rounded linear radiopacity (adventitial membrane) thickened. It occurs in chronically complicated or infected cysts.
Yes
Yes
Pleuroparenchymal complications
Pneumonitis or bronchoaspiration, Atelectasis, Bronchiectasis, Hydropneumothorax, Pleural thickening, lymphadenopathy.
Yes/No
Yes

Fig. 3. A relationship between the radiological findings and the status of the hydatid cyst and the magnitude of the symptoms is shown.

Thoracic ultrasound shows if the cyst is complicated or not, if it is above or below the diaphragm, or if is in the process of migration from the abdomen to the chest.

In a noncontrast *computed tomography (CT) of the chest*, the same signs described in the radiograph are observed, but it has better sensitivity and specificity.[11,21,22] The usefulness of CT scans lies in the following:

- Determining the number of cysts and the extent of lung, pleural, mediastinal, diaphragmatic damage, and so forth.
- Diagnostic uncertainty or difficulty localizing the cyst.
- Suspicion of complications or presence of other concomitant pathologic conditions
- Surgical planning

Immunologic tests, including the enzyme-linked immunosorbent assay (ELISA) and Western blot tests, are the most widely used for diagnosis owing to their high efficiency and ease of use. ELISA detects specific circulating antibodies against parasite antigens (immunoglobulin G), although the sensitivity in pulmonary hydatidosis (50%–60%) is lower than in the liver. ELISA is used as a screening or initial test as well as for postoperative follow-up (10 days, 30 days, 3 months and 6 months, normally negative 30 days after surgery). Western blot detects immune complexes and serves to confirm the diagnosis after the ELISA test. In both tests, there may be false positives and false negatives, depending on the release of antigens from the cyst into the bloodstream. Therefore, the results will be more satisfactory in ruptured or complicated cysts. If these tests are negative, the diagnosis of hydatidosis should not be ruled out.[23–26]

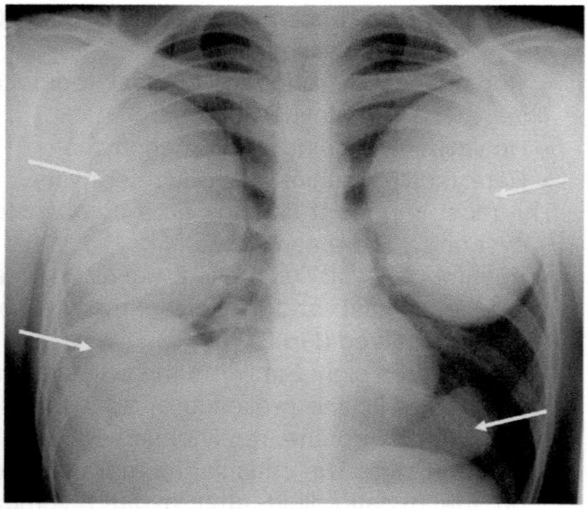

Fig. 4. Frontal CXR shows 4 uncomplicated hydatid cysts (*arrows*), 2 giant cysts found in the infraclavicular areas of both hemithorax that occupy a large area of the lung fields, and the other two are seen in the lower third of both lungs, the one on the right side larger than the left. Uncomplicated cysts are characterized by being round or oval homogeneous radiopaque images, with defined borders and generally normal lung parenchyma.

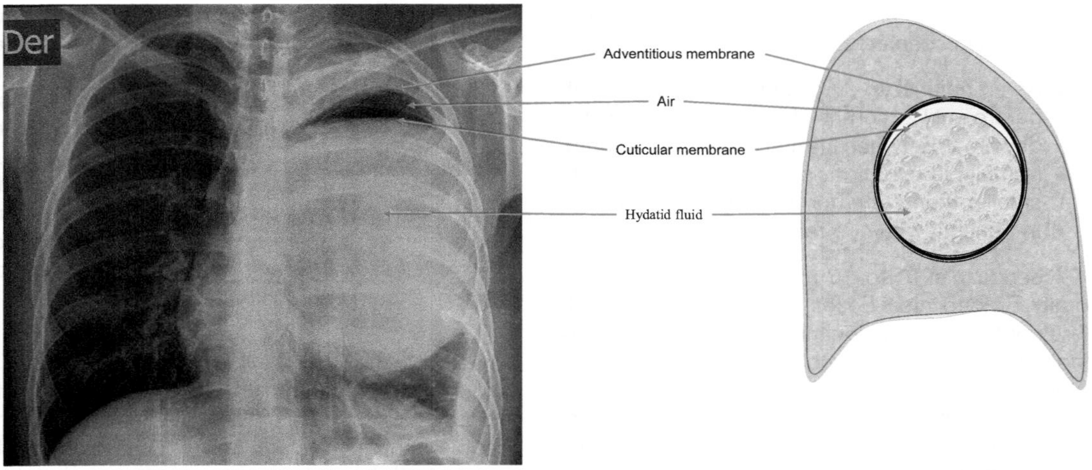

Fig. 5. Frontal CXR shows a giant hydatid cyst, which occupies 80% of the entire left hemithorax, with the sign of pneumopericyst, which consists of the presence of radiolucency (air) between the adventitial and cuticular membrane, within this membrane is the hydatid fluid, which on the radiograph is shown as a homogeneous oval radiopacity. In addition, there is a slight deviation of the mediastinum to the right and a slight left pleural effusion.

Sputum examination is indicated in patients who have had hydatid vomica. Through direct microscopic examination or staining, cuticle fragments, scolices, hooks, or daughter vesicles are searched for, confirming the diagnosis in 100% of cases. The absence of this does not rule out the clinical diagnosis.[11,13]

In the differential diagnosis, there should be a high index of suspicion for pulmonary hydatidosis in patients who come from endemic areas; however, the differential diagnosis includes bronchogenic cysts, lung abscess, lung cancer, sarcoma, hematoma, tuberculosis, mesothelioma, and granuloma, all of which must be taken into account.[21]

Treatment

Surgical management of pulmonary hydatidosis is the treatment of choice in low-resource settings because it provides the definitive cure.[1–3,11,18,27]

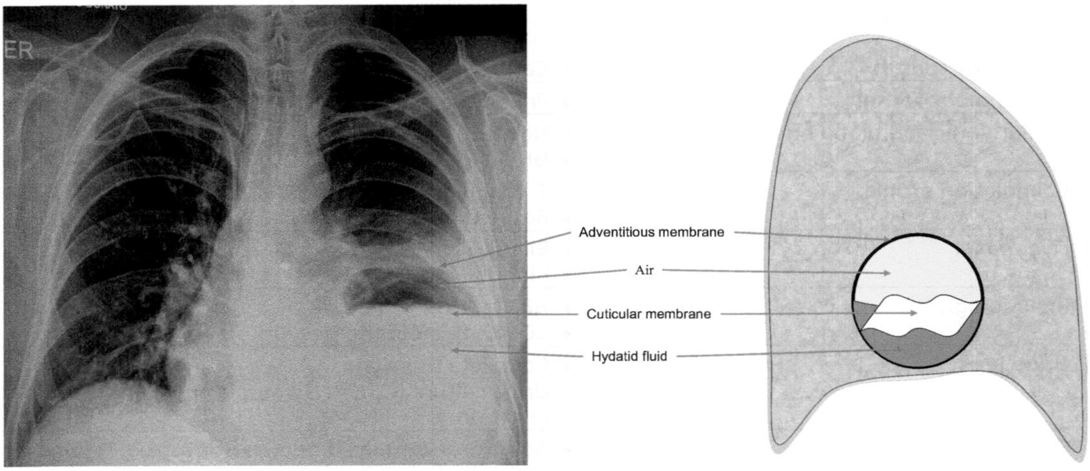

Fig. 6. The frontal CXR and the graph on the right show a complicated hydatid cyst with the sign of the chamalot in the lower third of the left hemithorax. This radiological characteristic is due to the presence of air inside the adventitial cavity with the cuticular membrane supernatant in the hydatid fluid that has remained there after hydatid vomiting. This radiological sign is characterized by presenting a sinuous line that is between the radiolucency corresponding to air and the homogeneous radiopaque image corresponding to the hydatid fluid and the cuticular membrane, all within the adventitial cavity.

Treatment with antiparasitics is indicated under the following scenarios[1,2,11,26]:

- As an adjunct to surgical treatment: 1 month before until 2 months after surgery, with a 15-day break between the first and second month.
- In multiple hydatidosis: Uncomplicated cysts smaller than 7 cm, for 3 months or more.
- In patients with contraindication to surgery.

Albendazole 10 to 15 mg/kg per day is used, orally, divided into 3 doses, with food; in case of allergy or toxicity, Praziquantel 40 mg/kg per day is indicated. Treatment is monitored with a complete blood count and liver function tests every 2 months to detect hematopoietic or hepatic side effects; radiological controls every 6 months for 2 years and then once a year for 5 years are also recommended.[1,2,11,26].

The goals of the surgery are as follows[3,18]:

- Remove the parasite
- Close the bronchial communications and treat the cystic bed
- Avoid complications
- Preserve as much lung parenchyma as possible because some patients return with new community-acquired cysts

Preoperative preparation Presurgical examinations are requested on an outpatient basis (**Table 1**) to detect comorbidities. In the case of cysts complicated by aspiration and/or atelectasis, bronchoscopy is useful to aspirate secretions. In pericystic pneumonitis, broad-spectrum antibiotic treatment is indicated, preferably first-generation cephalosporins administered intravenously (IV). If a patient presents with spontaneous hydropneumothorax owing to rupture of a cyst into the pleural cavity, a pleural drain should be urgently placed; if there is a high-output bronchopleural fistula with respiratory failure, emergency surgery should be considered.

Anesthetic procedure Inhaled general anesthesia should be used and may be combined with epidural anesthesia. The placement of the double-lumen endotracheal tube is essential to isolate both lungs to avoid aspiration and atelectasis and to facilitate surgical maneuvers.

Surgical approach Surgery should preferably be elective and consists of the 3 following critical steps (**Fig. 7**):

1. Incision:
   a. *Posterolateral thoracotomy* is the most widely used and safest incision, as it allows wide access to the entire hemithorax, which permits removal of large cysts, allows exploration of the entire lung, mediastinum, diaphragm, and chest wall in search of other cysts, and gives control of the pulmonary

Table 1
The preoperative tests necessary to find out what clinical conditions the patient has in order to proceed with surgery

Cardiology consult	• Cardiovascular surgical risk assessment
Pulmonology consult	• Pneumologic surgical risk assessment
Hematologic and blood biochemistry tests	• Hct, Hb • Glucose, BUN, creatinine
Coagulation profile	• T. coagulation y sangria, TP, TTPA, TTP ratio, INR • Recuento de Plaquetas
Liver panel	• Bilirubin, alkaline phosphatase, TGO, TGP • Blood proteins
Inmunologic tests	• HBsAg, HIV • COVID-19 molecular testing
Urine tests	• Complete urinalysis • Urine culture if there is a suspicion of urinary infection
Others	• Additional consults if necessary: Gastroenterology, endocrinology, psychiatry, nutrition (BMI)
Drug availability	• It must be ensured that the patient has the full treatment

Note: If any alteration is detected that endangers the life of the patient or the adequate intraoperative or postoperative evolution, other previously scheduled examinations or respective treatments will be carried out to ensure that the patient enters the operating room in the best of conditions.

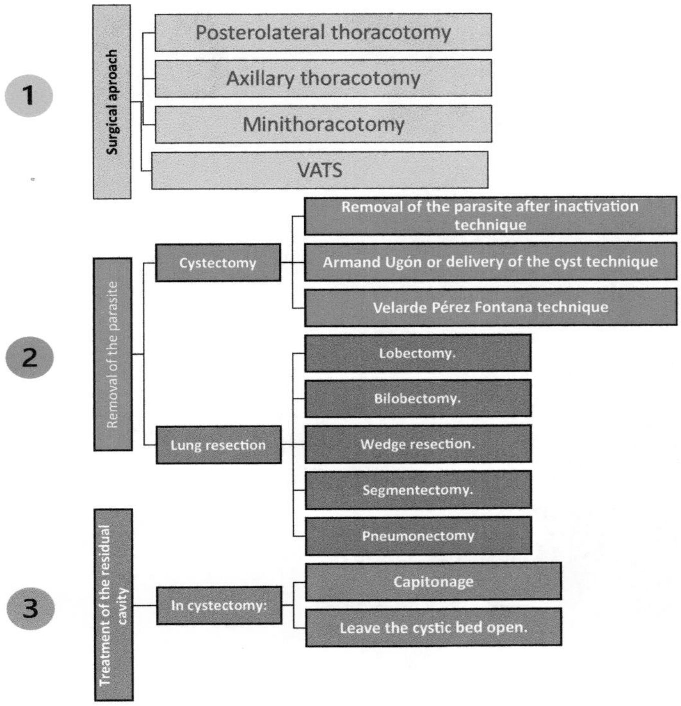

Fig. 7. The 3 steps that are recommended for a proper surgical procedure and the surgical techniques that can be performed. VATS, video-assisted thoracoscopic surgery.

hilum and the heart; its disadvantage is the high postoperative pain.

b. *Axillary thoracotomy, minimal thoracotomy, and video-assisted thoracoscopic surgery* are used in patients with peripheral cysts near the pleura that are less than 5 cm in diameter. These surgical approaches are less painful and produce a shorter hospital stay, but they provide less exposure of the operative field.

2. *Removal of the parasite* may be accomplished by cystectomy or lobectomy, depending on the degree of involvement with the surrounding lung tissue and cyst size.[1,3,18,20,27] Should the patient experience anaphylaxis owing to spillage of the parasite, the anesthesiologist will administer epinephrine in boluses of 100 to 200 μg (every 1–2 minutes) followed by an infusion of 0.05 to 0.1 μg/kg per minute IV. In cases of refractory hypotension (at doses >2 mg of adrenaline), infusion of vasopressin or norepinephrine should be used. In bronchospasm without hypotension, inhaled bronchodilators (1–2 puffs of salbutamol) or epinephrine nebulization is recommended.

   a. *Cystectomy* consists of removing only the hydatid cyst without pulmonary parenchyma. In all cases, the cyst is first surrounded with gauze soaked in hypertonic sodium chloride or povidone iodine and then the following techniques are applied:

      i. *Excision of the cyst after puncture, aspiration, and inactivation*: The most visible area the cyst is punctured with a 16- to 18-gauge needle and a 20- to 50-cc syringe coupled to a triple-way valve connected to a system of drainage, and the hydatid fluid is drawn into a container. An external aspirator will suck up the liquid in cases of leakage. Then, without removing the needle, 20% hypertonic sodium chloride is injected in a volume similar to that extracted, so that the parasites die because of dehydration. Eight to 10 minutes later, all the liquid is aspirated, and the needle is withdrawn. The adventitia is opened, and then the cuticular membrane is excised with Foerster forceps. This technique provides better postoperative results and low complications (**Fig. 8**).

      ii. *Armand Ugón technique or cyst delivery*: This technique is indicated in peripheral cysts smaller than or equal to 5 cm in diameter. It consists of removing the entire cyst without aspirating its contents and without removing the adventitial membrane. The adventitial membrane is

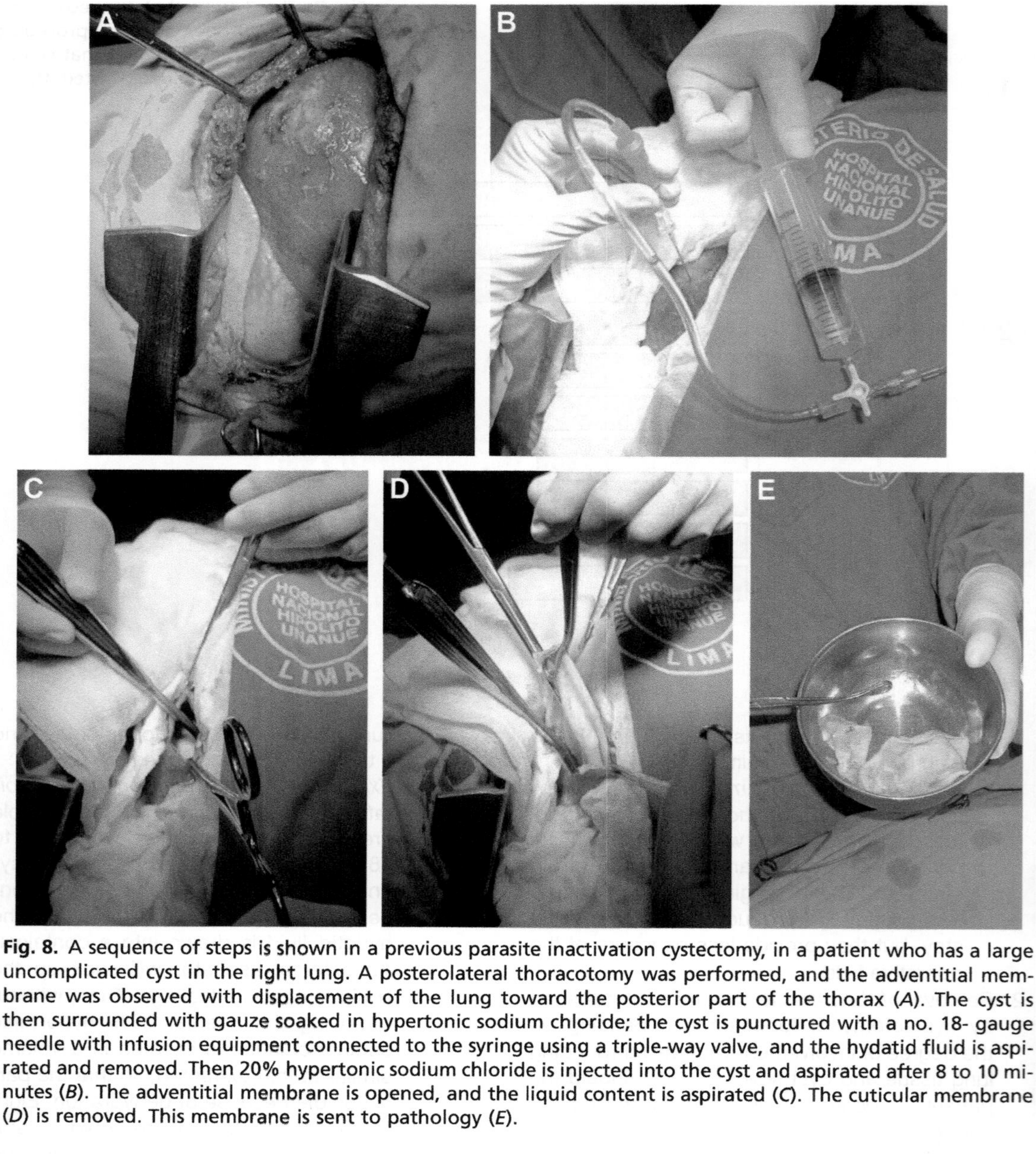

Fig. 8. A sequence of steps is shown in a previous parasite inactivation cystectomy, in a patient who has a large uncomplicated cyst in the right lung. A posterolateral thoracotomy was performed, and the adventitial membrane was observed with displacement of the lung toward the posterior part of the thorax (*A*). The cyst is then surrounded with gauze soaked in hypertonic sodium chloride; the cyst is punctured with a no. 18- gauge needle with infusion equipment connected to the syringe using a triple-way valve, and the hydatid fluid is aspirated and removed. Then 20% hypertonic sodium chloride is injected into the cyst and aspirated after 8 to 10 minutes (*B*). The adventitial membrane is opened, and the liquid content is aspirated (*C*). The cuticular membrane (*D*) is removed. This membrane is sent to pathology (*E*).

opened with a scalpel, and with digital or instrumental maneuvers, the cuticular membrane is exposed, separating it from the adventitia; then the anesthesiologist inflates the lung, and the surgeon expels the cyst with delicate manual pressure directly into a container or in the assistant's hands. The disadvantage is that the cyst may rupture, and hydatid seeding may occur in the pleural cavity.

iii. *Velarde Pérez Fontana technique:* This technique consists of removing the entire cyst, including the adventitial membrane, without aspirating the content. It is indicated in peripheral cysts smaller than 5 cm in diameter. With electrocautery or digital maneuvers, the lung parenchyma around the adventitia is cut, and the hydatid cyst is removed. Hemostasis and pneumostasis are done. The most important complications are hemorrhage and postoperative bronchopleural fistula.

b. *Lung resection* consists of removing part of the lung parenchyma along with the cyst. It is indicated when the hydatid cyst is infected or the adjacent lung parenchyma is hepatized, infected, with functionally unrecoverable atelectasis, or the adventitia is friable with multiple bronchial communications. Lobectomy is indicated when the lung damage encompasses one lobe, bilobectomy if it reaches 2 lobes, and pneumonectomy when giant cysts are found and make the entire lung unviable. Segmentectomy is performed if only one segment is involved. Before performing lung resection, the cuticular membrane and its contents are first excised to avoid atelectasis and aspiration. Wedge resection is performed in small, peripheral cysts, infected or not, and smaller than 5 cm in diameter.

3. Treatment of residual cavity:
   a. Closure of bronchial communications to avoid postoperative bronchopleural fistulas, by placing "U" or "X" stitches with 3/0 or 4/0 polypropylene, and pledgets made with parietal pleura or Teflon if the cystic bed is friable, to avoid suture dehiscence.
   b. Capitonnage when the cystic bed is deep, and tobacco-pouch stitches are placed concentrically from the depth to the surface. Thus, their walls are plicated or brought together, avoiding leaving dead space and favoring healing. The redundant adventitia is trimmed, and the edges are sutured with mattress sutures with 4/0 polypropylene; if the cystic bed is superficial, it can be left open, making sure that the bronchial communications are hermetically closed.
4. *Closure*: The pleural cavity is washed with physiologic saline, and it is verified that there are no other cysts in the remaining lung parenchyma. Two thoracic drains are placed directly toward the pulmonary apex and over the diaphragm, which emerge 2 intercostal spaces below the incision at the level of the midaxillary line. In the case of pneumonectomy, one drain is placed, and it is kept clamped.

After the surgery, the patient goes to recovery, preferably awake and extubated, with morphine as an analgesic, prophylactic antibiotic, such as first-generation cephalosporin; in case of infection, an aminoglycoside is added, and nebulization every 4 to 6 hours with physiologic saline is indicated.

RESULTS

Cystectomy is the most frequently performed and recommended technique. In the reviewed literature, cystectomies are reported from 40.7% to 83.7% of operated cases and lung resections are reported from 10.6% to 54.9%; lobectomies are reported from 6.5% to 41.8%, segmentectomies are reported at 3.3%, and pneumonectomies are reported from 0.8% to 2.7%.[3,20,27,28] The investigators who report more radical surgeries operated on more complicated cysts, whereas those who did more conservative surgery had a higher proportion of uncomplicated cysts.

Postoperative Complications

Postoperative morbidity ranges between 6.5% and 39% and is higher in complicated cysts, according to the literature reviewed. The most frequent complication described by Gonzáles and colleagues[3] is bronchopleural fistula, atelectasis 15%, as described by Rafael and colleagues,[20] and finally, prolonged air leak 8.1%, as described by Aldahmashi and colleagues.[29]

Operative mortality ranges from 0% to 2.3% and is most often due to giant abscessed cysts or ruptured into the pleural cavity with bronchopleural fistula and pleural empyema.[3,20,25,27,29] Recovery is often favorable, and the patient is discharged after 5 to 10 days without postoperative complications.

Summary and Recommendations

Ingesting the eggs of the helminth *E. granulosus*, which is endemic in some agricultural areas, may cause lung cysts that can rupture and cause systemic illness and/or locally enlarged lung damage. The common clinical presentations can be further characterized by chest imaging findings. Surgical resection (cystectomy with or without parenchymal resection) is the mainstay of definitive treatment and is augmented to neo/adjuvant antiparasitic drugs.

In order to move treatment outcomes of pulmonary hydatidosis going forward, multicenter studies should be planned to standardize the types of surgeries to be performed for each presentation and therefore improve their results. There should be standardization of the use of immunologic tests for diagnosis and follow-up. Finally, policy changes should provide more strict regulations to prevent this disease, especially in endemic areas.

SURGICAL MANAGEMENT OF LUNG ABSCESS

Pathogenesis

Infection of the lung with bacterial, mycobacterial, fungal, or parasitic organisms can lead to destruction of the parenchyma and development of liquefactive collections.[30] This section focuses on bacteria, as other agents are covered elsewhere. The causative species vary depending on the risk factors of the patient and geography. The lower respiratory tract is colonized with anerobic (eg, *Prevotella* and *Veillonella*) and microaerophilic (eg, oral *Streptococcus*) species. However, lung abscesses are often polymicrobial, and the isolated organisms also may include gram-negative or gram-positive aerobes.[31] For example, in Peru, the most commonly observed organisms are *Pseudomona aeruginosa* and *Acinetobacter*, whereas in Taiwan *Klebsiella pneumoniae* predominated in one study.[32] The mechanism of abscess formation involves a local pneumonitis (owing to aspiration in primary lung abscess or obstruction/emboli in secondary lung abscess), followed by tissue necrosis owing to the etiologic organism or organisms.[33]

Patients who develop severe or necrotizing pneumonia should be followed closely clinically and/or with serial radiographs while receiving antimicrobial treatment because of the formation of an abscess, which may subsequently rupture and lead to empyema and associated complications, including bronchopleural fistula.

Epidemiology

The incidence of lung abscesses has decreased markedly after introduction of antibiotics, as well as morbidity and mortality. Lung abscess epidemiology varies by cause. Most abscesses are primary, whereby the host does not have an underlying condition, and aspiration is causative. Secondary lung abscesses in low-resource settings may be due to a structurally abnormal lung (eg, owing to bronchiectasis) and can be affected by risk factors, including an immunocompromised state (eg, HIV-AIDS), impaired clearance (eg, owing to poor cough), and increased aspiration (eg, in patients with poor dental hygiene).[33] Public health measures should be concentrated to mitigate these risk factors.

Clinical Presentation and Diagnosis

Patients with lung abscess typically present with systemic signs of infection, including fever, malaise, and weight loss, similar to patients with pneumonia. The time course is subacute (several weeks), although may become chronic (>4–6 weeks). The locale of primary lung abscess is the dependent lung segments (superior segment, posterior segment) and secondary, depending on the underlying cause. Cough may or may not be productive.

As with pulmonary hydatidosis, imaging can confirm the location and size of the abscess. CXR and ultrasound are often adequate to guide initial therapy, but chest CT scan should at least be obtained in patients without response and/or requiring surgical treatment (**Fig. 9**). Even then, the distinction between a peripheral lung abscess and empyema may not be clear. Additional diagnostic tests, such as bronchoscopy and aspiration, can be considered if empiric therapies fail.

Treatment

Before the 1950s, surgery for drainage of abscesses was commonly used. However, currently, the first-line treatment is directed or empiric antibiotics, depending on the type of abscess, patient risk factors, and location of acquisition. For example, in Peru, the treatment for community-acquired abscesses is a third-generation cephalosporin or a quinolone plus amikacin (for gram-negative aerobes), and clindamycin (as in general anaerobes also coinfect lung abscesses). The empirical treatment for hospital-acquired abscesses is ceftazidime and imipenem.

Abscesses that do not respond to antibiotics after 1 week, that evade microbial characterization, or that lead to complications, such as hemoptysis or rupture, warrant drainage or surgery. In low-resource settings where percutaneous image-guided drains are less available, abscesses greater than 5 cm may undergo resection. In one hospital in Brazil, of 252 patients with lung abscess, surgery was required in 52 (20.6%), including drainage of empyema (n = 24), pulmonary resection (n = 22), and drainage of the abscess (n = 6).[34] Resection is typically done as segmentectomy or lobectomy, taking care not to spill the abscess contents to prevent the postoperative complication of pneumonia or empyema. The surrounding tissue is often quite inflamed and, as described in the prior article on empyema, the timing of surgery is critical to ensure an optimal outcome and avoid bronchopleural fistula formation. Wide-bore drainage tube or tubes should be left and antibiotics continued until the pleural space drainage normalizes. Consideration should be given to sending abscess tissue for pathologic examination, particularly when there are risk factors to ensure there is no underlying tumor.

Data on operative results are limited by the rarity of lung abscesses in the present era and the high cure rates of nonoperative therapy (>90%). However, the increasing numbers of patients worldwide with risk for secondary abscesses (eg, those undergoing cancer chemotherapy or stem-cell transplants) may increase the need for

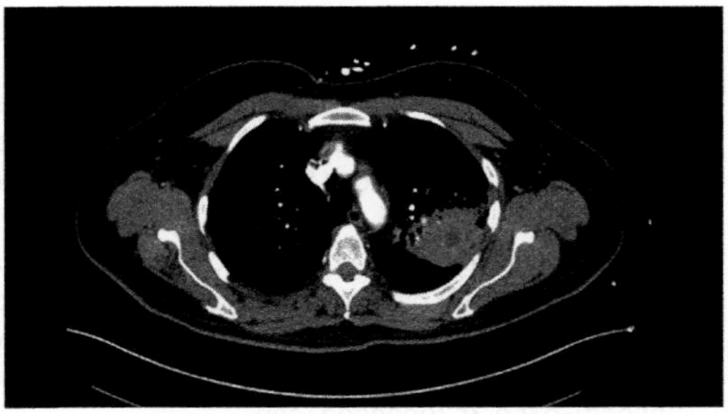

Fig. 9. Left upper lobe posterior apical segment pulmonary abscess on chest CT scan shows liquefactive component surrounded by consolidation.

operative interventions for this disease. In one single-center case series of 75 patients undergoing thoracoscopic drainage of lung abscesses, complications (13%) largely entailed local site issues (infection, subcutaneous emphysema), bleeding, pneumothorax, and one death.[35] In another large multicenter study of outcomes of segmentectomy (n = 18), lobectomy (n = 58), and pneumonectomy (n = 15), 30-day mortality following surgery was 15%, suggesting the high-risk nature of these cases.[36]

SUMMARY

Lung resection is used to manage lung abscesses in low-resource settings if size or lack of improvement suggests future complications. In general, with adequate surgical selection, outcomes of operative therapy are anticipated to be good.

CLINICS CARE POINTS

- Chest x-ray, ultrasound, and computed tomographic scan as well as serology are used as adjuncts to the clinical presentation to diagnose and determine treatment for hydatid cyst.
- Perioperative antimicrobial therapy should be directed by microbiology results for hydatid cysts and lung abscesses.
- Coordinated care between surgery and anesthesia is required for safe resection of pulmonary cysts and abscesses. If resection is required, hilar structures may be inflamed and pose technical challenges.
- Pleural complications may occur and cause systemic illness in the case of rupture or bronchial fistula formation from large cysts or abscesses.

DISCLOSURE

The authors declare no commercial or financial conflicts of interest.

REFERENCES

1. Guerra L, Ramírez M. Hidatidosis Humana en el Perú. Apunt Cienc Soc 2015;5(01):94–101.
2. Zuñiga E, Terashima A, Falcon N. Características epidemiológicas de pacientes con equinococosis quística humana en el Hospital Nacional Cayetano Heredia, Lima-Perú. Periodo 2008-2012. Salud Tecnol Vet 2015;1:37–43.
3. González R, Riquelme A, Reyes R, et al. Hidatidosis pulmonar: características, manifestaciones clínicas y tratamiento en pacientes hospitalizados en Concepción, Región de Biobío, Chile. Rev Med Chile 2020;148:762–71.
4. Armiñanzas C, Gutierrez-Cuadra M, Fariñas M. Hidatidosis: aspectos epidemiológicos, clínicos, diagnósticos y terapéuticos. Rev Esp Quimioter 2015; 28(3):116–24.
5. World Health Organization. Equinococcosis. 2021. Available at: https://www.who.int/news-room/fact-sheets/detail/echinococcosis. Accessed May 30, 2021.
6. Salazar P, Cabrera M. Hidatidosis. In: Becerril M, editor. Parasitología Médica. . México: McGraw Hill; 2014. p. 187–95.
7. Instituto Nacional de Seguridad y Salud en el Trabajo. Echinococcus spp. insst.es. 2018. Available at: https://www.insst.es/documents/94886/354041/Echinococcus+spp+-+A%C3%B1o+2019.pdf/13eea2d3-cd42-4830-a08d-39033a2e41ec?version=1.0&t=1601421536628. Accessed October 23, 2021.
8. Murray P, Rosenthal K, Pfaller M, editors. Microbiología Médica. 7th edition. Barcelona: Elsevier; 2014.
9. Botero D, Restrepo M, editors. Parasitosis Humanas. 5th edition. Medellín: Corporación para Investigaciones Biológicas; 2012.
10. Paho.org. Hidatidosis/Equinococosis - OPS/OMS | Organización Panamericana de la Salud. 2021. Available at: https://www.paho.org/es/temas/hidatidosis-equinococosis. Accessed October 23, 2021.
11. Somocurcio J, Álvarez G, Sotomayor A. Hidatidosis pulmonar. In: Cirugía de Tórax y cardiovascular. Lima (Peru): Universidad Nacional Mayor de San Marcos Fondo Editorial; 2000. p. 233–55.
12. Tay J. Microbiología y Parasitología Médicas de Tay. 5th edition. Ciudadde, México: Méndez editores; 2019. p. 960.
13. Sapunar J. Hidatidosis y equinococosis. In: Werner L, editor. Parasitología Humana. México: Mc Graw Hill; 2013. p. 427–46.

14. Budke C, Deplazes P, Torgerson P. Global Socio-economic Impact of Cystic Echinococcosis. Emerging Infect Dis J 2006;12:296–7. Available at: http://www.cdc.gov/eid. Accessed October 23, 2021.
15. Torgerson PR, Budke CM. Echinococcosis – an international public health challenge. Res Vet Sci 2003;74(3):191–202.
16. Organización Panamericana de la Salud. Equinococosis: informe epidemiológico en la región de América del Sur - 2018, n.4, 2020. iris.paho.org. 2020. Available at: https://iris.paho.org/handle/10665.2/51942. Accessed November 7, 2021.
17. Pacífico J, Cabrera R, Salgado-Díaz S, et al. Factores asociados a complicaciones prequirúrgicas en pacientes con equinococosis quística de áreas endémicas del Perú. Revista Peruana de Medicina Experimental y Salud Pública 2021;38(1):33–40.
18. Tercero MJ, Olalla R. Hidatidosis Una Zoonosis de Distribución Mundial. OFFARM 2008;27(9):88–94. Available at: https://www.elsevier.es/es-revista-offarm-4-articulo-hidatidosis-una-zoonosis-distribucion-mundial-13127387. Accessed August 11, 2021.
19. Soledad JS, Rodríguez V, Candia M, et al. Hidatidosis pulmonar. Revista de postgrado de la VI Cátedra de Medicina 2005;152:16–8. Available at: https://med.unne.edu.ar/revistas/revista152/5_152.htm. Accessed October 25, 2021.
20. Rafael A, Ramos W, Peralta J, et al. Hidatidosis pulmonar en un hospital de Lima, Perú: experiencia en 113 pacientes. Rev Peru Med Exp Salud Publica 2008;25(3):285–9.
21. Durhan G, Tan AA, Düzgün SA, et al. Radiological manifestations of thoracic hydatid cysts: pulmonary and extrapulmonary findings. Insights into Imaging 2020;11(1). https://doi.org/10.1186/s13244-020-00916-0.
22. Emlik D, Ödev K, Poyraz N, et al. Radiological Characteristics of Pulmonary Hydatid Cysts. Curr Top Echinococcosis 2015. https://doi.org/10.5772/60884.
23. Pinto GPP. Diagnóstico, tratamiento y seguimiento de la hidatidosis. Revista Chilena de Cirugía 2017; 69(1):94–8.
24. Miranda-Ulloa E, Ayala-Sulca E, Flores-Reátegui H. Evaluación del Western blot con cinco antígenos hidatídicos para el diagnóstico de equinococosis humana. Revista Peruana de Medicina Exp y Salud Pública. 2014;30(2). https://doi.org/10.17843/rpmesp.2013.302.224.
25. Sarkar M, Pathania R, Jhobta A, et al. Cystic pulmonary hydatidosis. Lung India 2016;33(2):179.
26. Simao Ferreira M, Gonzaga E, Rausch R. Hidatidose equinococoses. In: Focaccia R, editor. Tratado de Infectología.. 5th edition. Sao Paulo: Editora Atheneu; 2015. p. 290–1.
27. González LR, Riquelme UA, Ávalos TM, et al. Hidatidosis pulmonar: hallazgos y tratamiento quirúrgico en quistes complicados versus no complicados. Revista de Cirugía. 2020;72(4). https://doi.org/10.35687/s2452-45492020004609.
28. Sadrizadeh A, Dalouee M, Haghi S, et al. Evaluation of the effect of pulmonary hydatid cyst location on the surgical technique approaches. Lung India 2014;31(4):361–5.
29. Aldahmashi M, Alassal M, Kasb I, et al. Conservative Surgical Management for Pulmonary Hydatid Cyst: Analysis and Outcome of 148 Cases. Can Respir J 2016;2016:1–6.
30. Kuhajda I, Zarogoulidis K, Tsirgogianni K, et al. Lung abscess-etiology, diagnostic and treatment options. Ann Transl Med 2015;3(13):183.
31. Surana NK, Kasper DL. Infections Due to Mixed Anaerobic Organisms. In: Jameson J, Fauci AS, Kasper DL, et al, editors. Harrison's Principles of Internal Medicine, 20e. New York: McGraw Hill; 2018. p. 1227–35. Available at: https://accessmedicine.mhmedical.com/content.aspx?bookid=2129&sectionid=192023257. Accessed January 03, 2022.
32. Wang JL, Chen KY, Fang CT, et al. Changing bacteriology of adult community-acquired lung abscess in Taiwan: Klebsiella pneumoniae versus anaerobes. Clin Infect Dis 2005;40(7):915–22.
33. Baron RM, Barshak M. Lung Abscess. In: Jameson J, Fauci AS, Kasper DL, et al, editors. Harrison's Principles of Internal Medicine, 20e. New York: McGraw Hill; 2018. p. 919–21. Available at: https://accesspharmacy-mhmedical-com.libproxy.lib.unc.edu/content.aspx?bookid=2129&sectionid=183880727. Accessed January 03, 2022.
34. Moreira Jda S, Camargo Jde J, Felicetti JC, et al. Lung abscess: analysis of 252 consecutive cases diagnosed between 1968 and 2004. J Bras Pneumol 2006;32:136–43.
35. Akopov A, Egorov V, Deynega I, et al. Awake video-assisted thoracic surgery in acute infectious pulmonary destruction. Ann Transl Med 2015;3(8):100.
36. Schweigert M, Solymosi N, Dubecz A, et al. Predictors of outcome in modern surgery for lung abscess. Thorac Cardiovasc Surg 2017;65:535–41.

Management of Empyema Thoracis in Low-Resource Settings

Abebe Bekele, MD, FCS (ECSA), FACS[a,b,*],
Barnabas Tobi Alayande, MBBS, MBA, FMCS[a,c]

KEYWORDS

• Empyema thoracis (thoracic empyema) • Low-resource settings (LRS) • Chest tube • Thoracotomy • Decortication

KEY POINTS

- Most cases of empyema thoracis are sequelae of severe pneumonia, but chest trauma and complications of chest tube insertion as cause are not uncommon in low-resource settings.
- The diagnosis is usually late due to delayed presentation to health care facilities, low index of suspicion among health care professionals, and inability to properly stage the disease with the available diagnostic tools.
- Early use of antibiotics and appropriate-sized and well-placed chest tube drainage is associated with good outcomes at a decreased cost.
- Surgical management of empyema thoracis is indicated when chest tube drainage and antibiotic treatment fails to achieve complete resolution.
- The decision to operate on patients with thoracic empyema in an LRS should not be taken lightly due to the risks of bleeding, incomplete expansion, and lung injury.

INTRODUCTION

Pleural effusions and empyema thoracis are common diseases globally. The clinical presentation of this spectrum of disease, alongside attempts at their management, has been described since the Hippocratic era, and still has contemporary implications.[1] The specifics of the practice in low- and middle-income countries (LMICs) and the challenges in managing this continuum of chest pathologies requires a contextualized approach. The characteristics of the patient population, limited number of thoracic specialists (specialist and pulmonologists) in LMIC settings, the lack of advanced imaging techniques, and challenges of postprocedure care are but a few considerations in the management of effusions and empyema in resource-limited settings.[2] The main purpose of this review is to update the reader regarding the diagnostic approach and appropriate treatment of thoracic empyema in resource-constrained settings.

ANATOMY OF THE PLEURAL SPACE

The pleural cavity is a 20-μm-wide potential space located between the parietal and the visceral pleura (**Fig. 1**), and both pleural surfaces are lined by a special type of simple squamous epithelium known as the mesothelium.[3] The mesothelium lining the lungs is the visceral pleura, whereas the mesothelium lining the thoracic cavity is called the parietal pleura. In normal circumstances, the pleural space is filled with a thin fluid known as pleural fluid, which

[a] University of Global Health Equity Kigali Heights, Plot 772, KG 7 Avenue, 5th floor, PO Box 6955, Kigali, Rwanda; [b] Addis Ababa University, School of Medicine, Addis Ababa, Ethiopia; [c] Program in Global Surgery and Social Change, Harvard Medical School, Boston, MA, USA
* Corresponding author. University of Global Health Equity Kigali Heights, Plot 772, KG 7 Avenue, 5th floor, PO Box 6955, Kigali, Rwanda.
E-mail address: abekele@ughe.org

Thorac Surg Clin 32 (2022) 361–372
https://doi.org/10.1016/j.thorsurg.2022.02.004

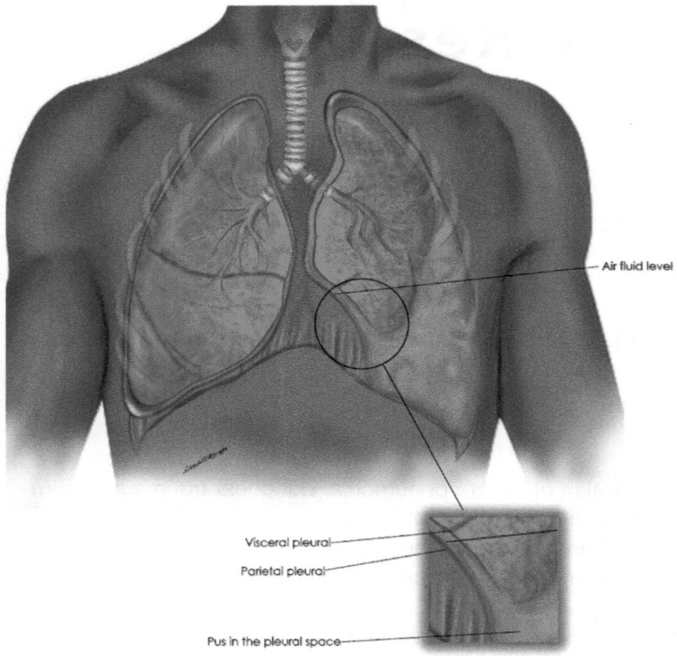

Fig. 1. The pleural space and pleural collections.

is mainly a transudate from systemic vessels that supply the parietal pleura. This fluid is important to minimize friction between the 2 pleural surfaces during respiration. The negative pressure inside the pleural cavity creates a vacuum that keeps the airways open at all times.[3]

The parietal pleura is innervated by somatic fibers from the intercostal nerves and by the phrenic nerves. Hence, it is able to sense the classical pleuritic type of pain when irritated.[3] However, the visceral pleura is not supplied by somatic nerves and is thus insensitive to pain, touch, or pressure. The visceral pleura receives its blood supply from the bronchial circulation, and the parietal pleura receives its blood supply from the chest wall. The right and left pleural cavities have no anatomic connection.[3]

EPIDEMIOLOGY

In the United States, up to 1.5 million cases of pleural effusion occur yearly.[4] China records up to 4684 effusions per million adults.[5] Many LMICs lack comprehensive data on the local incidence and epidemiology of pleural effusions and empyema. Epidemiology varies globally based on the prominent locoregional underlying cause. Both uncomplicated parapneumonic effusions and empyema are common at the extremes of age: in the very young and in the elderly.[6,7] In addition, various risk factors contribute to the development of empyema in LMICs. These risk factors include comorbidities (cancer, tuberculosis, malnutrition, diabetes), immunosuppressants (human immunodeficiency virus/AIDS, chronic steroid use), alcohol and intravenous (IV) abuse, and underlying structural lung disease.[6,8,9] The epidemiology and cause of post-chest tube empyema is usually underreported in low-resource contexts; however, substandard care for chest tubes after insertion, duration of the chest tube in situ, retained hemothorax or chylothorax, and the presence of pulmonary contusions increase the incidence of post–chest tube empyema.[10]

CAUSES

Thoracic empyemas are always secondary—infectious agents need to get access to the normally sterile pleural cavity (**Fig. 2**). Empyemas occur when infections spread to the pleural cavity from the lung, mediastinum, chest wall, diaphragm; from the external environment; or from circulation.[11] These infections may be bacterial, viral, or atypical; however, bacterial infections are the most common. Pneumonia is the single most significant cause because more than 50% of empyemas result from infected parapneumonic effusions.[12]

Empyema also results from penetrating or blunt chest injuries where undrained hemothorax subsequently gets infected.[13] One of the most underrecognized and underreported causes of empyema

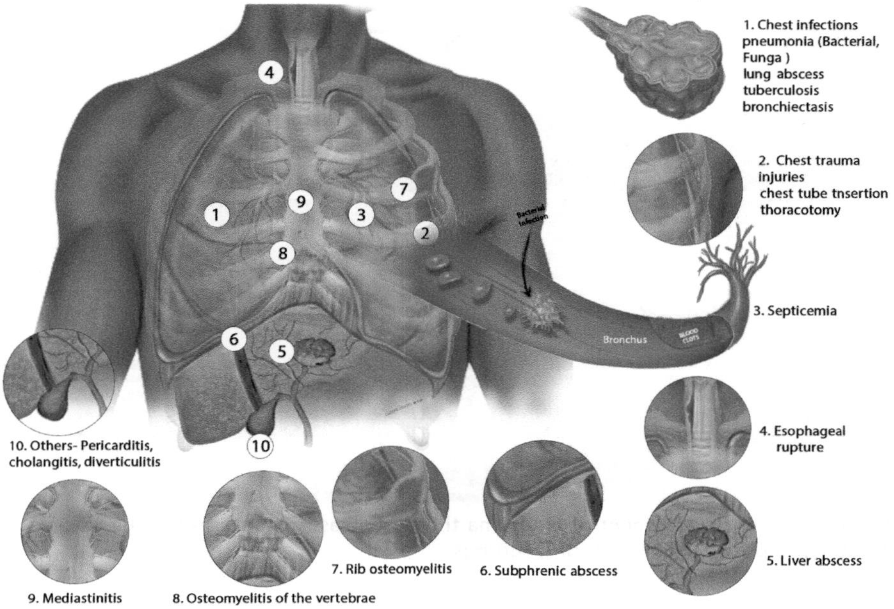

Fig. 2. Causes of empyema thoracis.

are complications of chest tubes and needle thoracentesis procedures.[10,14] Pleural infections also occur after thoracic or esophageal surgery especially if associated with esophageal anastomosis leak. However, a bronchopleural fistula should be assumed when empyema occurs after thoracic surgery. In addition, mediastinitis, pericarditis, ruptured esophagus, pancreatitis, and subdiaphragmatic abscesses have been identified as causes.[12]

The exact infectious cause of empyema cannot be identified in most cases because culture results are negative in about 40% of aspirates.[15] In about 13%, cultures are polymicrobial.[15] Streptococci are common pathogens. In Africa, Asia, and the Middle East, however, *Staphylococcus aureus* is responsible for most (20% to 77%) empyema cases[15] and bacteria from the *Streptococcus milleri* group (*Streptococcus intermedius*, *Streptococcus constellatus*, and *Streptococcus anginosus*) are the predominant organisms cultured in adults with underlying comorbidities.[16] Tuberculous empyema is also a very common finding in low-resource settings (up to 29%).[15,17] A recent review of 10,241 patients showed that *S aureus* is the predominant cause of pleural effusion in adults globally; however, there are variations in microbiology according to the geographic location and setting of infections.[15]

In children, complicated community-acquired pneumonia secondary to *Streptococcus pneumoniae* is the predominant pathogen, and together with *S aureus* are responsible for up to 70% of aerobic gram-positive infections.[18]

In hospital-acquired infections, methicillin-resistant *S aureus* (MRSA) accounts for about 60% of the cases, whereas gram-negative aerobic organisms account for most of the remainder (37%).[15] MRSA and a variety of gram-negative organisms and anaerobes (*Klebsiella, Pseudomonas,* and *Haemophilus sp*) are also identified causes in children.

Other uncommon causes of empyema include enterococci, *Entamoeba histolytica,* and complicated pulmonary *Echinococcus granulosus* (hydatid cysts).[15]

Postthoracotomy empyemas are usually caused by *S aureus* followed by *Streptococcus*. However, delayed empyemas occurring after 14 days of thoracotomy and postesophagectomy empyema are usually polymicrobial. Fungal empyema (*Candida* sp) has been described following esophagectomy and typically results in high mortality rates.[19] Empyema secondary to chest tube insertion from high-income settings suggests an incidence ranging from 1% to 25% with predominantly staphylococcal or streptococcal bacteriology. Very rarely coronavirus disease 2019 can result in loculated empyema.[20]

STAGES OF EMPYEMA

Over a period of 4 to 6 weeks, the classical thoracic empyema passes through 3 stages of development (**Fig. 3**).[21,22]

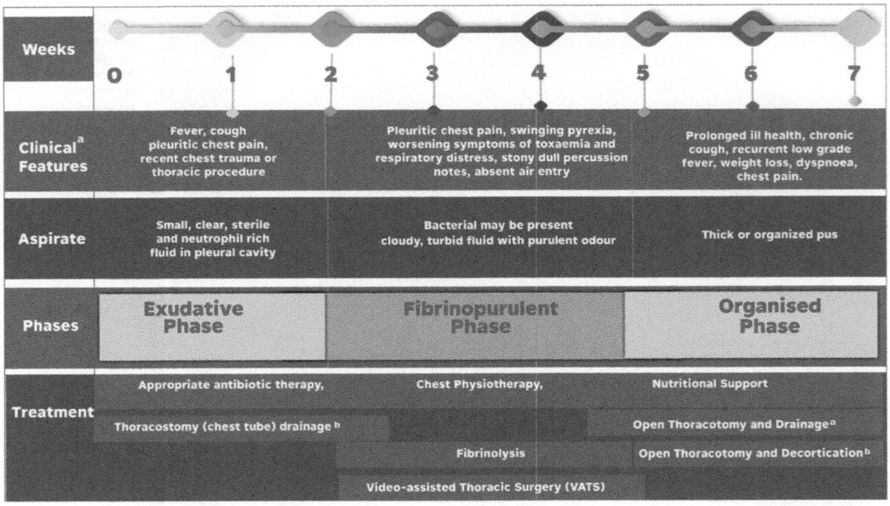

Fig. 3. Classical stages of development of empyema thoracis. [a]Classical features may be masked by antibiotics. [b]Practical treatment options for low-resource settings.

The Exudative Phase

This phase, synonymous with the parapneumonic phase, is characterized by the accumulation of clear, sterile, and neutrophil-rich fluid in the pleural cavity. The collection is usually small in amount and occupies the most dependent area of the pleural cavity (costophrenic recess usually). Aspiration and laboratory analysis of the fluid reveal an exudative fluid free of any organisms. Simple drainage at this stage results in the complete evacuation of the fluid and reexpansion of the underlying lung without any sequel (**Table 1**).[21]

The Fibropurulent Phase

At this stage, bacterial invasion of the collection occurs. This invasion results in several biochemical, microbiologic, and pathologic changes. The fluid collection becomes cloudy, even turbid, sometimes with a clear purulent odor. The fluid collection also becomes more exudative and acidic, and the white blood cell count increases. The amount of fluid significantly increases and occupies a significant portion of the pleural cavity. As the inflammation continues, fibrous strands and septa begin to develop inside the pleural cavity, hence leading to the development of a complex multiloculated purulent fluid collection.[21] Initially, the septa are flimsy and incomplete, hence chest tube drainage may be effective in complete evacuation. However, as the pathologic condition worsens, the septa become tough and may result in the complex multiloculated collections. If chest tube drainage fails to resolve the collection, fibrinolytics and DNase can be used to dissolve the septa and facilitate drainage.[23] However,

Table 1
Pleural fluid characteristics: Parapneumonic effusion versus empyema

Plural fluid characteristics	Parapneumonic effusion	Empyema
Appearance	Clear, or slightly turbid	Cloudy, turbid, or frank pus
Biochemistry		
pH	>7.3 (normal)	<7.2 (more acidic)
Glucose level	>60 mg/dL	<40 mg/dL
LDH	<700 U/L	>1000 U/L
WBC count	<15,000 count/μL	>15,000 count/μL
Microbiology	Always negative	May be negative

Abbreviations: LDH, lactate dehydrogenase; WBC, white blood cell.

Adapted from Sahn SA. Diagnosis and management of parapneumonic effusions and empyema. Clin Infect Dis. 2007 Dec 1;45(11):1480-6.

complete drainage in such situations may require video-assisted thoracoscopic surgery (VATS) or open thoracotomy drainage.

The Organized (Fibrous) Phase

Approximately at 6 weeks, the collected pus becomes very thick pus and the septa become very tough. Granulations start to occur all over the pleural space, and both the parietal and the visceral pleura thicken.[21] The thickened pleura become apparent in radiological imaging. Thickening of the visceral pleura and the large amount of pus collection result in the collapse of the adjacent lung, and expansion of the lung is significantly restricted. Thickening of the parietal pleura leads to a frozen chest wall and rib crowding hence impairing the physiologic chest wall mechanics during respiration. Thickening of the diaphragmatic pleura can also restrict the diaphragmatic movement. If left untreated, the thickened pleura can become calcified, hence further worsening the restriction to lung expansion, chest wall mechanics, and diaphragmatic movement. The pus can spontaneously burst through the chest wall (empyema necessitans) and fistulize toward the lung (bronchopleural fistula) or into any of the mediastinal structures adjacent to it.[24]

CLINICAL FEATURES

Clinical presentation of patients with empyema depends on the stage of the disease, age of the patients, associated comorbidities, treatment history, and the health-seeking behavior of patients. The symptoms of acute empyema and parapneumonic effusion are usually similar to those of uncomplicated pneumonia, including features of acute febrile illness, cough, pleuritic chest pain, and respiratory distress. However, these symptoms can be masked or significantly altered in cases of partial treatment with antibiotics, in patients with comorbidities such as immunocompromised patients, and in the elderly. Patients may also have a suggestive recent history of tube thoracostomy or thoracotomy. Recent chest trauma with gradual worsening respiratory symptoms and fever is also suggestive.

As the pleural fluid collection worsens, the classical pleuritic pain improves; however, the respiratory symptoms (cough, respiratory distress), the fever with a swinging pattern, and the general features of toxemia persist or worsen. A physical examination will show an acutely sick patient with tachycardia, tachypnea, pyrexia, and features of dehydration. The effusion in the pleural space will be characterized by stony dull percussion notes on the affected hemithorax, diminished breath sounds, and sometimes mediastinal displacement to the opposite side.

Chronic empyema is characterized by a prolonged history of deteriorating general health status, recurrent and intermittent low-grade fever, weight loss, dyspnea, chest tightness and pain, and chronic cough. Examination will reveal a chronically sick and malnourished patient with features of respiratory distress. The affected chest shows reduced movement with breathing, and its size may be contracted; intercostal space may be narrowed. In some instances, patients may present with empyema necessitans in which an undrained empyema ruptures to the skin. Occasionally, the empyema persists to involve the ribs giving features of rib chronic osteomyelitis. Breath sounds may be absent or reduced, and all sorts of respiratory sounds may be present. Clinical findings of underlying or associated abdominal diseases like pancreatitis, subdiaphragmatic abscess, and amebic liver abscesses may be present.

APPROACH TO DIAGNOSIS

The diagnosis of empyema thoracic in low-resource countries should be mainly clinical and established by plain chest radiograph and microscopy, culture, and sensitivity. Hence, practitioners in such situations should have a high index of suspicion when faced with such patients.

Needle Aspiration

Needle thoracocentesis is a safe bedside procedure that should be performed under sterile techniques, and the use of wide-bore needle is advised. In some instances, the procedure is important to relieve life-threatening collections under tension.[25] In addition, the procedure should be carried out with caution in the presence of uncontrolled coughing, bleeding disorders, and altered chest wall anatomy. Image-guided aspiration is advised in cases of uncertain fluid locations and minimal volumes. Cellulitis at the potential needle insertion site and overlying herpes zoster are contraindications.

The needle insertion site is typically the midscapular line at the upper border of the sixth or seventh rib (or at least 1 intercostal space below the top of the effusion if image guided). The preferred site is the triangle of safety. Local anesthesia should be used, and the large needle is advanced till the pleural space is entered. Aspiration of pleural fluid or pus is thus attained (**Table 2**).[25]

Table 2
Characteristics of pleural aspirate

Characteristic	Transudate	Exudate
Protein concentration	<30 g/L	>30 g/L
Total protein:serum ratio	<1.016	>0.5
Lactate dehydrogenase	<0.51 IU/L	>20 IU/L
LDH fluid:serum ratio	<20	>0.6
Specific gravity	<0.6	>1.016

Data from Refs[5] and[39]

Chest Radiograph

Plain chest radiographs are important in the diagnosis and follow-up of patients with empyema.[26] Posteroanterior views (P/A chest radiograph) are the most frequently used. However, it should be noted that a negative P/A chest radiograph does not rule out the presence of empyema because the volume of the pleural collection must be more than 250 mL before becoming detectable on an erect chest radiograph. A lateral decubitus view, ultrasound scan, in this case, is sensitive for collections as small as 50 to 200 mL. In contrast, supine chest radiographs can mask large quantities of fluid.[26]

The typical radiologic features include blunting of the costophrenic and cardiophrenic angles, presence of fluid within the lung fissures, and a typical air fluid level. In large-volume collections, a mediastinal shift from the side of the effusion to the contralateral aspect can be observed. (**Figs. 4** and **5**).[26]

Ultrasound Scan

An ultrasound scan can be used to detect minimal amounts of fluid, as small as 3 to 5 mL, and is significantly more sensitive than a plain chest radiograph. Ultrasound scan is very effective in guiding aspiration of small pleural volumes and collections located in unusual sites.[26] The ultrasound appearance of an empyema depends on the composition of the collection. Typical findings are of collections that are not uniformly anechoic and are often septate.[27]

However, in low-resource settings), ultrasound scans may not be considered as a first-line investigation for thoracic empyema diagnosis but can be used to define complex collections, or to make diagnoses especially in the absence of radiography or computed tomography (CT). Therefore, it is imperative that health facilities and institutions embark on expansion of training programs and increased access to relevant diagnostic devices to help overcome the barriers of not having reliable CT scanning in these settings.

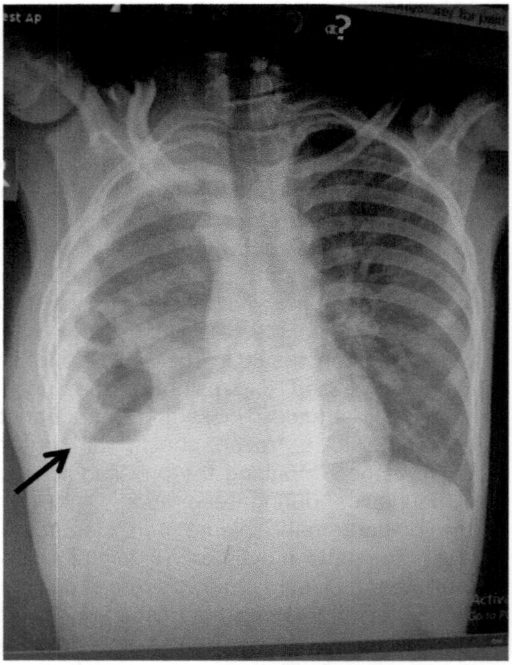

Fig. 4. Posteroanterior chest radiograph from a 37-year-old male, showing right-sided pleural collection. Arrow shows blunting of right costophrenic angle and fluid levels.

Computed Tomographic Scan

The use of CT scan for the diagnosis of pleural collections in low-resource settings is often not routine mainly due to unavailability of the CT scans and radiologists in LIC settings, and emphasis

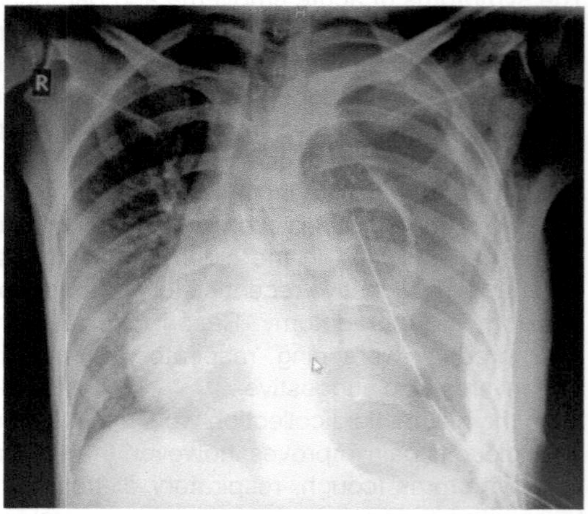

Fig. 5. Posteroanterior chest radiograph from a 22-year-old male patient taken 6 h after insertion of a chest tube for left-sided empyema. Note the significant postprocedure pneumothorax, deviation of the mediastinum to the right side despite the correctly placed chest tube, and the trapped lung.

should be on clinical diagnosis and judicious use of plain chest radiographs and ultrasonography. However, CT provides the best diagnostic opportunity to precisely characterize the location and stage of the disease.[26] CT is also very useful in the identification of small-volume collections and the detection of underlying intrathoracic or abdominal pathologic conditions.

Typical findings include an enhancing thickened pleura known as the split pleural sign, which is due to fibrin coating of both parietal and visceral pleural surfaces and ingrowth of blood vessels.[28] Both layers of the pleura are visualized as linear regions of enhancement that meet at the margins of the collection.[28] This sign is the most reliable one used to distinguish empyema from a peripheral pulmonary abscess. Other findings during CT scan include visible septations, distortion and compression of adjacent lung, associated consolidation, presence or absence of gas locules, and adjacent infections like subdiaphragmatic abscess (**Figs. 6** and **7**).[26]

PRINCIPLES OF TREATMENT

There are 3 objectives in the treatment of thoracic empyema. These objectives include[29]:

1. Control of ongoing infection (sepsis)
2. Evacuation of infected material from the pleural space
3. Reexpansion of the lung

The aforementioned objectives can be achieved by:

1. Appropriate antibiotic therapy with specific emphasis on selection, route of administration, and duration of treatment
2. Drainage of the intrapleural collection
3. Supportive measures to improve patient's general condition (pulmonary physiotherapy, nutritional support and rehabilitation, correction of anemia, and treatment of underlying medical conditions)

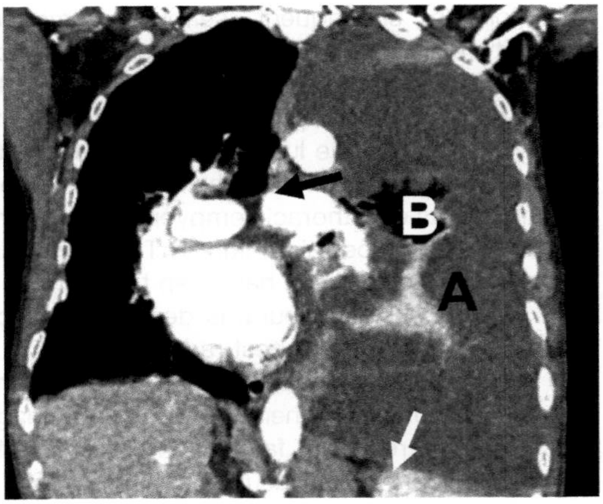

Fig. 6. Coronal section of a chest computed tomographic scan showing left-sided empyema (A) under tension associated with almost complete lung collapse (B), mediastinal deviation to the right (*black arrow*), and depression of the left diaphragm (*white arrow*).

Antibiotic Therapy

All patients with thoracic empyema should receive antibiotic therapy. The choice of antibiotics is best guided by the availability of Gram stain and culture results.[30] In addition, the local antibiotic sensitivity and resistance pattern should be used when decisions are made.[30] When microbiology results are not available or take long time to organize, a combination of third-generation cephalosporin (cefuroxime or ceftriaxone) and metronidazole, or amoxicillin/clavulanic acid and metronidazole should be considered for community-acquired empyema.[30] In hospital-acquired cases, vancomycin plus meropenem is an appropriate choice. The selected antibiotics should be administered IV and converted to oral antibiotics once patients are symptomatically well improved (fever controlled, respiratory rate normalized, feeding well). Antibiotics should also be continued until the chest drainage returns to normal (pus fully drained) and the chest tubes are removed. Antibiotics are to be continued for a total duration of 14 days.[30]

Pleural Space Drainage

Surgical interventions used in the treatment of thoracic empyema include the insertion of a thoracostomy tube (chest tube), simple open drainage (thoracotomy or VATS assisted), thoracotomy with decortication, and thoracic window procedures.

CHEST TUBES

The best way to completely drain the pleural space is by the insertion of a chest tube. Chest tubes are most effective in the exudative and early fibropurulent stage of the empyema. If available, 10F to 14F Seldinger drains can also be tried as first-line treatment in simple exudative effusions. However, larger-sized (28F–32F) chest drains are preferred.[31] The authors discourage the practice of repeated needle thoracentesis because it rarely results in a complete evacuation of the pleural space, is very painful, and predisposes patients to complications. In addition, the exudative stage of empyema is very short and cannot always be detected even during hospital treatment of pneumonia, hence proper chest tube insertion is more favorable than multiple thoracentesis.[25]

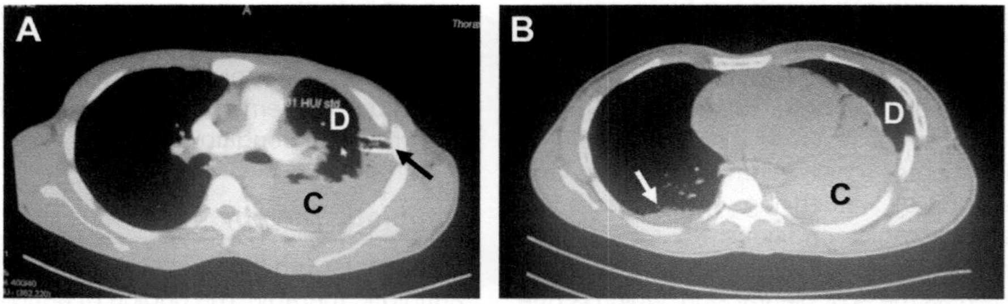

Fig. 7. (*A,B*) Contrast-enhanced axial computed tomographic scan of a young male showing left-sided empyema with significant collection posteriorly (C), and reduced lung volume (D). Note the chest tube on the left side (*arrow*). Minimal collection on the right side is also noted (*arrow*).

Clear indications of chest tube insertion include the presence of purulent, turbid, or cloudy fluid in the pleural cavity, pleural fluid pH less than 7.2, a positive Gram stain or microbiological culture, or the presence of loculations on ultrasonography. Poor progress with antibiotic therapy alone is also another indication. The authors also recommend that a collection of a parapneumonic effusion of more than 500 mL should be drained by chest tube insertion. Chest tubes can be inserted at the bedside or more preferably through the guidance of ultrasonography.[32] However, care must be taken to avoid injury to the lung parenchyma and the diaphragm because chronicity of the condition makes the procedure difficult and risky.

Chest tubes should be kept in situ until there is clinical and radiological evidence of evacuation lung expansion. Evidence of complete evacuations include:[32]

- complete resolution of the patient signs and symptoms (no fever, normal respiratory rate, controlled pleuritic chest pain, and general recovery of patient),
- physical examination evidence of full lung expansion (normal percussion note and audible air entry on the affected side),
- radiologic (chest radiograph) evidence of complete lung expansion, and
- drainage of clear pleural fluid, which is less than 50 to 100 mL, over 24 hours.[32]

It should be recognized that post-chest tube care is as important as the insertion procedure because chest tubes are associated with the development of empyemas.[10,14] Various underwater seal drainage tube improvisations such as the use of intravenous fluid bags and plastic water bottles have been described for low-resource settings; however, improvised drainage systems must be proved to be effective via randomized trials before they are adopted.

Fibrinolysis or Enzymatic Decortication

Fibrinolysis refers to the administration of fibrinolytics through the chest tube into the pleural cavity to facilitate the breakdown of septa in the empyema cavity.[33,34] The enzymes will also help to degrade the necrotic tissue mass. The most commonly used enzyme is streptokinase, which is a proteolytic enzyme that converts plasminogen to plasmin, leading to the breakdown of fibrin in the pleural cavity. Cost, availability, and expertise are limitations to the common use of fibrinolytics in low-income settings.[35,36]

Pleural Space Drainage: Surgical Drainage Procedures

The timing and extent of surgical management of thoracic empyema is still a point of contention and remains controversial.[35] On one hand, early surgical intervention can result in the complete evacuation of the pleural cavity, hence promoting control of sepsis, reduced hospital stays, and reduction in subsequent serious pulmonary morbidity. On the other hand, surgical intervention before an adequate trial of tube drainage and antibiotics could result in significant bleeding, inability to fully decorticate the lung, and serious injury to the lung parenchyma. Hence, the decision to operate on patients with thoracic empyema at the early stage should not be taken lightly. The traditional approach to the decision has been to wait until a clear peel (thickened pleura) is demonstrable on either chest radiograph chest radiograph or CT.

In general, surgical management of empyema thoracis is indicated when chest tube drainage and antibiotic treatment fail to achieve complete resolution,[25,29,30] which usually coincides with a case history of more than just 6 weeks, equivalent to the last stage of the empyema process. The ultimate aim of surgical intervention is to control sepsis and allow complete expansion of the trapped lung.

The techniques used during surgical intervention are the evacuation of all necrotic and purulent materials from the pleural space, decortication or peeling of the organized parietal and visceral pleura, and complete separation of the diaphragm from the lung. Empyemectomy, or the complete enucleating of the infected sac, can also be attempted.[29]

Thoracotomy With or Without Decortication

In low-resource settings, in the absence of advanced surgical techniques such as VATS, open thoracotomy is the best option to achieve complete resolution of the disease.[37] Thoracotomy should be performed when antibiotic therapy and chest tube drainage fail to achieve the desired goal.[37] This usually coincides with the end of the second or the third stage of the disease.

The procedure is performed under general anesthesia (single- or double-lumen intubation), and access to the chest cavity is through a classical posterior lateral incision.[38] However, the incision can be planned preoperatively in cases in which the empyema is loculated to a specific site. Rib resection may sometimes be needed to access the pleural cavity but should be done only if necessary.

Once the cavity is entered, frank pus, debris, fibrinous peel, and dirty tissue should be completely evacuated. All loculi and pockets in the pleural cavity, including sequestered fluid between the lung fissures, should be removed. The cavity must then be thoroughly lavaged and mopped. In most cases, this is sufficient. However, visibly thickened, and restrictive abscess walls can be peeled from the lung and the chest wall, hence allowing the lung to fully expand. However, care must be taken to identify the correct plane between the abscess cavity and the underlying visceral pleura. An unnecessarily aggressive attempt to separate the poorly developed visceral pleura from the lung will result in significant bleeding and the development of several fistulas from the lung surface.

It is highly recommended to submit the pus or fibrinous peel for microbiological study (stain and cultures) to guide postoperative antibiotic use. However, this depends on the availability of such diagnostic facilities.

Lung expansion is considered complete when the lung can come in contact with the chest wall and the diaphragm during positive pressure ventilation. Chest drain, usually 2, should be left in situ after the procedure in all patients and can be removed once air leak stops and daily drainage volume reduces significantly and becomes clean.

It should be noted that the late third stage of the disease that is associated with a fibrothorax, significant trapping of the lungs and significant chest wall deformity, needs the attention of a thoracic surgeon.[29,30,37]

Box 1
Suggested supplies for chest tube insertion

Patient preparation

- Consent forms
- Intravenous canula
- Intravenous fluid
- Infusion giving set

Site and skin preparation

- Sterile gloves
- Sterile gown (optional)
- Sterile drapes
- Skin preparatory antiseptic (chlorhexidine, methylated spirit, or povidone iodine)
- Sterile gauze

Access

- 1% or 2% Lignocaine (combination with longer-acting bupivacaine an advantage for postprocedure analgesia)
- 10-mL syringe with 2 needles for drawing (21G) and infiltrating (23G)
- Surgical blade (scalpel—with blade and handle—preferable)
- Suture set (with hemostats, stitch scissors, needle driver)
- Medium-sized curved artery forceps (or any instrument suitable for blunt dissection)

Insertion

- Chest drain or appropriate improvisation
- Connecting tubing
- Closed drainage system
- Sterile water for underwater seal
- 2 curved clamps
- Gauze piece for padding the tube from clamps
- Closure
- Suture: nylon/silk 0 or 1/0 (any sturdy suture type can be adapted)
- Nonadherent dressing
- Plaster

Box 2
List of equipment needed for open thoracotomy

Patient preparation

- Double lumen endotrachealEndotracheal tube
- General anesthesia
- IV access and IV fluids
- Cross-matched blood
- Antibiotics
- Urinary catheter
- Povidone iodine solution

Thoracotomy and drainage

- Scalpel and scalpel holder
- Artery forceps (different sizes)
- Dissecting forceps
- Scapular retractor
- Finocchio retractors (rib spreader)
- Vascular clamps
- Rib approximator
- Silk, vicryl, and proline sutures

SUMMARY

Empyema thoracis or thoracic empyema is defined as the accumulation of purulent material (usually pus) in the pleural cavity. Pus accumulates between the parietal and the visceral layers of the pleura, hence replacing the normal pleural fluid with such another substance. Most cases of empyema are sequelae of severe pneumonia and often begin as parapneumonic effusion. However pulmonary tuberculosis, chest trauma, and complications of chest tube insertion contribute to a nonnegligible number of cases.

The diagnosis of the disease is usually delayed due to delayed presentation to health care facilities, low index of suspicion among health care professionals, and inability to make a proper diagnosis with the available diagnostic tools, especially in low-resources settings. High prevalence of malnutrition and anemia among patients and lack of proper follow-up of chest tubes contribute to the frequently noted advanced state of the disease in low-resource settings.

If treated early and appropriately, the chances of cure are very high. However, delayed diagnosis and treatment is associated with high morbidity and mortality. Most cases respond well to early initiation of antibiotic therapy with or without drainage; however, close to one-third require surgical intervention. Surgical interventions used in the treatment of thoracic empyema include the insertion of a thoracostomy tube (chest tube), simple open drainage (thoracotomy or VATS assisted), thoracotomy with decortication, and thoracic window procedures. Early use of appropriate-sized and well-placed chest tube drainage is associated with early recovery, decreased hospital stay, decreased cost of treatment, and increased chances of cure. However, chest tubes must be properly followed and removed on time to avoid the dreadful complications of empyema.

The review was written to update the reader on the diagnostic approach and appropriate treatment of thoracic empyema in resource-constrained settings (**Boxes 1** and **2**).

CLINICS CARE POINTS

- The diagnosis of empyema thoracic and pleural effusions in low-resources settings needs a high index of suspicion.
- Clinicians should rely on detailed history, thorough physical examination, prompt chest radiograph, and needle aspiration to make a diagnosis, but pleural collections and thoracic empyema may occur in the absence of the classical symptoms of cough, fever, and pleuritic chest pain.
- A properly performed chest radiograph and chest ultrasonography is very important to support the diagnosis.
- A negative P/A chest radiograph does not rule out the presence of small-volume empyema (250 mL and less); lateral decubitus view or ultrasonography is sensitive for small collections.
- Key principles of treatment are control of ongoing infection (sepsis), evacuation of infected material from the pleural space, and ensuring reexpansion of the lung.
- Repeated needle thoracocentesis should be avoided because it rarely results in a complete evacuation of the pleural space, is very painful, and predisposes patients to complications.
- Early appropriate antibiotics and timely placement of a chest tube are often sufficient treatment of pleural collections in low-resource settings.
- Local microbial sensitivity patterns should always be considered for antibiotic selection; however, a combination of third-generation cephalosporin and metronidazole, or

amoxicillin/clavulanic acid and metronidazole should be considered for community-acquired empyema.

- The decision to operate on patients with thoracic empyema at the early stage should not be taken lightly.
- On one hand, early surgical intervention can result in the complete evacuation of the pleural cavity, hence promoting control of sepsis, reduced hospital stays, and reduction in subsequent serious pulmonary morbidity.
- On the other hand, too aggressive surgical intervention could result in significant bleeding, inability to fully decorticate the lung, and serious injury to the lung parenchyma.
- The traditional approach to the decision for thoracotomy and decortication has been to wait until a clear peel (thickened pleura) is demonstrable on either chest radiograph or CT scan (usually at about 6 weeks of pathology).

DISCLOSURE

The authors declare no commercial or financial conflicts of interest.

REFERENCES

1. Tsoucalas G, Sgantzos M. Hippocrates (ca 460-375 bc), introducing thoracotomy combined with a tracheal intubation for the parapneumonic pleural effusions and empyema thoracis. Surg Innov 2016; 23(6):642–3.
2. Hassan MY, Elmi AM, Baldan M. Experience of thoracic surgery performed under difficult conditions in Somalia. East Cent Afr J Surg 2004;9(1). https://doi.org/10.4314/ecajs.v9i1.
3. Charalampidis C, Youroukou A, Lazaridis G, et al. Pleura space anatomy. J Thorac Dis 2015;7(Suppl 1):S27–32.
4. Light RW. Pleural effusions. Med Clin North Am 2011;95(6):1055–70.
5. Tian P, Qiu R, Wang M, et al. Prevalence, causes, and health care burden of pleural effusions among hospitalized adults in China. JAMA Netw Open 2021;4(8):e2120306.
6. Bobbio A, Bouam S, Frenkiel J, et al. Epidemiology and prognostic factors of pleural empyema. Thorax 2021;76(11):1117–23.
7. Kuti BP, Oyelami OA. Risk factors for parapneumonic effusions among children admitted with community- acquired pneumonia at a tertiary hospital in south-west Nigeria 2014;10(1):9.
8. Risk factors for complicated parapneumonic effusion and empyema on presentation to hospital with community-acquired pneumonia | Thorax. Available at: https://thorax-bmj-com.ezp-prod1.hul.harvard.edu/content/64/7/592. Accessed October 25, 2021.
9. Cargill TN, Hassan M, Corcoran JP, et al. A systematic review of comorbidities and outcomes of adult patients with pleural infection. Eur Respir J 2019;54(3). https://doi.org/10.1183/13993003.00541-2019.
10. Kesieme EB, Dongo A, Ezemba N, Irekpita E, Jebbin N, Kesieme C. Tube Thoracostomy: Complications and Its Management. Pulm Med 2011;2012: e256878.
11. Alfageme I, Muñoz F, Peña N, Umbría S. Empyema of the Thorax in Adults: Etiology, Microbiologic Findings, and Management. Chest 1993;103(3):839–43.
12. Shebl E, Paul M. Parapneumonic pleural effusions and empyema thoracis. In: StatPearls. StatPearls Publishing; 2021. Available at: http://www.ncbi.nlm.nih.gov/books/NBK534297/. Accessed October 25, 2021.
13. Karmy-Jones R, Holevar M, Sullivan RJ, Fleisig A, Jurkovich GJ. Residual hemothorax after chest tube placement correlates with increased risk of empyema following traumatic injury. Can Respir J J Can Thorac Soc 2008;15(5):255–8.
14. Kwiatt M, Tarbox A, Seamon MJ, et al. Thoracostomy tubes: A comprehensive review of complications and related topics. Int J Crit Illn Inj Sci 2014;4(2):143–55.
15. Hassan M, Cargill T, Harriss E, et al. The microbiology of pleural infection in adults: a systematic review. Eur Respir J 2019;54(3):1900542.
16. Maskell NA, Batt S, Hedley EL, Davies CWH, Gillespie SH, Davies RJO. The bacteriology of pleural infection by genetic and standard methods and its mortality significance. Am J Respir Crit Care Med 2006;174(7):817–23.
17. Wen P, Wei M, Han C, He Y, Wang M-S. Risk factors for tuberculous empyema in pleural tuberculosis patients. Sci Rep 2019;9(1):19569.
18. Burgos J, Falcó V, Pahissa A. The increasing incidence of empyema. Curr Opin Pulm Med 2013; 19(4):350–6.
19. Senger SS, Thompson GR, Samanta P, Ahrens J, Clancy CJ, Nguyen MH. Candida Empyema Thoracis at Two Academic Medical Centers: New Insights Into Treatment and Outcomes. Open Forum Infect Dis 2021;8(4):ofaa656.
20. Ayad S, Gergis K, Elkattawy S, et al. Loculated Empyema and SARS-CoV-2 Infection: A Report of Two Cases and Review of the Literature. Eur J Case Rep Intern Med 2021;8(7):002706.
21. Light RW. Parapneumonic effusions and empyema. Proc Am Thorac Soc 2006;3(1):75–80.
22. Andrews NC, Parker EF, Shaw RP, et al. Management of non-tuberculous empyema. Am Rev Respir Dis 1962;85:935–6.

23. Intrapleural Use of Tissue Plasminogen Activator and DNase in Pleural Infection | NEJM. Available at: https://www.nejm.org/doi/full/10.1056/NEJMoa1012740. Accessed November 2, 2021.
24. Pugh CP. Empyema necessitans a rare complication of methicillin-resistant staphylococcus aureus empyema in a child. Pediatr Infect Dis J 2020;39(3): 256–7.
25. Havelock T, Teoh R, Laws D, Gleeson F. Pleural procedures and thoracic ultrasound: British Thoracic Society pleural disease guideline 2010. Thorax 2010;65(Suppl 2):i61–76.
26. Hallifax RJ, Talwar A, Wrightson JM, Edey A, Gleeson FV. State-of-the-art: Radiological investigation of pleural disease. Respir Med 2017;124:88–99.
27. King S, Thomson A. Radiological perspectives in empyema: childhood respiratory infections. Br Med Bull 2002;61(1):203–14.
28. Kraus GJ. The Split Pleura Sign. Radiology 2007; 243(1):297–8.
29. Scarci M, Abah U, Solli P, et al. EACTS expert consensus statement for surgical management of pleural empyema. Eur J Cardiothorac Surg 2015; 48(5):642–53.
30. Shen KR, Bribriesco A, Crabtree T, et al. The American Association for Thoracic Surgery consensus guidelines for the management of empyema. J Thorac Cardiovasc Surg 2017;153(6):e129–46.
31. Porcel JM. Chest tube drainage of the pleural space: a concise review for pulmonologists. Tuberc Respir Dis 2018;81(2):106–15.
32. Chest-Tube Insertion | NEJM. Available at: https://www.nejm.org/doi/full/10.1056/nejmvcm071974. Accessed October 25, 2021.
33. Idell S, Rahman NM. Intrapleural fibrinolytic therapy for empyema and pleural loculation: knowns and unknowns. Ann Am Thorac Soc 2018;15(5):515–7.
34. Maskell NA, Davies CWH, Nunn AJ, et al. U.K. Controlled Trial of Intrapleural Streptokinase for Pleural Infection. N Engl J Med 2005;352(9):865–74.
35. Raveenthiran V. Empyema thoracis: controversies and technical hints. J Indian Assoc Pediatr Surg 2005;10(3):191.
36. Pediatric empyema thoracis management: should the consensus be different for the developing countries? - Journal of Pediatric Surgery. Available at: https://www.jpedsurg.org/article/S0022-3468(19)30516-0/fulltext. Accessed October 25, 2021.
37. Gupta DK, Sharma S. Management of empyema - role of a surgeon. J Indian Assoc Pediatr Surg 2005;10(3):142.
38. Kaufman AJ, Flores RM. Technique of pleurectomy and decortication. Oper Tech Thorac Cardiovasc Surg 2010;15(4):294–306.
39. Light RW, Macgregor MI, Luchsinger PC, Ball WC Jr. Pleural effusions: the diagnostic separation of transudates and exudates. Ann Intern Med 1972;77(4): 507–13. Unpublished others.

Tracheobronchial Surgery in Emerging Countries

Benoit Jacques Bibas, MD[a,b,c], Paulo Henrique Peitl-Gregorio, MD[a], Mariana Rodrigues Cremonese, MD[a], Ricardo Mingarini Terra, MD, PhD[a,b,*]

KEYWORDS

• Tracheal diseases • Airway surgery • Tracheal stenosis • Developing countries • Tracheostomy

KEY POINTS

- The real incidence of postintubation tracheal stenosis in developing countries is probably underrated.
- The high incidence of tracheal diseases in emerging countries has allowed for great expertise in the surgical field and high-volume scientific research.
- Improvement of airway management in intensive care units is mandatory and must be promoted.
- Inclusion of newer technologies, and techniques to prevent airway damage may reduce the incidence of postintubation tracheal stenosis.

INTRODUCTION

Tracheal stenosis is a complex surgical problem that is often mistaken and interpreted as being a simple structural disease. However, tracheal stenosis is a heterogeneous disease in its cause, natural history, and clinical outcome.[1] It derives from various clinical entities, such as iatrogenic airway injuries (ie, postintubation, posttracheostomy), autoimmune diseases (ie, granulomatosis with polyangiitis, relapsing polychondritis, sarcoidosis, amyloidosis), congenital, primary and secondary neoplastic diseases, and idiopathic.[1,2]

Despite improvements in technology, such as low cuff pressure and percutaneous dilation tracheostomy approaches, postintubation tracheal stenosis (PITS) continues to be a major burden, especially in emerging countries.[3] Studies have suggested that some degree of stenosis develops in up to 20% to 30% of patients with tracheostomy, and 1% to 7% of patients develop symptoms with the need for invasive procedures. This results in frequent visits to the emergency department, increased health care costs, and reduced health-related quality of life for the patients.[3,4]

PITS still represents the most common indication for tracheal resection worldwide,[5–8] and airway resection with primary reconstruction remains the definitive treatment modality for benign and malignant tracheal diseases.[6–11]

REGIONAL INCIDENCE

According to Hagmeyer and colleagues,[12] PITS is estimated to occur in 1.8% to 12% of patients after prolonged orotracheal intubation. However, reviews with regional data from emerging countries suggest a higher prevalence of stenosis, which can vary from 2.3% to 17%.[13,14] In fact, the real incidence of PITS in Brazil, as well as in other emerging countries is probably underrated. In Brazil, the proportion of hospitalizations owing to external causes, such as traffic accidents and violence, has increased steadily in recent years, unlike in the developed countries.[15] Pogorzelski

[a] Division of Thoracic Surgery, Instituto do Coracao, Hospital das Clinicas HCFMUSP, Faculdade de Medicina, Universidade de Sao Paulo, Rua Dr. Eneas de Carvalho Aguiar 44, bloco 2, 2° andar, Sala 9, Secretaria de Cirurgia Torácica, São Paulo, São Paulo CEP 05403-904, Brazil; [b] Hospital Israelita Albert Einstein, São Paulo, São Paulo, Brazil; [c] Hospital Municipal Vila Santa Catarina, São Paulo, São Paulo, Brazil
* Corresponding author. Division of Thoracic Surgery, Instituto do Coracao, Hospital das Clinicas HCFMUSP, Faculdade de Medicina, Universidade de Sao Paulo, Rua Dr. Eneas de Carvalho Aguiar 44, bloco 2, 2° andar, Sala 9, Secretaria de Cirurgia Torácica, São Paulo, São Paulo CEP 05403-904, Brazil.
E-mail address: rmterra@uol.com.br

Thorac Surg Clin 32 (2022) 373–381
https://doi.org/10.1016/j.thorsurg.2022.04.004

and colleagues[16] analyzed the trauma patients admitted in the intensive care unit (ICU) of a tertiary healthy public system hospital. They reported that 48.2% of patients had a Glasgow Coma Score $\leq$8 at the trauma site, where the conditions of laryngoscopy and intubation are not ideal and can result in laryngotracheal lesions. At the authors' institution, most patients with postintubation stenosis are trauma victims with head injuries that are often submitted to tracheostomy at the primary care center before they are referred to the authors' center. At present, more than 80% of the authors' patients with subglottic or tracheal stenosis have a tracheostomy tube when referred to their institution.[4,7,9]

The high number of surgical resections for PITS can be seen as a surrogate of the total number of cases. Farzanegan and colleagues[14] reported a total of 2167 operated patients in Iran over the course of 24 years. At the authors' institution, for the last 12 years, they have constantly operated on 20 to 30 patients each year.[1,7,9,17–19] Such high numbers reflect a breach in the proper airway care of mechanically ventilated patients. The culprit for such "epidemic" is probably multifactorial, and a thorough analysis of the predictors for development would be important. Unfortunately, the incidence of PITS will not decrease in the upcoming years because the COVID-19 pandemic has put a severe strain on the health care systems, with thousands of patients submitted to prolonged mechanical ventilation.

CLINICAL RELEVANCE

Patients with laryngotracheal stenosis often experience dyspnea, stridor, phonation ablation, dysphonia, and dysphagia. It can lead to significant morbidity and may progress to acute airway compromise if not properly managed.[6,7] Furthermore, benign tracheal stenosis with tracheostomy is associated with an overall poor health-related quality of life, with severe physical and mental impact.[4]

Moreover, the costs associated with tracheal injuries are overwhelming. Bhatti and colleagues[20] performed a cost analysis using the Agency for Healthcare Research and Quality 2006 National Inpatient Sample and compared patients with tracheal injury coded during the medical or surgical stay for length of stay (LOS) and mean hospital cost with diagnosis-related matched controls. A total of 3232 discharge records met criteria for tracheal injury from within the index hospital stay. Average LOS for patients with tracheal injury (6.3 days) exceeded LOS in the uncomplicated sample (5.2 days) by 1.1 days. The average hospital cost was US$1888 higher with tracheal injury ($10,375 [confidence interval (CI), $9762-$10,988] vs $8487 [CI, $8266-$8669]). LOS for procedures treating prior tracheal injury averaged 4.7 days, and cost averaged $11,025 per discharge.

SURGICAL RESEARCH IN EMERGING COUNTRIES

The high incidence of tracheal diseases in emerging countries has allowed for great expertise in the surgical field, as well as opportunity for high-volume scientific research. Over the last 2 decades, the experience of institutions from Brazil and other emerging countries has been published. Nevertheless, scientific evidence in this area relies mainly on retrospective single-center studies.

The authors' experience with airway surgery began in the early 2000s, and they published their first article in 2008.[21] In this report, the authors presented the case of a patient with symptomatic idiopathic stenosis that had multiple endoscopic dilations. After the diagnosis of gastroesophageal reflux disease (GERD) was established, she was treated accordingly, and all her respiratory symptoms subsided. A close relationship between anti-GERD therapy and the clinical outcome was noted.

This led the authors to investigate the role of GERD in the pathogenesis of tracheal stenosis. In 2019, Bianchi and colleagues[19] published a large retrospective study with 175 patients with benign tracheal stenosis. The patients were submitted to esophageal manometry and dual-probe 24-hour ambulatory esophageal pH study. Patients with an abnormal pH study were managed with laparoscopic-modified Nissen fundoplication or medical treatment (omeprazole 80 mg/d, orally). Patients with normal pH study results were observed. After propensity score matching, the outcome of tracheal stenosis in the fundoplication group was similar to that of the observation group (odds ratio [OR], 1; P = .99) and better than that of the omeprazole group (OR, 5.31; P = .03). The observation (no gastroesophageal reflux) group had a better outcome of stenosis than those treated with omeprazole (OR, 3.54; P = .02). This is relevant information because GERD may have a negative impact on the outcome after tracheal resection and reconstruction, which is a subject of great interest at the authors' division.

In 2009, the authors published a case series of 20 patients with severe glottic/subglottic stenosis that was submitted to laryngeal split with anterior and posterior interposition of a rib cartilage graft, with a final decannulation of 80%, with low morbidity and no mortality. Even though the series demonstrated good surgical results, the authors sought to investigate if predictors for complications in Brazil were the same as the ones published in the developed countries.[6] The authors conducted a retrospective analysis that encompassed 94 patients with tracheal stenosis that were operated on during a 7-year period.[7] Of those who underwent surgery during the study period, 42 (44.6%) had some sort of complication. Twenty patients (21%) had anastomotic complications. The most common complication was restenosis, which occurred in 16% of the patients. The presence of comorbidities (OR, 7.0; P = .013), previous tracheal resection (OR, 49.9; P = .012), and the length of tracheal resection greater than 4 cm (OR, 5.1; P = .001) were the statistically significant factors for the onset of complications.

Benign postintubation tracheoesophageal fistulas (TEF) have also been a subject of study.[9,11] In 2016, the authors retrospectively analyzed the charts of 20 patients that were operated on with this diagnosis over a 10-year period.[9] Although surgical results were good, the procedure had a high morbidity, and nonnegligible mortality. There was 1 dehiscence of the tracheal anastomosis, and 1 procedure-related death (5%). Closure of the TEF occurred in 95% of cases. Two patients had tracheal stenosis recurrence, and 1 patient had both TEF and tracheal stenosis recurrence. The complexity of this treatment is depicted in **Table 1**. It is also worth mentioning the contribution to this topic by Camargo and colleagues.[22] In a retrospective analysis, the investigators question the use of the muscle flap to buttress the esophageal suture from leakage. In their experience, the use of the muscle flap is not necessary and could, in theory, reduce the lumen of the airway anastomosis. Also of interest is the report of Gurram and colleagues,[23] from India. The investigators reported an innovative technique to staple the TEF with the use of an endostapler and interposition with sternocleidomastoid muscle flap through a cervical approach, with good results. Nonetheless, this requires a normal airway lumen. Otherwise, a formal airway resection and reconstruction will be required.

Currently, at the authors' institution, every patient with tracheal stenosis, or other airway diseases, is evaluated at the outpatient clinic. It is mandatory to perform a larynx and trachea computed tomographic scan and an airway endoscopy before resection procedures. Those examinations are complementary and provide different information regarding the areas affected by the stenosis. It is of utmost importance to clearly define the target area to be operated on, and to understand the level of the stenosis. The authors categorize the affected airway into the 3 following subgroups:

1. No laryngeal involvement: Surgery will consist of a primary airway end-to-end anastomosis
2. Involvement of the anterior plate of the cricoid cartilage without glottic stenosis: Surgery will consist of a primary airway anastomosis (tracheal-thyroid cartilage). This may or not be accompanied by a protective tracheostomy, at the surgeon's intraoperative judgment.
3. Involvement/destruction of the posterior plate of the cricoid cartilage with high laryngotracheal stenosis (<10 mm from the vocal folds): Surgery will consist of laryngeal split and rib cartilage interpositional grafting.

Other rarer conditions are more frequent in developing countries, such as blind-end subglottic stenosis (Myer-Cotton IV) and tracheobronchial stenosis due to tuberculosis. The Myer-Cotton grading system is used to measure the severity of subglottic or tracheal stenosis.[30] The grading system is as follows: grade 1: 0% to 50% obstruction; grade 2: 51% to 70% obstruction; grade 3: 71% to 99% obstruction; and grade 4: no detectable airway lumen. Recently, the authors proposed a method for managing long-segment blind-end subglottic stenosis with a hybrid (endoscopic-surgical) approach.[10] The technique is innovative in that the surgeon can safely place a silicone T-tube in a Myer-Cotton IV stenosis without exposing the patient to a high-risk operation. This allows immediate return of nasal breathing and voice, which is highly beneficial (**Fig. 1**).

An equally interesting article was published by Pulle and colleagues,[31] which reported a retrospective analysis of a prospectively maintained database at a dedicated thoracic surgical unit in New Delhi, India, regarding patients with tracheal and tracheobronchial stenosis owing to tuberculosis infection. It included 20 patients with very complex diseases. In most patients, the left main bronchus was involved. Cases were managed with intricate lung-preserving operations that involved the main carina (bronchial sleeve resection and sleeve lobectomy), whereas some cases required pneumonectomy, with good surgical outcomes.

CURRENT CONTROVERSIES

Airway Management in Intensive Care Units

Providing the best available resources for procedures like endotracheal intubation or tracheostomy and delivering high-quality care during the use of airway devices are pivotal in preventing

Table 1
Complications and recurrence after surgical treatment of benign tracheoesophageal fistula

Studies	N	Morbidity (%)	Mortality (%)	TEF Recurrence (%)
Baisi et al,[24] 1999	29	NR	3.4	0
Macchiarini et al,[25] 2000	32	22	3.1	3.2
Camargo et al,[22] 2010	16	25	0	0
Shen et al,[26] 2010	21	54.3	5.7	8.6
Muniappan et al,[27] 2013	74	56	2.8	11
Bibas et al,[9] 2016	20	55	5	5
Puma et al,[28] 2017	10	50	10	10
Qureshi et al,[29] 2018	8	37.5	12.5	0
Gurram et al,[23] 2020	11	27.2	0	0

Abbreviation: NR, not reported.

undesirable airway diseases that pose a challenge for thoracic surgeons to treat in developing countries. The use of videolaryngoscopes for endotracheal intubation is an example of a resource that has still not been widely implemented in emerging countries owing to financial restrictions. Unfortunately, the price of many devices used for airway management, not limited to videolaryngoscopes, discourages most hospitals from acquiring them despite the undeniable benefits. Also, routine practices that mitigate the risk of laryngotracheal complications, such as repeated measurement of the cuff pressure, appropriate endotracheal tube fixation, and decannulation protocols, are far from being standardized, resulting in an abnormally high rate of tracheobronchial complications.[32]

Sadly, the association of all those factors leads to an elevated rate of complications related to airway management in ICUs that include TEF, postintubation tracheal rupture, and acquired laryngotracheal stenosis. The repair of those lesions frequently involves using scarce resources in most hospitals in developing countries, like tracheal stents and/or extracorporeal membrane oxygenation. For example, Grewal and colleagues[33] in 2019 reviewed the main articles concerning tracheal rupture and proposed a treatment algorithm including the use of the abovementioned devices. The fulfillment of all the proposed recommendations is probably intangible in several institutions, which usually only have more common tools for approaching those complications, including ordinary silicon stents and adjustable flange/double-lumen tracheostomy tubes. A case of a long-segment tracheal laceration that was treated with direct suture through a cervical tracheostomy incision is depicted in **Fig. 2**.

Surgical Outcomes in Developed versus Emerging Countries

PITS accounts for most of the cases of benign tracheal stenosis around the world. However, in North America and Europe, this predominance is less pronounced and, recently, a slow shift may

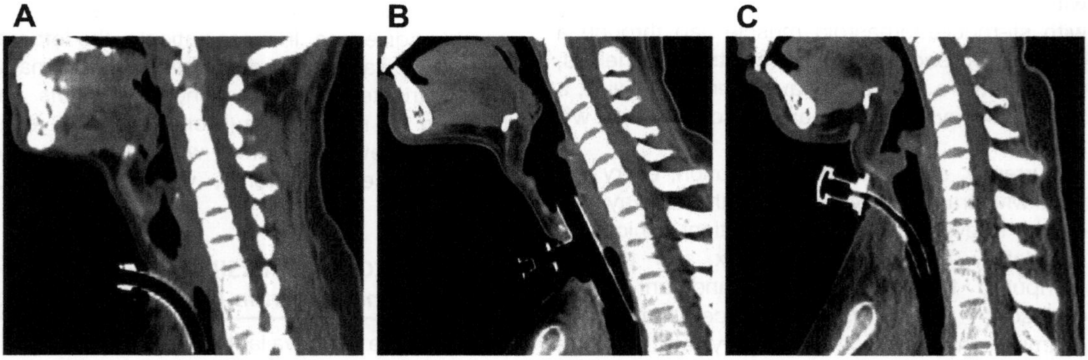

Fig. 1. (*A*) Long-segment (3.5 cm) blind-end tracheal stenosis. (*B*) T-tube in place after hybrid desobstruction technique. (*C*) Patient was submitted to tracheal resection and reconstruction with a protective tracheostomy. He was decannulated 10 days after surgery.

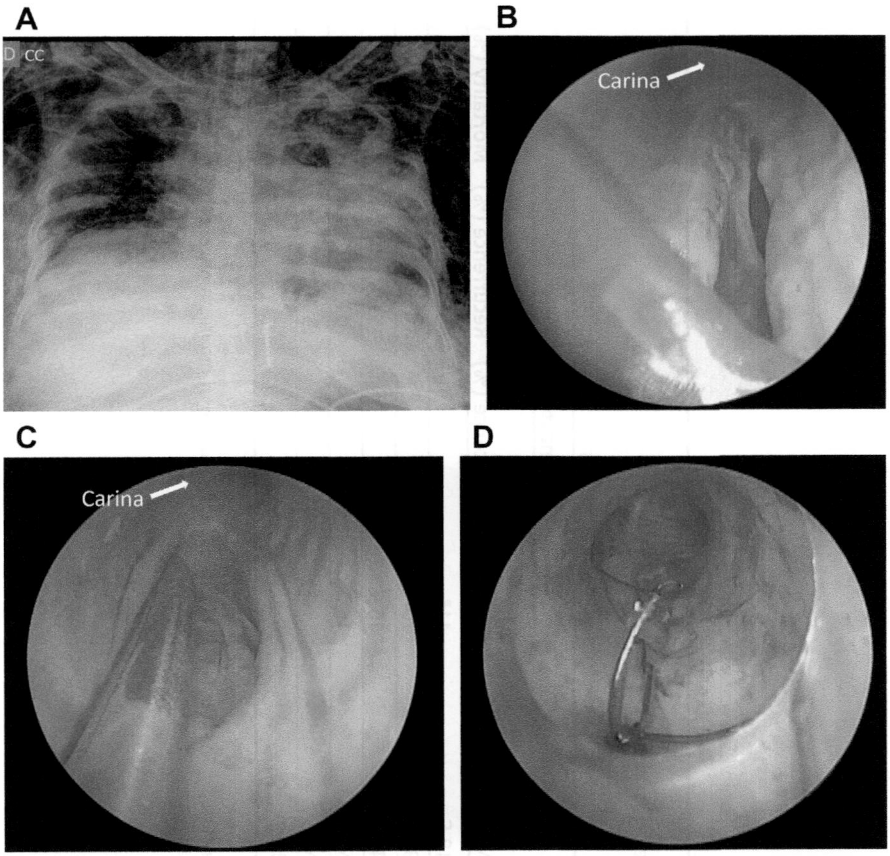

Fig. 2. (*A*) A 62-year-old woman was intubated due to pulmonary sepsis and developed massive subcutaneous and mediastinal emphysema. (*B*) The patient underwent a flexible bronchoscopy that identified a long-segment airway laceration that extended down to the main carina. (*C*) A small cervicotomy and tracheotomy were performed to address the laceration. Upper gastrointestinal endoscopy did not show esophageal rupture. (*D*) Direct suture of the laceration was performed using a 5 mm/30° rigid scope and a long video-assisted thoracoscopic surgery needle holder. Airway suture was performed with a running suture of 4-0 PDS. A tracheostomy cannula was left in place and removed 15 days after.

be occurring toward other causes, such as idiopathic diseases.[5] In emerging countries, PITS is still responsible for more than 90% of the cases of tracheal stenosis. This number may increase following the COVID-19 pandemic, considering that thousands of patients were under prolonged invasive mechanical ventilation in hospitals where, because of insufficient resources, the best practices regarding endotracheal tube management and tracheostomy might not have been followed thoroughly.[34]

To date, there are no comparative studies between developed and emerging countries regarding demographics, perioperative/intraoperative characteristics, and surgical outcomes of patients submitted to tracheobronchial reconstruction. However, a brief review of the literature over the last 2 decades allows us to infer that those factors, which are summarized in **Table 2**, are quite different. A higher male predominance and younger patients are more frequent in developing countries, which may be due to the event that led to the intubation before the PITS. Abbasidezfouli and colleagues[35] and Mohsen and colleagues[36] found that trauma was the cause of intubation in 66.8% and 40.3% of their PITS patients, respectively. In the authors' center, trauma is also the leading cause of referred patients with tracheal stenosis with a large margin.

Socioeconomic variables, including the access to health care in emerging countries, also have a putative role in the challenging treatment of tracheal diseases. The time between intubation and definitive surgery may reach almost 2 years in locations where access to specialized centers is poor.[6] During this period, the individual may be

Table 2
Patient characteristics, stenosis cause, and surgical outcomes of tracheal resection

						Complications				
							Anastomotic			
Country	PITS (%)	Men (%)	Age (y)	Previous Tracheostomy	Lesion Length (cm)	Nonanastomotic (%)	Total (%)	Dehiscence (%)	Recurrence (%)	Mortality (%)
USA[6]	85.0	53.3	42.6	42.6%	3.3	18.5	11[a]	—	—	1.4
Italy[5]	80.3	57.4	44.8	NA	3.5	9.6	7.4	1.3	6.1	0
Brazil[7]	91.3	81	31.2	72%	2.9	44	16.9	1.0	15.9	0
Iran[35]	86.6	72.2	25.4	60.7%	3.8	NA	16.2	6.0[a,b]	10.2	NA
Egypt[36]	86.5	71.1	34.5	NA	4.4	NA	13.4	0	13.4	NA
India[37]	96.9	75.3	31.0	29.2%	3.3	12.3	6.1	3	NA	1.5

Abbreviation: NA, not applicable.
[a] This proportion has not been divided in dehiscence and recurrence in the original study. The number also includes the formation of granulation tissue.
[b] Originally reported as anastomosis infection.

submitted to several procedures, which delay a definitive treatment, and which could make it more challenging. Tracheostomy before tracheal resection, which some investigators have suggested as a risk factor for anastomotic complications, exceeds rates of 60% and 70% in studies published in Iran and Brazil, respectively.[6,7,35]

The criteria for a general postoperative complication or a successful tracheobronchial reconstruction depend on several parameters that vary across different studies. For this reason, anastomotic complications, which are usually reported, might be regarded as a surrogate when comparing the surgical outcomes in tracheobronchial surgery. The rates of anastomotic complications, also described in **Table 2**, in developed countries are commonly lower than 10%. For example, Maurizi and colleagues[5] recently published a series with 228 subjects, on which they achieved an impressive low proportion (7.4%) of anastomosis dehiscence and/or stenosis recurrence. Unfortunately, in emerging countries, anastomotic complications commonly may affect up to 16.9% of the surgical patients, with particular emphasis on stenosis recurrence that accounts for most of those cases.

Role of Genotype in the Development of Postintubation Tracheal Stenosis

In the era of personalized medicine, discovering genetic profiles that pose an increased risk of developing tracheal stenosis might be a turning point in how to deal with this condition. The first studies searching for genetic markers associated with acquired stenosis were only published in the last decade. Anis and colleagues[38] compared 53 patients with PITS versus 85 control subjects that did not develop stenosis after intubation and sought to analyze if single nucleotide polymorphisms of specific wound healing genes could be associated with the development of PITS. Although no differences were found in the overall group, a subgroup analysis showed an increased frequency of a specific genetic maker among African Americans with PITS.

Indirect signs of abnormal wound healing have also been investigated as a risk factor for developing tracheal stenosis after intubation. A Chinese study reviewed 133 patients with subglottic stenosis and grouped them as those with a previous history of keloid and those who had not (nonkeloid).[39] Patients with keloid had a higher proportion (83.3% vs 25.7%) of lesions classified as Myer and Cotton grading III/IV, and the time to develop stenosis after intubation was shorter (27 days vs 41 days) in this group as well. Also, the incidence of stenosis was higher in the keloid group (19.4% vs 1.82%, $P < .001$), and a significantly lower cure rate was observed.

Establishing genetic or clinical signs that turn an intubated patient into a potential candidate for the development of tracheal stenosis is still incipient. Nevertheless, the progress on those discoveries may soon provide new tools to overcome the current limitations and drawbacks on tracheal stenosis treatment, such as recurrent restenosis after several tries of endoscopic and/or surgical procedures some patients experience.

FUTURE PERSPECTIVES

International Databases in Tracheal Diseases

Considering the peculiarity of tracheal diseases as well as the evolving scenario of tracheal surgery characterized by high complexity and rapid technical advances, the need of a multi-institutional database for tracheal operative procedures is clear. During the last 4 years, the European Society of Thoracic Surgeons (ESTS) and the Brazilian Society of Thoracic Surgery started a joint project to create a registry for collecting information about airways surgery. The final goal of this international project is the creation of a dedicated airways surgery registry that could contribute to extract information, standardize practice, and increase the quality of care for patients affected by tracheal diseases and submitted to operative treatments.[40,41]

In January 2018, the ESTS Laryngotracheal Database was officially announced by the ESTS as an international registry, co-chaired by Brazil and Europe. It was formally presented during the symposium "Management of Laryngotracheal Problems III," held in Vienna in March 2018. Currently, final arrangements are still underway. Once the database is ready, it will be launched to the entire ESTS and BSTS membership. Thus, relevant and quality information will be available in order to advance the knowledge in airway surgery and perhaps compare the differences between tracheal diseases in emerging and developed countries.[40,41]

Early Diagnosis and Tracheal Replacement

Murgu and colleagues[42] showed that the addition of radial probe Endobronchial Ultra-sound and optical coherence tomography to the standard bronchoscopy might help identify in vivo real-time changes in airway wall structures and hypertrophic stenotic tissues. The multimodality imaging could potentially assist in treatment plan, providing a precise and objective evaluation and replacing the subjective visually assessment of the extent of stenosis and avoiding collateral damage to airway mucosa and airway cartilage.

Extensive tracheal replacement remains one of the greatest challenges in thoracic surgery when direct end-to-end anastomosis is impossible or has failed. Different attempts to achieve it using diverse approaches have been made, including synthetic prosthesis, allografts, autologous tissue composite, tracheal transplantation, and tissue engineering. None of them has been shown to be the ideal tracheal replacement. However, promising results have been obtained with some of them, as shown by tracheal transplantation and free forearm flap reinforced with cartilage struts. Compared with tracheal transplantation, indications for autologous replacement can be extended to malignant tumors, as no immunosuppressive therapy is required. The absence of a mucociliary respiratory epithelium is the main limitation for autologous reconstruction, requiring aggressive management of postoperative secretions. Further research in tracheal replacement is necessary in order to optimize existing techniques, discover new ones, and understand the complex physiopathology behind tissue regeneration and stem cell use.[43]

SUMMARY

In conclusion, PITS is still widely common in developing countries. The high incidence is multifactorial, but probably related to a high number of severe traumas and inadequate airway management in ICUs. The challenge for thoracic surgeons in developing countries is to reduce the number of airway-related complications and to diagnose lesions before significant scarring occurs. Incorporation of newer technologies and better understanding of the scarring process will lead to better outcomes.

DISCLOSURE

The authors have no conflict of interest to report regarding this article.

REFERENCES

1. Cardoso PFG, Bibas BJ, Minamoto H, et al. Prophylaxis and treatment of complications after tracheal resection. Thorac Surg Clin 2018;28(2):227–41.
2. Tamagno M, Bibas BJ, Minamoto H, et al. Subglottic and mediastinal hemangioma in a child: treatment with propranolol. J Bras Pneumol 2011;37(3):416–8. English, Portuguese.
3. Bibas BJ, Cardoso PFG, Hoetzenecker K. The burden of tracheal stenosis and tracheal diseases healthcare costs in the 21st century. Transl Cancer Res 2020;9(3):2095–6.
4. Bibas BJ, Cardoso PFG, Salati M, et al. Health-related quality of life evaluation in patients with non-surgical benign tracheal stenosis. J Thorac Dis 2018;10(8):4782–8.
5. Maurizi G, Vanni C, Rendina EA, et al. Surgery for laryngotracheal stenosis: Improved results. J Thorac Cardiovasc Surg 2021;161(3):845–52.
6. Wright CD, Grillo HC, Wain JC, et al. Anastomotic complications after tracheal resection: prognostic factors and management. J Thorac Cardiovasc Surg 2004;128(5):731–9.
7. Bibas BJ, Terra RM, Oliveira Junior AL, et al. Predictors for postoperative complications after tracheal resection. Ann Thorac Surg 2014;98(1):277–82.
8. Hoetzenecker K, Schweiger T, Roesner I, et al. A modified technique of laryngotracheal reconstruction without the need for prolonged postoperative stenting. J Thorac Cardiovasc Surg 2016;152(4):1008–17.
9. Bibas BJ, Guerreiro Cardoso PF, Minamoto H, et al. Surgical management of benign acquired tracheoesophageal fistulas: a ten-year experience. Ann Thorac Surg 2016;102(4):1081–7.
10. Rodrigues Cremonese M, Bibas BJ, Minamoto H, et al. Hybrid desobstruction of blind-end subglottic stenosis with long-term stenting. Ann Thorac Surg 2021;112(6):e393–5.
11. Bibas BJ, Cardoso PFG, Minamoto H, et al. Surgery for intrathoracic tracheoesophageal and bronchoesophageal fistula. Ann Transl Med 2018;6(11):210.
12. Hagmeyer L, Oesterlee U, Treml M, et al. Successful weaning and decannulation after interventional bronchoscopic recanalization of tracheal stenosis. J Crit Care 2014;29(4):695 e9-14. https://doi.org/10.1016/j.jcrc.2014.03.023. PMID: 24793660.
13. Forte V. Ressecção da estenose traqueal pós-intubação com reconstrução da traqueia por anastomose laríngeo, crico ou traqueotraqueal: análise clínica e cirúrgica. [Tese Livre-Docência]. São Paulo: Universidade Federal de São Paulo, Escola Paulista de Medicina; 1996. p. 206.
14. Farzanegan R, Zangi M, Abbasidezfouli A, et al. Postintubation multisegmental tracheal stenosis: a 24-year experience. Ann Thorac Surg 2021;112(4):1101–8.
15. GBD 2015 Disease and Injury Incidence and Prevalence Collaborators. Global, regional, and national incidence, prevalence, and years lived with disability for 310 diseases and injuries, 1990-2015: a systematic analysis for the Global Burden of Disease Study 2015. Lancet 2016;388(10053):1545–602. Erratum in: Lancet. 2017;389(10064):e1. PMID: 27733282; PMCID: PMC5055577.
16. Pogorzelski GF, Silva TA, Piazza T, et al. Epidemiology, prognostic factors, and outcome of trauma

patients admitted in a Brazilian intensive care unit. Open Access Emerg Med 2018;10:81–8.
17. Terra RM, Minamoto H, Carneiro F, et al. Laryngeal split and rib cartilage interpositional grafting: treatment option for glottic/subglottic stenosis in adults. J Thorac Cardiovasc Surg 2009;137(4):818–23.
18. Terra RM, Bibas BJ, Minamoto H, et al. Decannulation in tracheal stenosis deemed inoperable is possible after long-term airway stenting. Ann Thorac Surg 2013;95(2):440–4.
19. Bianchi ET, Guerreiro Cardoso PF, Minamoto H, et al. Surgery of the Digestive Tract Group. Impact of fundoplication for gastroesophageal reflux in the outcome of benign tracheal stenosis. J Thorac Cardiovasc Surg 2019;158(6):1698–706.
20. Bhatti NI, Mohyuddin A, Reaven N, et al. Cost analysis of intubation-related tracheal injury using a national database. Otolaryngol Head Neck Surg 2010;143(1):31–6.
21. Terra RM, de Medeiros IL, Minamoto H, et al. Idiopathic tracheal stenosis: successful outcome with antigastroesophageal reflux disease therapy. Ann Thorac Surg 2008;85(4):1438–9.
22. Camargo JJ, Machuca TN, Camargo SM, et al. Surgical treatment of benign tracheo-oesophageal fistulas with tracheal resection and oesophageal primary closure: is the muscle flap really necessary? Eur J Cardiothorac Surg 2010;37(3):576–80.
23. Gurram RP, Gnanasekaran S, Kalayarasan R, et al. Stapled Repair of Benign Acquired Tracheoesophageal Fistula: Description of Novel Technique and Assessment of Outcomes. Cureus 2020;12(8): e9854.
24. Baisi A, Bonavina L, Narne S, et al. Benign tracheoesophageal fistula: results of surgical therapy. Dis Esophagus 1999;12(3):209–11.
25. Macchiarini P, Verhoye JP, Chapelier A, et al. Evaluation and outcome of different surgical techniques for postintubation tracheoesophageal fistulas. J Thorac Cardiovasc Surg 2000;119(2):268–76.
26. Shen KR, Allen MS, Cassivi SD, et al. Surgical management of acquired nonmalignant tracheoesophageal and bronchoesophageal fistulae. Ann Thorac Surg 2010;90(3):914–8 [discussion: 919].
27. Muniappan A, Wain JC, Wright CD, et al. Surgical treatment of nonmalignant tracheoesophageal fistula: a thirty-five-year experience. Ann Thorac Surg 2013;95(4):1141–6.
28. Puma F, Vannucci J, Santoprete S, et al. Surgery and perioperative management for post-intubation tracheoesophageal fistula: case series analysis. J Thorac Dis 2017;9(2):278–86.
29. Qureshi YA, Muntzer Mughal M, Markar SR, et al. The surgical management of non-malignant aerodigestive fistula. J Cardiothorac Surg 2018;13(1):113.
30. Myer CM 3rd, O'Connor DM, Cotton RT. Proposed grading system for subglottic stenosis based on endotracheal tube sizes. Ann Otol Rhinol Laryngol 1994;103(4 Pt 1):319–23.
31. Pulle MV, Asaf BB, Puri HV, et al. Surgical intervention is safe, feasible, and effective in tubercular tracheobronchial stenosis. Lung India 2021;38(3): 245–51.
32. Stauffer JL, Olson DE, Petty TL. Complications and consequences of endotracheal intubation and tracheotomy. A prospective study of 150 critically ill adult patients. Am J Med 1981;70(1):65–76.
33. Grewal HS, Dangayach NS, Ahmad U, et al. Treatment of Tracheobronchial Injuries: A Contemporary Review. Chest 2019;155(3):595–604.
34. Piazza C, Filauro M, Dikkers FG, et al. Long-term intubation and high rate of tracheostomy in COVID-19 patients might determine an unprecedented increase of airway stenoses: a call to action from the European Laryngological Society. Eur Arch Otorhinolaryngol 2021;278(1):1–7.
35. Abbasidezfouli A, Akbarian E, Shadmehr MB, et al. The etiological factors of recurrence after tracheal resection and reconstruction in post-intubation stenosis. Interact Cardiovasc Thorac Surg 2009;9(3): 446–9.
36. Mohsen T, Abou Zeid A, Abdelfattah I, et al. Outcome after long-segment tracheal resection: study of 52 cases. Eur J Cardiothorac Surg 2018; 53(6):1186–91.
37. Puri HV, Asaf BB, Mundale VV, et al. Predictors of Anastomotic Complications After Resection and Anastomosis for Tracheal Stenosis. Indian J Otolaryngol Head Neck Surg 2021;73(4):447–54.
38. Anis MM, Krynetskaia N, Zhao Z, et al. Determining Candidate Single Nucleotide Polymorphisms in Acquired Laryngotracheal Stenosis. Laryngoscope 2018;128(3):E111–6.
39. Chang E, Wu L, Masters J, et al. Iatrogenic subglottic tracheal stenosis after tracheostomy and endotracheal intubation: A cohort observational study of more severity in keloid phenotype. Acta Anaesthesiol Scand 2019;63(7):905–12.
40. Ruiz Tsukazan MT, Terra RM, Bibas BJ, et al. An adaptation of the Hungarian model: the Brazilian model. J Thorac Dis 2018;10(Suppl 29):S3511–5.
41. Salati M, Bibas BJ. Databases in tracheal diseases. Transl Cancer Res 2020;9(3):2149–53.
42. Murgu SD, Colt HG, Mukai D, et al. Multimodal imaging guidance for laser ablation in tracheal stenosis. Laryngoscope 2010;120(9):1840–6.
43. Etienne H, Fabre D, Gomez Caro A, et al. Tracheal replacement. Eur Respir J 2018;51(2):1702211.

Lung Cancer Management in Low and Middle-Income Countries

Sabita Jiwnani, MCh, MRCS[a,*], Prasanth Penumadu, MS, MCh[b], Apurva Ashok, MS[c], C.S. Pramesh, MS, FRCS[d]

KEYWORDS

• Low- and middle-income countries • Lung cancer • Disparities • Tobacco • Advanced stage

KEY POINTS

- Increasing tobacco usage and high prevalence of air pollution are chief etiologic factors.
- Most patients present in advanced stage due to misdiagnosis, lack of screening programs, and inequitable access to health care.
- Low and middle-income countries need to develop accessible and low-cost, high-quality programs to strengthen cancer prevention, early detection, treatment, and palliation.

INTRODUCTION

Low- and middle-income countries (LMICs)[1] have witnessed a rise in mortality due to noncommunicable diseases in the last 2 decades.[2] Although cancer accounted for 9.3 million annual deaths globally, most of these deaths occurred in LMICs. Even though high-income countries (HICs) have a higher incidence of cancer, cancer-related mortality is significantly higher in LMICs. It is expected that by 2030, cancer-related mortality in LMICs will account for 75% of global cancer deaths.[3] Factors for the increase in cancer worldwide are an aging population, tobacco and alcohol use, increasing obesity, sedentary lifestyles, and dietary factors.[4] LMICs are facing a burgeoning of these risk factors and are unable to manage the rising cancer burden due to lack of awareness, late presentation and limited resources for diagnosis and treatment.[5,6] The Global Adult Tobacco Survey conducted in 2016 to 2017 in India showed that close to 30% of Indians consume tobacco, either smoked or smokeless.[7] To compound the problem, scarce health care resources which include not only diagnostic modalities such imaging and pathology but also preventive and primary care services and specialized cancer centers are often inequitably distributed.[4]

Worldwide, lung cancer constitutes 11.4% of the total cancers making it the second most frequently diagnosed cancer and the leading cause of cancer death (18% of the total cancer deaths).[8] The highest incidence of lung cancer is seen in Micronesia/Polynesia, Eastern and Southern Europe, Eastern Asia, and Western Asia, whereas Africa has a low incidence rate.[8] China has a high incidence of lung cancer, including Chinese women, due to smoking, air pollution and use of household cooking fuel.[8,9] Lung cancer is the third most common cancer in Latin America and

[a] Division of Thoracic Surgery, Department of Surgical Oncology, Tata Memorial Centre, Homi Bhabha National Institute, India; [b] Department of Surgical Oncology, Jawaharlal Institute of Medical Education and Research, JIPMER, 5343, 3rd Floor, SSB, Gorimedu, Pondicherry 605006, India; [c] Division of Thoracic Surgery, Department of Surgical Oncology, Tata Memorial Centre, Homi Bhabha National Institute, Tata Memorial Hospital, 3rd Floor, Dr. E. Borges Road, Parel, Mumbai 400012, India; [d] Division of Thoracic Surgery, Department of Surgical Oncology, Tata Memorial Centre, Homi Bhabha National Institute, Tata Memorial Hospital, Main Building, Ground Floor, Dr. E. Borges Road, Parel, Mumbai 400012, India
* Corresponding author. 1217, 12th floor, Homi Bhabha Block, Tata Memorial Hospital, Dr. E. Borges Road, Parel, Mumbai 400012, India
E-mail address: sabitajiwnani@gmail.com

Thorac Surg Clin 32 (2022) 383–395
https://doi.org/10.1016/j.thorsurg.2022.04.005

Caribbean Region.[8] It is the fourth most common cancer in India, causing 6% of all cancers and the third most common cause of cancer-related mortality. The highest incidence of lung cancer in India is found in the north-eastern region, according to population-based cancer registries.[10]

Smoking remains the most common cause of lung cancer; however, 40% of lung cancer occurs in nonsmokers.[11] Primary prevention through legislation and awareness regarding tobacco control and smoking cessation remain the most effective measures for decreasing mortality due to lung cancer.[12] Screening with low dose computed tomography (LDCT) has shown significant mortality reduction in large randomized controlled trials.[13,14] Several barriers exist to the adoption of screening in LMICs, such as lack of infrastructure and risk of overdiagnosis due to high prevalence of granulomatous diseases.[9,15] (**Box 1**) Screening has been evaluated in LMICs such as Brazil, Taiwan and China with promising results.[16,17] In spite of the Brazilian Lung Cancer Screening Trial (BRELT1)[18] showing equivalent rates of invasive procedures for a higher number of positive screens in high-risk individuals, screening is not recommended in these settings due to long waiting periods for imaging and widespread unavailability of procedures such as biopsy and surgery.

The further increase in lung cancer incidence and mortality will be driven by LMICs where smoking rates are increasing.[8] WHO introduced a cost-effective and evidence-based six-point package to counter the tobacco epidemic utilizing measures such as monitoring the use of tobacco and prevention policies, Protection from tobacco smoke, Offering help to quit tobacco use, Warning about dangers of tobacco, Enforcing bans on advertisements, and Raising taxation. Adoption of the MPOWER package interventions by WHO may be helpful to reduce tobacco use and limit initiation.[12] Tobacco control mass media campaigns on national television and/or radio have helped increase the awareness about the harms of tobacco, and the recent legislation requiring large printed health warnings on tobacco products have also proved to be deterrents to the initiation and continued use of cigarettes. A 10% increase in value-added taxation on cigarettes in India has led to a 6.5% decrease in cigarette and bidi smoking in adult males.[19]

There is a scarcity of published literature on the management of lung cancer in LMICs.[20,21] A tertiary center reviewed the management of patients with nonsmall cell lung cancer (NSCLC) receiving curative treatment and found that 70% (261 out of 370 patients) of the diagnosed cases received anticancer treatment, of which 26% (n = 68) of the cases were in stage I–III.[22] Another study from South India reported outcomes of over a thousand patients with lung cancer treated over a period of 9 years and reported dismal overall survival.[23]

Box 1
Challenges with screening in LMICs

Disease-related

- High prevalence of Tuberculosis
- High false-positive rate due to various granulomatous diseases
- Comparatively low prevalence of smoking
- Increasing incidence of lung cancer among non-smokers

Infrastructure & Manpower

- Limited number of CT scans and PET CT facilities
- Limited number of Radiologists for interpretation and intervention
- Limited resources to manage false-positive lesions
- Limited centres and trained surgeons to treat screen-detected lung cancers
- Challenges in procuring annual/biennial screening scans and follow up of participants
- Economic challenges and feasibility to implement on a large population

This article covers the practices followed in LMICs for the surgical management of lung cancer with the available evidence. We also briefly discuss other modalities, such as neoadjuvant and adjuvant strategies, the role of radiation, chemotherapy, and immunotherapy.

Diagnosis and Staging

The diagnostic and staging strategy in LMICs is similar to those in HICs with minor differences. Treatment decisions are usually made following multidisciplinary discussions in dedicated cancer centers and individualized for better patient outcomes.[24] A Computed tomography (CT) scan is routinely conducted for both diagnosis and staging. Framing a diagnostic algorithm for screen-detected incidental solid and subsolid nodules is challenging. Nonsolid nodules, such as ground-glass opacities (GGOs) and ground glass nodules (GGNs), may resolve, and persistent ones may not develop into significant cancer.[25] Biopsy or surgery is considered for highly suspicious nodules, while surveillance is an option for nodules with low suspicion. Positron Emission Tomography (PET) scans are utilized for intermediate-risk nodules (ie, 40%–50% probability of cancer).[26,27] However, high false-positive rates are common in LMICs due to inflammatory and granulomatous lung lesions.

CT is commonly used to stage lung cancer in LMICs, while PET and PET-CT are primarily accessible in urban areas and private health care facilities. Whole-body PET-CT scan is essential for noninvasive staging of lung cancer, but it is neither widely available nor affordable. In Indian centers, where PET-CT is unavailable, a radionuclide bone scan with a contrast-enhanced CT scan of the chest and upper abdomen (including liver and adrenals) is usually conducted for staging.[28]

Disparities and inequity in access are major problems in LMICs. Among the 19 centers in Malaysia providing PET CT scanning, 75% are private health care facilities.[29] In South Africa, PET is recommended for staging patients being considered for curative surgery, early-stage cancer, or for an inconclusive CT.[30] In a survey from Brazil, the number of CT scanners per one million population in public and private sector was 4.9 and 30.8, respectively.[31] Sistema Nico de Saúde (Brazilian Unified Health Care System) public health care system integrated PET CT for staging only in 2014.[31] In a recent study in China of over 500 patients with solitary pulmonary nodules, where FDG PET was correlated with histologic diagnosis, the authors concluded that FDG PET has low specificity and high false positives in a tuberculous endemic country.[32]

In patients with suspected NSCLC, many techniques are available for tissue diagnosis, including sputum cytology, bronchoscopy with biopsy and transbronchial needle aspiration (TBNA), image-guided transthoracic core needle biopsy, mediastinoscopy, open surgical biopsy and video-assisted thoracic surgery (VATS). The most common approaches remain a bronchoscopy or CT-guided trucut biopsy. Recent techniques include Endobronchial Ultrasound (EBUS) guided biopsy, Endoscopic Ultrasound (EUS) guided biopsy and navigational bronchoscopy, are available in limited centers. When distant metastasis is excluded, mediastinal staging is recommended before surgical resection (**Fig. 1**), except in peripheral tumors with no nodes on imaging.[33]

In LMICs, the method used for invasive mediastinal staging varies. Despite its cost-effectiveness and superior safety to mediastinoscopy or VATS, EBUS-TBNA invites considerable expenses and requires special expertise, resulting in limited utilization in LMICs.[34] In LMICs, the most common diagnosis following an EBUS-TBNA is granulomatous inflammation.[35,36] In India, bronchoscopy utilization has expanded, although concentrated in metropolitan cities. In a recent survey, only 27% of respondents preferred EBUS-FNA over TTNA (74%).[37]

Endobronchial ultrasound (EBUS) and image-guided transthoracic sampling are being used at several centers in India. However, these facilities are available in less than 1% of centers in other LIMCs.[38] Endobronchial biopsy is widely available in Malaysia in almost all public and private sector health care, while electromagnetic navigational bronchoscopy is available only in 2 hospitals.[29] From a survey conducted in Brazil by The Socieda de Brasileira de Pneumologia e Tisiologia, 19.2% of pulmonologists were familiar with both flexible and rigid bronchoscopy.[39] After 2010, endobronchial ultrasound was launched in large institutions in Brazil. In 76% of patients, endobronchial ultrasound was used for diagnostic purposes, yielding sufficient specimens in 74%.[40] In Mexican hospitals, patients who undergo surgery also undergo mediastinal lymphadenectomy, either by lymph node sampling or by systematic lymph node dissection.[41] in most LMICs, the indications for mediastinal staging are similar, but the availability of resource-dependent advanced technologies is uneven.

Overlap with Tuberculosis

Approximately 2% to 4% of patients with lung cancer have a concomitant infection with tuberculosis, and this incidence is higher in LMICs.[42,43] In India, due to a higher incidence of granulomatous diseases, including tuberculosis, on both the symptomatology and imaging, there can be substantial delays of more than 3 months from the onset of symptoms to a definite diagnosis and 4 months to treatment initiation, leading to a delay in the initiation of anticancer treatment with the upstaging of disease and poor outcomes.[43–45]

Lung cancer can develop in a background of healed tuberculosis scars and cavities. This has been attributed to chronic inflammation causing metaplastic changes in the bronchial and pulmonary alveolar epithelium. The proinflammatory state caused by mycobacteria with multiple cycles of inflammation and tissue repair has been proposed to increase the tumorigenic potential.[46] In a study evaluating biopsy slides and autopsy tissues, the incidence of tuberculosis was much higher in patients with lung cancer than the general population without lung pathology (24% vs 7%, respectively).[47] In China, whereby the incidence of tuberculosis among patients with cancer is as high as 12%, no serious adverse effects were

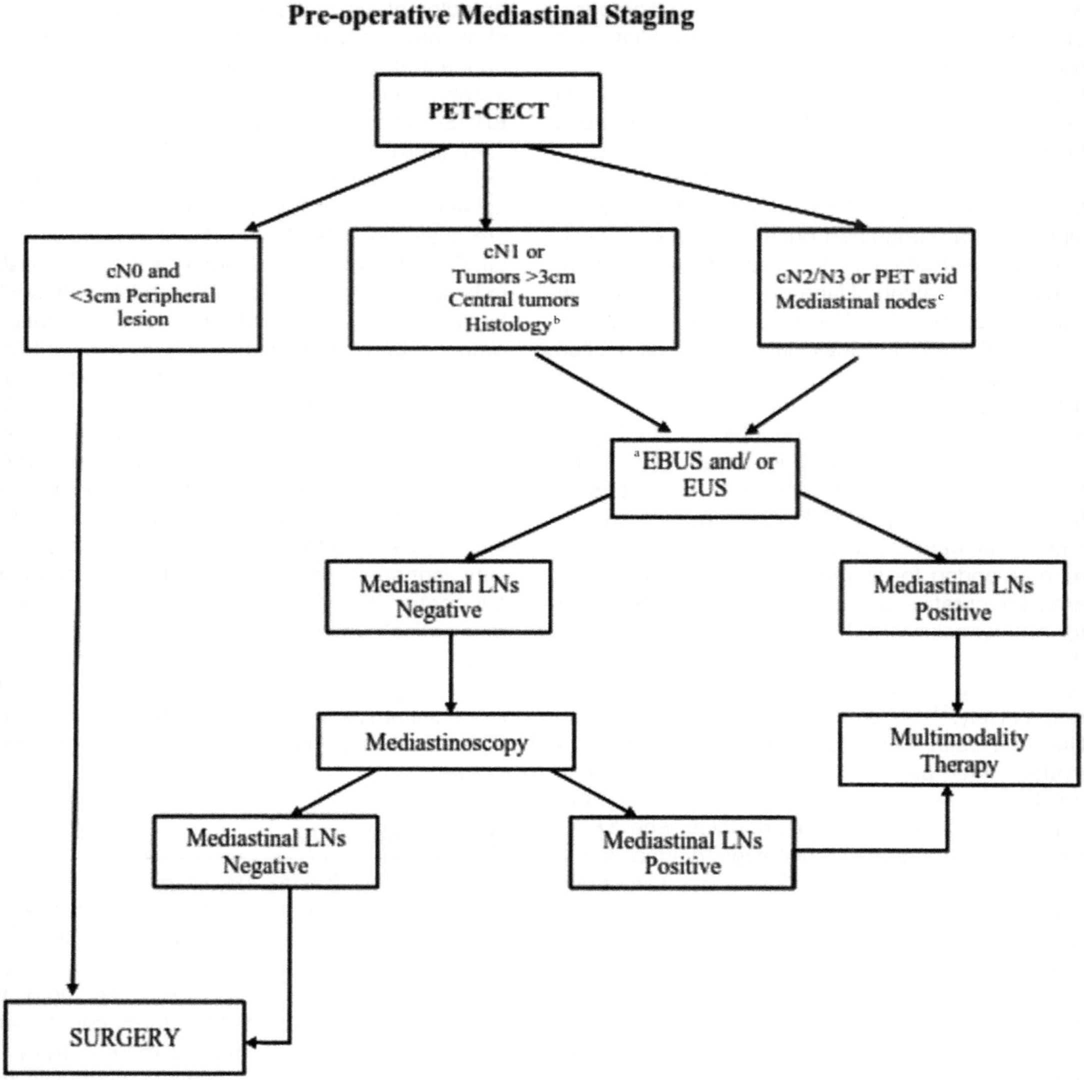

Fig. 1. Staging algorithm for mediastinal nodes. [a] The first choice of mediastinal nodal staging is always minimum invasive (EBUS-Endobronchial ultrasound & EUS–Endoscopic Ultrasound). [b] Adenocarcinoma histology with high uptake on PET should undergo further mediastinal staging. [c] Radiological assessment is sufficient in patients with nodal disease and extensive mediastinal infiltration.

noted while administering cisplatin-based chemotherapy for lung cancer along with antituberculous treatment. Radiation and targeted therapy were not used to avoid pneumonitis.[48] A retrospective study showed surgery performed after 3 weeks of antituberculosis treatment (ATT), with ATT and adjuvant therapy continued in the postoperative period, did not increase postoperative morbidity or mortality.[49]

Preoperative Evaluation and Prehabilitation

Preoperative evaluation for lung resection in LMICs is similar to those in HICs and usually follows one of the following combined guidelines: American College of Physicians, British Thoracic Society and European Respiratory Society(**Fig. 2**). Decisions on surgical resection are made after pulmonary functional evaluation depending on the patient's comorbid conditions, spirometry, and extent of resection.[50,51] Discussion of the high-risk surgical candidates, especially those with poor postoperative predicted lung functions and comorbid conditions in a multidisciplinary joint clinic consisting of thoracic surgeons, anesthetists, and pulmonary physicians has been followed for the last several years and found to be beneficial.[28]

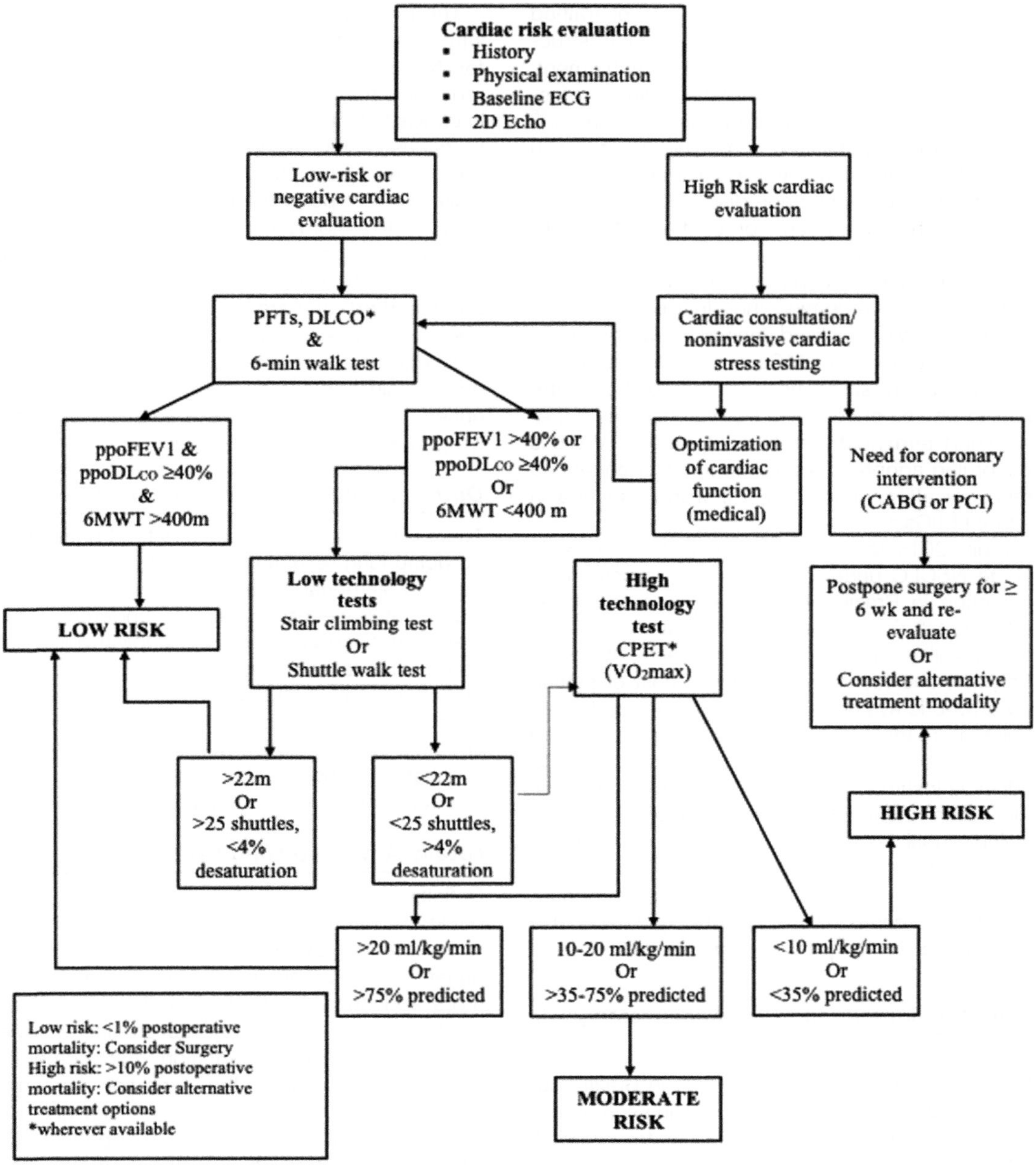

Fig. 2. Algorithm for preoperative functional evaluation for major lung resection.

Surgical Management in Low- and Middle-Income Countries

Most of the patients with lung cancer in LMICs are diagnosed either with locally advanced disease or with metastases, which reduces the chances of curative surgical resection. In the authors' center (the largest cancer center in India), less than 10% of all patients with NSCLC are operable. Lung resection rates for NSCLC in Malaysia are as low as 4.8%.[29] In tertiary care centers in India, the curative treatment option is exercised less often than it should (only 31.7% of the patients with stages I to IIIA treated with curative intent).[52] A study from Nepal looked at the causes for low resection rate (less than 3%) and found that delayed presentation and referral to a speciality unit were the main causes.[53]

The open thoracotomy approach remains the most common, although video-assisted thoracoscopic surgery (VATS) and Robotic-assisted thoracoscopic surgery (RATS) are gradually increasing.[54] Challenges to establish VATS as the standard of care include the lack of trained minimally invasive thoracic surgeons, infrastructure such as high-definition video equipment, specialized VATS instrumentation, allied professional and technical support, among others.[55] There are no established screening programs in most LMICs, and hence there is a small proportion of patients with early-stage disease (amenable to VATS). With most patients presenting with locally advanced tumors necessitating an open approach and extensive resections, surgeons are faced with difficulties in overcoming their learning curves.[55] There are few specialized general thoracic surgical training pathways in LIMCs, leading to a shortage of specialized surgeons and mentorship. After having proven oncological equivalence and superior short-term postoperative outcomes,[56] VATS is becoming adopted as a component of enhanced recovery after surgery (ERAS) worldwide and in some LMICs.[57,58]

From 2015 to 2016, 52% patients with early-stage NSCLC underwent minimally invasive lung resection in Brazil with a steady rise in robotic approach.[59] Ghazanfar and colleagues conducted a feasibility and cost-effectiveness study in Pakistan and found that the initial cost of setting up a robotic system and that of recurring disposables as roadblocks in broader adoption.[60] Since acquiring the first robotic system in 2006 at AIIMS (All India Institute of Medical Sciences), New Delhi, more than 12,000 robotic surgeries were performed in India until 2019, and there are more than 500 trained robotic surgeons in India.[52,61] An analysis by Bora has predicted a rapid surge in robotic-assisted surgeries and suggested judicious use and standardized reporting of outcomes.[62]

Extent of Surgery and Lymphadenectomy

Lobectomy remains the most commonly performed operation for NSCLC (80% in Brazil), but a recent study showed an increase in segmentectomies for early-stage from 2.67% to 7.11%.[16] Although the pneumonectomy rate is decreasing in HICs, due to screen detected lesions, and utilization of lung preservation techniques, pneumonectomy is unavoidable in LMICs due to patients presenting with advanced disease. Shah and colleagues showed a pneumonectomy rate of more than 40%, with many patients requiring neoadjuvant chemotherapy.[63] They did not find any difference in morbidity and mortality on comparing with patients who underwent lobectomy, and there was no difference in survival. Another study from Iraq reported outcomes after pneumonectomy for central tumors with acceptable rates of morbidity and mortality.[64]

The meta-analysis by Mokhles showed benefit with systematic mediastinal lymphadenectomy for NSCLC, but there is scarcity of literature regarding mediastinal lymph nodal management in LMICs.[65] In a survey conducted among thoracic surgeons in India, systematic mediastinal lymphadenectomy was performed in 14 out of 19 centers, while the rest performed mediastinal nodal sampling.[28] A randomized study from China demonstrated a superior overall survival with lymph node dissection over sampling, establishing it as the standard of care.[66] The number of lymph nodes harvested was predictors of survival and adjuvant therapy improved outcome in suboptimal nodal evaluation and T2 disease.[67] In most experienced thoracic centers, systematic mediastinal lymphadenectomy is performed.

Outcomes of Surgical Management

There is scarcity of outcomes data of patients undergoing lung resection from LMICs like India. At the Tata Memorial Center, we have been maintaining a database of all patients undergoing lung resection since 2004 and will publish our results soon. The National Cancer Grid of India is also planning a multicentric database of all patients undergoing lung resection in the near future. Prospective data collection from LMICs is important to measure perioperative and long-term oncological outcomes in these countries.

Locally Advanced Lung Cancer

Definitive concurrent chemoradiotherapy is the backbone of the treatment of locally advanced unresectable NSCLC. As more than 60% of the patients in LMICs present in stage III with large tumors and bulky mediastinal nodes, access and availability to radiotherapy are critical. A review article evaluating the radiation management of NSCLC in LMICs noted that expertise, personnel, and infrastructure for radiation are not uniformly available in LMICs, whereby 60% of patients with NSCLC are located with only one-third of the radiation machines available globally.[68,69] International efforts ongoing to facilitate the establishment of radiation centers in LMICs to enhance capacity and establish treatment programs using cobalt teletherapy machines or megavoltage linear accelerator machines.[70]

In an audit of medically inoperable or unresectable NSCLC treated with chemoradiation, radiation was delivered at a median dose of 60 Gy with weekly/3 weekly regimens of chemotherapy in 86% of the patients, with 95% of the patients completing the treatment, and 66% receiving concurrent treatment. The 2-year overall survival was

61%, with response to treatment being the most important factor for prognosis.[71]

Guidelines published for appropriate management of lung cancer in limited-resource settings advocate that concurrent chemoradiation for unresectable NSCLC should be undertaken only if there are facilities to manage the treatment-related toxicities.[21,72] Often, patients with very large tumors undergo sequential chemoradiation rather than concurrent due to anticipated treatment-related toxicities.[73] While there is no level I evidence supporting the use of adjuvant Durvalumab after chemoradiation in locoregionally advanced unresectable NSCLC, cost constraints result in few patients receiving immunotherapy in LMICs.[74]

Management of Oligometastatic Disease

Oligometastatic disease represents a state between localized disease and widespread extensive disease. Although there is a no generalized consensus on the number of metastases and sites that can be treated with a curative intent, there is growing evidence that local consolidative therapy in the form of radiation or surgery should be considered along with systemic therapy[75] Few reports from LMICs have added to the evidence of management of selected stage IV patients with NSCLC.[76] A randomized phase III trial evaluating systemic therapy with the addition of localized treatment versus systemic therapy alone for oligometastatic disease is ongoing at Tata Memorial Hospital in Mumbai.[77] Our approach is to consider radical surgery in oligometastatic disease only after invasive mediastinal staging has ruled out N2 disease(**Fig. 3**).

Choosing Systemic Therapy for Advanced Lung Cancer in Resource Constraint Settings

Breakthroughs in the management of advanced NSCLC in the last 2 decades have revolutionized the treatment of these patients. Adjuvant treatment following surgery is standard across LMICs (**Fig. 4**) but the affordability and use of adjuvant targeted therapy/Immunotherapy are doubtful. The advent of molecular-driven targeted therapy and immunotherapy has benefited many patients and resulted in a meaningful improvement in disease-free and overall survival as well as the quality of life. In LMICs, the nonavailability of biomarker testing and newer therapies has precluded the widespread implementation of these strategies. The frequency of Epidermal Growth Factor Receptor (EGFR) mutations ranges from 23% to 35% in Asian and Latin American countries, but information regarding other molecular markers is scarce. There are several barriers to the availability of diagnostics, infrastructure, trained personnel, and targeted therapies in this heterogeneous region, and there are ongoing efforts by the International Association for Study of Lung Cancer (IASLC) to scale up the utilization of precision medicine in this region.[78] A survey among oncologists regarding the highest priority drugs from WHO essential medicines showed that even older, generic cytotoxic drugs were not easily accessible in LMICs.[79]

A recent review on first-line systemic therapy for NSCLC in India showed that a platinum doublet was the standard of care in patients without activating mutations.[80] In patients with EGFR mutation, first-line targeted agents were commonly used. Data on treatment with immunotherapy in the first line were scarce. A multicentric study analyzed 88 patients who received immune checkpoint inhibitors from 2016 to 2018. Most of the patients were pretreated, the most commonly used drug was Nivolumab and the median number of cycles was 4.[81] High costs of Pembrolizumab and other immune checkpoint inhibitors preclude their routine use in patients with metastatic NSCLC.

Palliative care

Palliative care forms an extremely important aspect of cancer treatment and lung cancer in particular. This is even more important in LMICs whereby most patients present in advanced stages of disease and multiple comorbidities, and symptom control and supportive care are often the only treatment options possible. While there have been attempts to integrate palliative care referrals early in the course of disease,[82] it is not routine in most LMICs[83] The National Cancer Grid strongly advocates that all cancer centers should have well-established departments of palliative care, and has included the importance of palliative care provision in their "Choosing Wisely" recommendations.[84]

Implementation of Guidelines

An online survey conducted among oncologists with 139 respondents, from countries such as India, China, Thailand, the Philippines, Malaysia, Vietnam, Indonesia, Argentina, Brazil, Chile, and Mexico showed that 58% of the respondents used guidelines such as those by the American Society for Clinical Oncology (ASCO), National Comprehensive Cancer Network (NCCN), European Society for Medical Oncology (ESMO) in their practice, 92% using NCCN guidelines, and 55% utilizing ASCO and ESMO guidelines with only

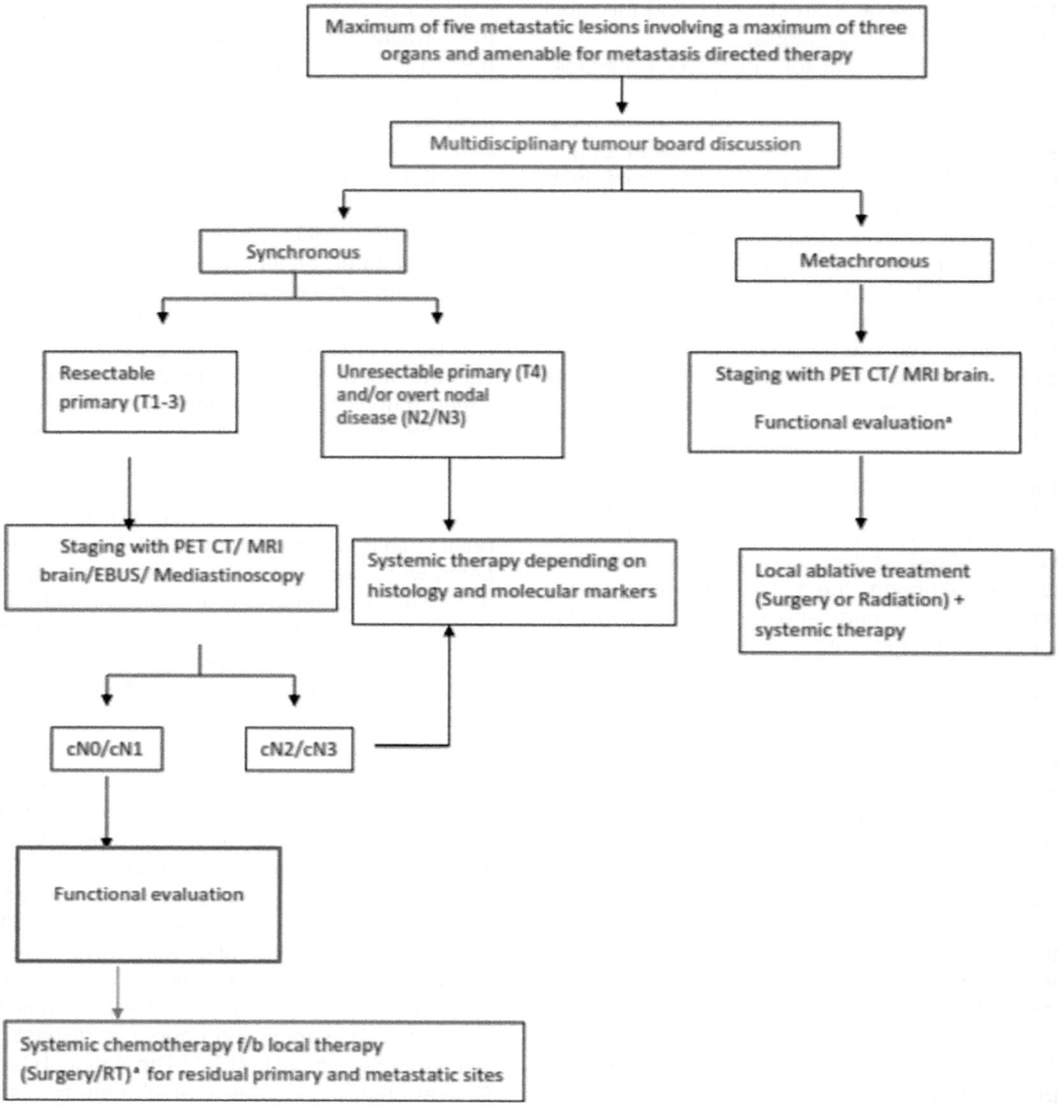

Fig. 3. Management of oligometastatic lung cancer. EBUS, endobronchial ultrasonography; MRI, magnetic resonance imaging; PET, positron emission tomography; RT, Radiotherapy. [a] Symptomatic primary or metastatic lesion may be treated with local therapy (sugery/radiation) before administering systemic therapy.

40% referring to national guidelines.[85] A review by Singh and colleagues emphasizes the importance of staging and investigations in advanced NSCLC based on availability and cost-effectiveness.[72] The authors reiterate that the systemic therapy regimen chosen should take into account the local context including the cost, insurance coverage, and frequency of treatments, especially for patients coming from remote places. The use of paclitaxel is advocated over pemetrexed, when the latter is not affordable and use of drugs such as gemcitabine should be advocated only after confirming the compliance in view of more frequent visits required. Many generic drugs, including cytotoxic chemotherapy and targeted agents, are available at lower prices in LMICs and their efficacy has been shown in other cancers.[86–88]

The National Cancer Grid (NCG) of India was formed in 2012 and has grown to more than 250 cancer centers, research institutes, patient groups, and professional societies, with the mandate of standardizing cancer care across the nation by formulating resource-stratified guidelines (with essential, optimal and optional criteria) and providing a platform for training and

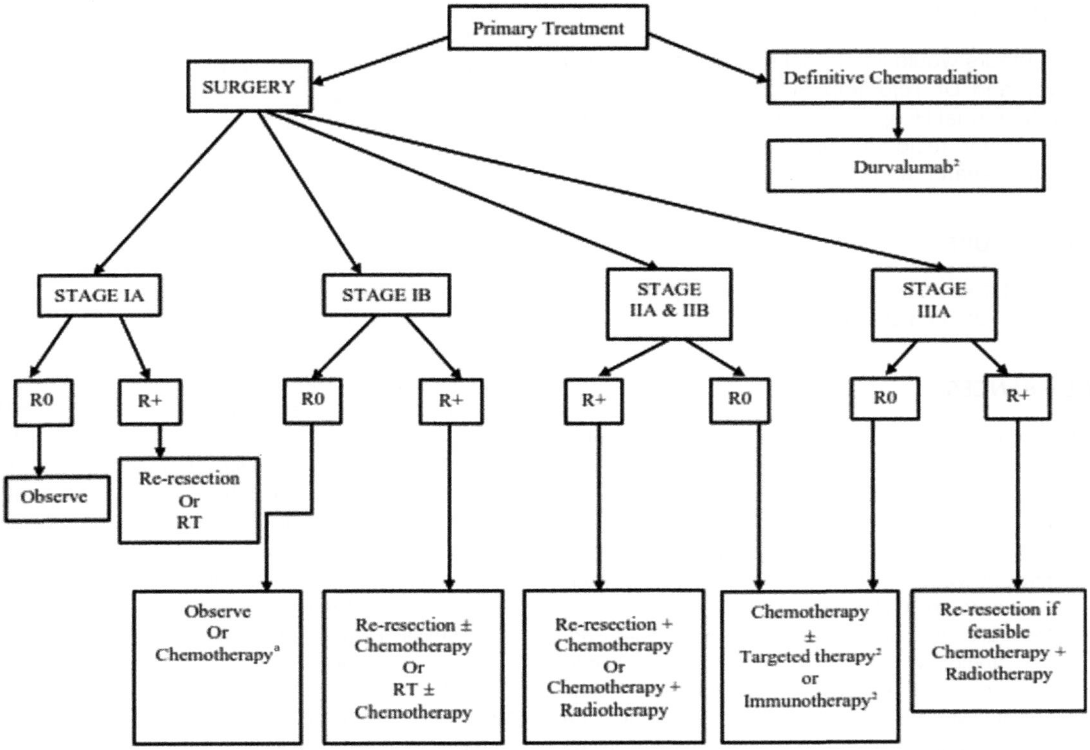

Fig. 4. Adjuvant treatment in lung cancer. [a] High risk features (size>4cms,visceral pleural involvement,poorly differentiate histology, LVI, wedge resection and Unknown nodal status). [b] May be considered in selected cases after discussing in a Multidisciplinary Tumor Board and with the patients.

collaborative research.[89,90] The NCG has played a major role in the adoption of these cancer treatment policies by the national government health insurance scheme[91] to dispel the inequity and disparities in health care across India. The consensus guidelines formulated by NCG are in the algorithmic format making them easy to follow and adapt to local conditions for most common cancers.[92] Such local and national guidelines, formulated keeping in perspective the local constraints, resources, and infrastructure, have the potential to transform cancer care accessibility in LMICs.

Value-based Cancer care

Cancer management has seen major breakthroughs in the past 2 decades. However, costs of cancer care have increased, and are not necessarily commensurate with the benefits the new interventions bring.[93,94] There is variation in health care spending by different countries, with little correlation to overall health outcomes in these countries.[95] Most LMICs have low governmental spending on health, resulting in heavy out of pocket expenses for patients, with catastrophic health care expenditure. While formal health technology assessment (HTA) initiatives like the NICE guidelines in the UK are ideal, these are difficult to create in LMICs and alternate options like Choosing Wisely or adaptive HTA mechanisms may need to be used in LMICs. Recommendations for treatment, including regional guidelines should consider value while evaluating new interventions, especially whereby benefits are marginal and come at high costs.[96]

SUMMARY

The current evidence shows that cancer awareness, prevention, diagnosis, and treatment are feasible in LMICs despite several challenges. To decrease global lung cancer-related mortality, cohesive efforts against the tobacco epidemic are essential along with detecting cancers early and ramping up training as well as infrastructure. Local as well as international collaboration for formulating guidelines and enhancing research can go a long way in this uphill task.

FUNDING SOURCES

None.

ACKNOWLEDGMENTS

The authors would like to acknowledge Dr Saiesh Reddy and Dr Tejpratap Singh, Senior resident, Tata Memorial Hospital, Mumbai and Dr Prosenjit Das, Senior resident, JIPMER, Pondicherry for literature search and algorithms.

DISCLOSURE

None of the above authors have any financial/ commercial conflicts of interest.

REFERENCES

1. World Bank Country and Lending Groups. Availabel at. https://datahelpdesk.worldbank.org/knowledgebase/articles/906519. Accessed on 30 November 2021.
2. WHO NCD mortality and morbidity. Availabel at. https://www.who.int/gho/ncd/mortality_morbidity/en. Accessed on 30 November 2021.
3. International Agency for Research on Cancer Cancer Tomorrow. Availabel at. https://gco.iarc.fr/tomorrow/home. Accessed on 30 November 2021.
4. Mallath MK, Taylor DG, Badwe RA, et al. The growing burden of cancer in India: epidemiology and social context. Lancet Oncol 2014;15(6): e205–12. https://doi.org/10.1016/S1470-2045(14)70115-9.
5. WHO fact sheet on cancer. Availabel at. https://www.who.int/news-room/fact-sheets/detail/cancer. Accessed on 30 November 2021.
6. Pramesh CS, Badwe RA, Borthakur BB, et al. Delivery of affordable and equitable cancer care in India. Lancet Oncol 2014;15(6):e223–33.
7. Global Adult Tobacco Survey-2 [GATS]-2.India fact sheet. 2016. Availabel at. http://gatsatlas.org. Accessed on 30 November 2021.
8. Sung H, Ferlay J, Siegel RL, et al. Global cancer statistics 2020: GLOBOCAN estimates of incidence and mortality worldwide for 36 cancers in 185 countries. CA Cancer J Clin 2021;71(3):209–49.
9. Shankar A, Saini D, Dubey A, et al. Feasibility of lung cancer screening in developing countries: challenges, opportunities and way forward. Transl Lung Cancer Res 2019;8(S1):S106–21.
10. Asthana S, Patil RS, Labani S. Tobacco-related cancers in India: A review of incidence reported from population-based cancer registries. Indian J Med Paediatr Oncol 2016;37(03):152–7.
11. Krishnamurthy A, Gadigi V, Sagar T, et al. The relevance of "Nonsmoking-associated lung cancer" in India: A single-centre experience. Indian J Cancer 2012;49(1):82.
12. WHO report on the global tobacco epidemic 2019: offer help to quit tobacco use. Availabel at. https://www.who.int/publications/i/item/9789241516204. Accessed on 30 November 2021.
13. Frille A, Hardavella G, Lee R. Lung cancer incidence and mortality with extended follow-up in the National Lung Screening Trial. Breathe 2020;16(1):190322.
14. Pastorino U, Silva M, Sestini S, et al. Prolonged lung cancer screening reduced 10-year mortality in the MILD trial: new confirmation of lung cancer screening efficacy. Ann Oncol 2019;30(7):1162–9.
15. Hammen I. Tuberculosis mimicking lung cancer. Respir Med Case Rep 2015;16:45–7.
16. de Sa V, Coelho J, Capelozzi VL, et al. Lung cancer in Brazil: epidemiology and treatment challenges. Lung Cancer 2016;7:141–8.
17. Hu P, Dai M, Shi J, et al. Abstract 1795: the feasibility study of a randomized cancer screening trial in China. In: Prevention research. American Association for Cancer Research; 2016. p. 1795. https://doi.org/10.1158/1538-7445.AM2016-1795.
18. Santos RS dos, Franceschini JP, Chate RC, et al. Do current lung cancer screening guidelines apply for populations with high prevalence of granulomatous disease? results from the first Brazilian lung cancer screening trial (BRELT1). Ann Thorac Surg 2016; 101(2):481–8.
19. Shang C, Chaloupka FJ, Fong GT, et al. The association between state value-added taxes and tobacco use in India—evidence from GATS and TCP India survey. Nicotine Tob Res 2018;20(11):1344–52.
20. Li X, Zhou Q, Wang X, et al. The effect of low insurance reimbursement on quality of care for non-small cell lung cancer in China: a comprehensive study covering diagnosis, treatment, and outcomes. BMC Cancer 2018;18(1):683.
21. Macbeth FR, Abratt RP, Cho KH, et al. Lung cancer management in limited resource settings: Guidelines for appropriate good care. Radiother Oncol 2007;82(2):123–31.
22. Malik PS, Sharma MC, Mohanti BK, et al. Clinicopathological profile of lung cancer at AIIMS: a changing paradigm in India. Asian Pac J Cancer Prev 2013;14(1):489–94.
23. Murali AN, Radhakrishnan V, Ganesan TS, et al. Outcomes in lung cancer: 9-year experience from a tertiary cancer center in India. J Glob Oncol 2017;3(5): 459–68.
24. Detterbeck FC, Lewis SZ, Diekemper R, et al. Executive summary. Chest 2013;143(5):7S–37S.
25. Yankelevitz DF, Yip R, Smith JP, et al. CT screening for lung cancer: nonsolid nodules in baseline and annual repeat rounds. Radiology 2015;277(2):555–64.
26. Deterbeck F, Khandani AH. The role of PET imaging in solitary pulmonary nodules. Clin Pulm Med 2009; 16:81–8.
27. Gould MK, Donington J, Lynch WR, et al. Evaluation of individuals with pulmonary nodules: when is it lung cancer? Chest 2013;143(5):e93S–120S.

28. Apurva A, Tandon SP, Shetmahajan M, et al. Surgery for lung cancer—the Indian scenario. Indian J Thorac Cardiovasc Surg 2018;34(S1):47–53.
29. Rajadurai P, How SH, Liam CK, et al. Lung cancer in Malaysia. J Thorac Oncol 2020;15(3):317–23.
30. van Eeden R, Tunmer M, Geldenhuys A, et al. Lung cancer in South Africa. J Thorac Oncol 2020;15(1):22–8.
31. Araujo LH, Baldotto C, Castro G de Jr, et al. Lung cancer in Brazil. J Bras Pneumol 2018;44(1):55–64.
32. Niyonkuru A, Chen X, Bakari KH, et al. Evaluation of the diagnostic efficacy of ^{18} F-Fluorine-2-Deoxy-D-Glucose PET/CT for lung cancer and pulmonary tuberculosis in a tuberculosis-endemic country. Cancer Med 2020;9(3):931–42.
33. Silvestri GA, Gonzalez AV, Jantz MA, et al. Methods for staging non-small cell lung cancer. Chest 2013;143(5):e211S–50S.
34. Harewood GC, Pascual J, Raimondo M, et al. Economic analysis of combined endoscopic and endobronchial ultrasound in the evaluation of patients with suspected non-small cell lung cancer. Lung Cancer 2010;67(3):366–71.
35. Srinivasan A, Agarwal R, Gupta N, et al. Initial experience with real time endobronchial ultrasound guided transbronchial needle aspiration from a tertiary care hospital in north India. Indian J Med Res 2013;137(4):803–7.
36. Madan K, Mohan A, Ayub II, et al. Initial experience with endobronchial ultrasound-guided transbronchial needle aspiration (EBUS-TBNA) from a tuberculosis endemic population. J Bronchol Interv Pulmonol 2014;21(3):208–14.
37. Madan K, Mohan A, Agarwal R, et al. A survey of flexible bronchoscopy practices in India: the Indian bronchoscopy survey (2017). Lung India 2018;35(2):98–107.
38. Singh N, Agrawal S, Jiwnani S, et al. Lung cancer in India. J Thorac Oncol 2021;16(8):1250–66.
39. Du Rand IA, Blaikley J, Booton R, et al. British thoracic society guideline for diagnostic flexible bronchoscopy in adults: accredited by NICE. Thorax 2013;68(Suppl 1):i1–44.
40. Tedde ML, Figueiredo VR, Terra RM, et al. Endobronchial ultrasound-guided transbronchial needle aspiration in the diagnosis and staging of mediastinal lymphadenopathy: initial experience in Brazil. J Bras Pneumol 2012;38(1):33–40.
41. Arrieta O, Zatarain-Barrón ZL, Aldaco F, et al. Lung cancer in Mexico. J Thorac Oncol 2019;14(10):1695–700.
42. Janjam H, Sukaveni V, et al. Cancer and tuberculosis. J Indian Acad Clin Med 2012;13:142–4.
43. Bhatt M, Kant S, Bhaskar R. Pulmonary tuberculosis as differential diagnosis of lung cancer. South Asian J Cancer 2012;01(01):36–42.
44. Zhou Y, Cui Z, Zhou X, et al. The presence of old pulmonary tuberculosis is an independent prognostic factor for squamous cell lung cancer survival. J Cardiothorac Surg 2013;8(1):123.
45. Leung CC, Hui L, Lee RSY, et al. Tuberculosis is associated with increased lung cancer mortality. Int J Tuberc Lung Dis Off J Int Union Tuberc Lung Dis 2013;17(5):687–92.
46. Fol M, Koziński P, Kulesza J, et al. Dual nature of relationship between mycobacteria and cancer. Int J Mol Sci 2021;22(15):8332.
47. Dacosta NA, Kinare SG. Association of lung carcinoma and tuberculosis. J Postgrad Med 1991;37(4):185–9.
48. Chai M, Shi Q. The effect of anti-cancer and anti-tuberculosis treatments in lung cancer patients with active tuberculosis: a retrospective analysis. BMC Cancer 2020;20(1):1121.
49. Evman S, Baysungur V, Alpay L, et al. Management and surgical outcomes of concurrent tuberculosis and lung cancer. Thorac Cardiovasc Surg 2017;65(07):542–5.
50. Roy PM. Preoperative pulmonary evaluation for lung resection. J Anaesthesiol Clin Pharmacol 2018;34(3):296–300.
51. Mathew B, Nag S, Agrawal A, et al. Comparison of predicted postoperative forced expiratory volume in the first second (FEV1) using lung perfusion scintigraphy with observed forced expiratory volume in the first second (FEV1) post lung resection. World J Nucl Med 2020;19(2):131–6.
52. Malik PS, Malik A, Deo SV, et al. Underutilization of curative treatment among patients with non small cell lung cancer: experience from a tertiary care centre in India. Asian Pac J Cancer Prev APJCP 2014;15(6):2875–8.
53. Thapa B, Sayami P. Low lung cancer resection rates in a tertiary level thoracic center in Nepal - where lies our problem? Asian Pac J Cancer Prev 2014;15(1):175–8.
54. Kumar A, Asaf B. Robotic thoracic surgery: the state of the art. J Minim Access Surg 2015;11(1):60.
55. Yendamuri S. Why India needs video-assisted thoracic surgery (VATS). Natl Med J India 2017;30(2):101–2.
56. Whitson BA, Groth SS, Duval SJ, et al. Surgery for early-stage non-small cell lung cancer: a systematic review of the video-assisted thoracoscopic surgery versus thoracotomy approaches to lobectomy. Ann Thorac Surg 2008;86(6):2008–18.
57. Smith A, Ramnarine I, Pinkney P. Evolution of video assisted thoracoscopic surgery in the caribbean. Int J Surg 2019;72:19–22.
58. Oparka J, Yan TD, Ryan E, et al. Does video-assisted thoracic surgery provide a safe alternative to conventional techniques in patients with limited pulmonary function who are otherwise suitable for

lung resection? Interact Cardiovasc Thorac Surg 2013;17(1):159–62.
59. Lim E, Batchelor TJ, Dunning J, et al. Video-assisted thoracoscopic or open lobectomy in early-stage lung cancer. NEJM Evid 2022;2100016.
60. Mathias C, Prado GF, Mascarenhas E, et al. Lung cancer in Brazil. J Thorac Oncol 2020;15(2):170–5.
61. Ghazanfar S, Qureshi S, Zubair M, et al. Feasibility of robotic surgery in a developing country, a public sector Perspective. J Pak Med Assoc 2019;69(1):44–8.
62. Kumar S, Saikia J, Kumar V, et al. Neoadjuvant chemotherapy followed by surgery in lung cancer: Indian scenario. Curr Probl Cancer 2020;44(3): 100563.
63. Bora GS, Narain TA, Sharma AP, et al. Robot-assisted surgery in India: A SWOT analysis. Indian J Urol 2020;36(1):1–3.
64. Shah S, Goel A, Selvakumar V, et al. Role of pneumonectomy for lung cancer in current scenario: an Indian perspective. Indian J Cancer 2017;54(1):236.
65. Baram A, Ramzi RM, Al Bermani S. Pneumonectomy for left-sided non-small cell lung cancer: analysis of 111 cases over 10 years. J Int Med Res 2020;48(1). 300060519889472.
66. Mokhles S, Macbeth F, Treasure T, et al. Systematic lymphadenectomy versus sampling of ipsilateral mediastinal lymph-nodes during lobectomy for non-small-cell lung cancer: a systematic review of randomized trials and a meta-analysis. Eur J Cardiothorac Surg 2017;51(6):1149–56.
67. Wu Y long, Huang Z fan, Wang S yu, et al. A randomized trial of systematic nodal dissection in resectable non-small cell lung cancer. Lung Cancer 2002;36(1):1–6.
68. Dai J, Liu M, Yang Y, et al. Optimal lymph node examination and adjuvant chemotherapy for stage i lung cancer. J Thorac Oncol 2019;14(7):1277–85.
69. Barton MB, Frommer M, Shafiq J. Role of radiotherapy in cancer control in low-income and middle-income countries. Lancet Oncol 2006;7(7):584–95.
70. Rodin D, Grover S, Xu MJ, et al. Radiotherapeutic management of non–small cell lung cancer in the minimal resource setting. J Thorac Oncol 2016; 11(1):21–9.
71. Page BR, Hudson AD, Brown DW, et al. Cobalt, linac, or other: what is the best solution for radiation therapy in developing countries? Int J Radiat Oncol 2014;89(3):476–80.
72. Agarwal J, Hotwani C, Prabhash K, et al. Optimizing treatment and analysis of prognostic factors for locally advanced nonsmall cell lung cancer in resource-limited population. Indian J Cancer 2016; 53(1):96.
73. Singh N, Aggarwal AN, Behera D. Management of advanced lung cancer in resource-constrained settings: a perspective from India. Expert Rev Anticancer Ther 2012;12(11):1479–95.
74. Aupérin A, Le Péchoux C, Rolland E, et al. Meta-analysis of concomitant versus sequential radiochemotherapy in locally advanced non–small-cell lung cancer. J Clin Oncol 2010;28(13):2181–90.
75. Dranitsaris G, Zhu X, Adunlin G, et al. Cost effectiveness vs. affordability in the age of immuno-oncology cancer drugs. Expert Rev Pharmacoecon Outcomes Res 2018;18(4):351–7.
76. Rim CH, Shin IS, Park S, et al. Benefits of local consolidative treatment in oligometastases of solid cancers: a stepwise-hierarchical pooled analysis and systematic review. NPJ Precis Oncol 2021; 5(1):2.
77. Thippeswamy R, Noronha V, Krishna V, et al. Stage IV lung cancer: is cure possible? Indian J Med Paediatr Oncol 2013;34(02):121–5. https://doi.org/10.4103/0971-5851.116207.
78. Tibdewal A, Agarwal JP, Srinivasan S, et al. Standard maintenance therapy versus local consolidative radiation therapy and standard maintenance therapy in 1–5 sites of oligometastatic non-small cell lung cancer: a study protocol of phase III randomised controlled trial. BMJ Open 2021;11(3): e043628.
79. Hirsch FR, Zaric B, Rabea A, et al. Biomarker testing for personalized therapy in lung cancer in low- and middle-income countries. Am Soc Clin Oncol Educ Book 2017;37:403–8.
80. Fundytus A, Sengar M, Lombe D, et al. Access to cancer medicines deemed essential by oncologists in 82 countries: an international, cross-sectional survey. Lancet Oncol 2021;22(10):1367–77.
81. Ghadyalpatil NS, Pandey A, Krishnamani I, et al. First-line management of metastatic non-small cell lung cancer: an Indian perspective. South Asian J Cancer 2019;08(02):073–9.
82. Kumar S, Joga S, Biswas B, et al. Immune checkpoint inhibitors in advanced non–small cell lung cancer: a metacentric experience from India. Curr Probl Cancer 2020;44(3):100549.
83. Ghoshal A, Deodhar J, Adhikarla C, et al. Implementation of an Early Palliative Care Referral Program in Lung Cancer: a quality improvement project at the Tata Memorial hospital, Mumbai, India. Indian J Palliat Care 2021;27:211–5.
84. Damani A, Salins N, Ghoshal A, et al. Provision of palliative care in National Cancer Grid treatment centres in India: a cross-sectional gap analysis survey. BMJ Support Palliat Care 2020. bmjspcare-2019-002152.
85. Pramesh CS, Chaturvedi H, Reddy VA, et al. Choosing Wisely India: ten low-value or harmful practices that should be avoided in cancer care. Lancet Oncol 2019;20(4):e218–23.
86. Kerr S, Jazieh AR, Kerr D. How useful are international treatment guidelines in low- and middle-income countries? J Glob Oncol 2017;3(5):441–3.

87. Wang KL, Yang YC, Cheng-Yen Lai J, et al. Comparison in purity and antitumor effect of brand and generic paclitaxel against human ovarian cancer cells by an in vitro experimental model. Drug Dev Ind Pharm 2010;36(10):1253–8.

88. Imai A, Ito N. Valid generic substitution of carboplatin for patients with gynecological cancer. Eur J Gynaecol Oncol 2009;30(4):435–6.

89. Fujii H, Iihara H, Yasuda K, et al. Evaluation of efficacy and safety of generic levofolinate in patients who received colorectal cancer chemotherapy. Med Oncol 2011;28(2):488–93.

90. Pramesh CS, Badwe RA, Sinha RK. The national cancer grid of India. Indian J Med Paediatr Oncol Off J Indian Soc Med Paediatr Oncol 2014;35(3):226–7.

91. Ranganathan P, Chinnaswamy G, Sengar M, et al. The international collaboration for research methods development in oncology (CReDO) workshops: shaping the future of global oncology research. Lancet Oncol 2021;22(8):e369–76.

92. Caduff C, Booth CM, Pramesh CS, et al. India's new health scheme: what does it mean for cancer care? Lancet Oncol 2019;20(6):757–8.

93. Chopra SJ, Mathew A, Maheshwari A, et al. National cancer grid of india consensus guidelines on the management of cervical cancer. J Glob Oncol 2018;4:1–15.

94. Monthly and median costs of cancer drugs at the time of FDA approval 1965-2016. J Natl Cancer Inst 2017;109(8).

95. Del Paggio JC, Sullivan R, Schrag D, et al. Delivery of meaningful cancer care: a retrospective cohort study assessing cost and benefit with the ASCO and ESMO frameworks. Lancet Oncol 2017;18(7):887–94.

96. Sullivan R, Pramesh CS, Booth CM. Cancer patients need better care, not just more technology. Nature 2017;549(7672):325–8.

Management of Esophageal Cancer Treatment in Resource-Limited Settings

Michael Mwachiro, MBChB, MPH[a,*], Russell White, MD, MPH[a,b]

KEYWORDS

• Esophageal cancer • Esophagectomy • Esophageal squamous cell carcinoma • SEMS

KEY POINTS

- Esophageal cancer care involves a multi-disciplinary approach.
- Access to supporting services such as endoscopy, critical care units, oncology units, and imaging services is key to offering comprehensive care.
- Surgery for esophageal cancer should be domiciled in high-volume centers due to the morbidity and mortality associated with it.
- Palliation for dysphagia in unresectable disease can be achieved with self-expanding metal stents (SEMS) placed endoscopically.
- Training and mentorship are key for capacity building in resource-limited settings.

INTRODUCTION

Esophageal cancer is the seventh most common cancer in the world.[1] Esophageal squamous cell carcinoma is the most common histologic variant and is found in Africa, the Middle East, and Far East.[2] Esophageal cancer in the early stages is asymptomatic and by the time the patient has dysphagia the disease has usually become more advanced. The care for esophageal cancer faces challenges globally. There are multiple treatment modalities available for esophageal cancer. Treatment is also dependent on the stage at the time of diagnosis. In this review, we look at care provision for esophageal cancer in resource-limited settings based on experience at our site.

MANAGEMENT STRATEGY?

Role of Endoscopy in the Management of Esophageal Cancer

Endoscopy is one of the critical components of care for esophageal cancer. Endoscopy is key for the diagnosis of disease and assessment of the extent of involvement as plans for treatment are being made. Endoscopic therapy is also available for very early disease through endoscopic resection techniques as well as ablative techniques.[3,4] Ablative techniques have so far been used in our setting in research studies and have not found their way to regular use due to the high cost of the probes and generator. In addition, endoscopy is currently the gold standard for screening through Lugol's chromoendoscopy.[5] Placement of self-expanding metal stents (SEMS) also needs endoscopy. We have also used endoscopy and CT evaluation as perioperative assessment tools to reassess the tumor before commencing surgery.[6] Endoscopic Ultrasound is largely unavailable, costly, and only found in a few centers and is therefore not used commonly. In the postoperative period, access to endoscopy is also key for dealing with issues like questionable viability of the conduit or dealing with complications. Esophageal stent placement also can provide a bridge to surgery for patients with poor nutrition.

[a] Tenwek Hospital, Bomet, Kenya; [b] Warren Alpert School of Medicine, Brown University, Providence, RI, USA
* Corresponding author.
E-mail address: deche2002@yahoo.com

Thorac Surg Clin 32 (2022) 397–404
https://doi.org/10.1016/j.thorsurg.2022.04.007

Patient Navigation

There are many challenges that patients face as they go through the esophageal cancer treatment journey. In many resource-limited settings, these may start as early as getting the diagnostic procedure performed. This is due to a few areas having endoscopy services.[7] In addition, there are myths and other gaps in knowledge that affect health-seeking behavior. This leads to patients either adopting a fatalistic attitude or not following through on treatment plans. With few areas being able to offer therapeutic services for esophageal cancer it also means that there ends up being a waiting list. Tumor progression can occur leading to inoperability as they wait. Patient navigation has been shown to help improve outcomes.[8] It is dependent on there being a system of being able to recall patients to the clinics. Two decades ago, this was more of a challenge, but with the advent and ubiquity of the mobile phone globally, this has become much easier. Some facilities have made use of a patient passport to help track this and we have made use of a simple registry/ledger to keep track of the patients. Integrated tumor board discussions help decide on the best mode and sequence of care.

Neoadjuvant Therapy

Chemo- and radiation therapy is available in limited numbers of LMICs for neoadjuvant therapy before resection or for curative intent.[9,10] Outcomes for patients who had received neoadjuvant therapy are much better compared with surgery alone or surgery and then adjuvant therapy.[9] Historically, due to lack of access to neoadjuvant therapy, we had been doing surgery only at our site as the mainstay therapy for many years. However, in recent years chemotherapeutic agents have become more available. At our institution, we recommend dual therapy with platinum and taxol-based neoadjuvant chemotherapy for patients with esophageal cancer before surgical resection. Studies on outcomes and complications in these groups are ongoing. Radiation therapy is only available in select facilities, which are centered in the capital of our country, and this requires a well-choreographed referral.

Surgical Resection

Surgical resection for esophageal cancer though not available in many resource-limited settings has been the mainstay of care in our setting. It is the preferred treatment option in our setting given the lack of other therapies and availability of surgery due to the local mentorship and training program. This is mainly driven by the lack of other treatment options. Currently, only a small percentage of patients present with resectable disease due to the nature of disease progression. While esophagectomy is associated with high morbidity and mortality rates even in the best of settings, there are now a number of studies from the region that were focused on surgery with curative intent.[11] Esophageal surgery outcomes have continued to improve over time as more patients are offered surgery. More staff have become familiar with esophageal surgery, and more intensive care units (ICU) have become available.

Patient selection is a key component of surgical resection. Nutrition has been shown to be an important predictor of survival and in our setup, this is one of the areas that we focus on. Body mass index is used to assess this and a cut-off of 18.5 kg/m^2 has been used. In addition, there are other factors at play including tumor length that is, we have seen that longer tumors correspond to more local advanced diseases. Patient preoperative functional status is also important.[6] Absence of metastatic disease is also an important component and CT scan evaluation is a key component. Positron Emission Tomography scans are now more available in our setup and are in use for initial assessment and to follow-up for tumor recurrence. These indications are summarized in **Table 1** later in discussion:

Perioperative Considerations

Provision of surgery is a multi-disciplinary process. Involving the anesthesiology team from the onset is important. The patient's ASA score is obtained as part of routine preparations. In addition, it is important to do a thorough evaluation of the patient's current health status, any preexisting comorbid conditions as well as talk them through what to expect before, during, and after the surgery. Baseline laboratory investigations and imaging are also obtained at this time.

Operative Considerations

Essentially, there are 5 different operative approaches used for the surgical resection of the esophagus.

McKeown or Three-field Esophagectomy

This operation involves 3 separate incisions in 2 separate stages. The procedure begins with a right thoracotomy with complete mobilization of the esophagus and tumor, along with a thorough lymphadenectomy. The chest is closed with appropriate drainage and the patient is placed in the supine position. An upper midline laparotomy is

Table 1
Current Indications for the surgical resection of esophageal cancer at Tenwek Hospital

Current Indications for the Surgical Resection of Esophageal Cancer	
Indications for surgical resection	• Absence of M1 disease on imaging: CT scan, Abdominal US or Chest X-ray • Albumin >3 g/dL • Age <70 y • Tumor Length <8 cm • SEMS in place for <8 wk • Completion of neoadjuvant therapy and endoscopic confirmation of tumor with no M1 disease
Absolute Contraindications for surgical resection	• Metastatic disease confirmed on imaging: liver, lung, presence of ascites and malignant pleural effusion • Recurrent laryngeal nerve paralysis • Presence of trachea-esophageal fistula • Cervical esophageal lesions
Relative Contraindications (Patient needs further review)	• Tumor >9 cm • Extreme cachexia (BMI<18.5) • Poor exercise tolerance (inability to walk up the flight of stairs • Comorbid conditions that are poorly controlled diabetes, hypertension • HIV positive with low CD4 and cachexia

performed for complete mobilization of the stomach and upper abdominal lymphadenectomy. Many surgeons perform a pyloromyotomy at this time. Hiatal dissection is carried out so that the entire esophagus is mobilized. Attention is then turned to a left cervical incision anterior to the sternocleidomastoid muscle. The esophagus is mobilized in this region to the level of the previous thoracic dissection. The esophagus is divided leaving an adequate length of esophagus distal to the cricopharyngeus muscle to comfortably perform an anastomosis. Most surgeons suture some type of flexible tube or umbilical tape to the distal portion of the divided esophagus to serve as a leader to guide the conduit through the posterior mediastinum. The entire esophagus is then delivered through the diaphragmatic hiatus into the abdomen (**Fig. 1**). The cardia of the stomach is usually divided with a stapling device and the specimen is removed from the field.

There is quite a bit of variability in the degree of tubularization that is created in the gastric conduit, which is then passed through the posterior mediastinum to the cervical region. An anastomosis is created between the gastric conduit and the esophageal remnant via a variety of different techniques. Before the completion of the anastomosis, a nasogastric tube is generally placed. Most surgeons place a feeding jejunostomy tube before the closure of the abdominal and cervical incisions.

Ivor Lewis Esophagectomy

This procedure involves 2 separate incisions in 2 separate stages. The operation begins with an upper midline laparotomy and the abdominal part of the procedure is essentially identical to that of the McKeown esophagectomy. After the completion of the abdominal portion, the patient is turned to the lateral decubitus position and a right thoracotomy is performed. Again, the thoracic portion is very similar to the McKeown procedure regarding the extent of dissection. However, in the Ivor Lewis approach, the esophagus is divided high in the thorax. The previously mobilized stomach is delivered into the thoracic cavity and the cardia of the stomach is divided as previously described. The esophagogastric anastomosis is performed high in the thorax via a number of different techniques, and the chest is closed.

Transhiatal Esophagectomy

This procedure involves 2 separate incisions in a single stage. An upper midline incision is performed and the stomach is mobilized as in the other procedures. The esophageal hiatus is fully mobilized and the esophageal dissection continues into the posterior mediastinum via a combination of sharp dissection under direct vision when possible, and blunt dissection using the surgeon's hand. This dissection is continued to a point well above the tracheal bifurcation. A separate incision is made in the cervical region and esophageal dissection is continued until the surgeon's 2 hands—generally the right in the cervical region and the left in posterior mediastinum via the abdomen—meet. When the surgeon is assured that circumferential dissection of the esophagus has been achieved from the diaphragmatic hiatus to the cervical incision, the remainder of the

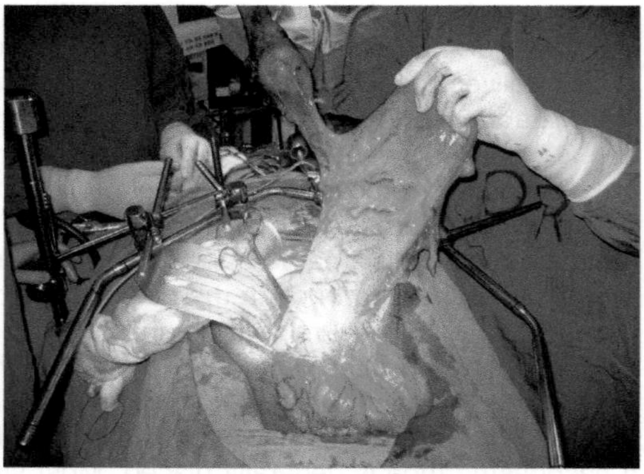

Fig. 1. Mobilized esophagus and stomach in abdominal phase of esophagectomy.

operation is completed in a fashion similar to the completion of the McKeown esophagectomy. The blunt mediastinal dissection causes significant compression of the right ventricle of the heart. It is advisable to use arterial pressure monitoring and to limit mediastinal blunt dissection to multiple short periods.

Left Thoracoabdominal Esophagectomy

This is a rarely used procedure. It involves a single left thoracoabdominal incision. Gastric mobilization is carried out as previously described. The gastric conduit is delivered in the left chest and the esophagus is divided inferior to the level of the aortic arch. The esophagogastric anastomosis is completed in the left chest. This procedure is only possibly applicable to distal lesions, as the approach to the esophagus in the left chest is hindered by the aortic arch.

Minimally Invasive Esophagectomy

Minimally invasive esophagectomy (MIE) is currently not widely used in LMICs due to a combination of equipment, t and patient-related issues (advanced stage). MIE involves a wide variety of combinations of thoracoscopic, laparoscopic, and robotic approaches that generally equal what either the McKeown or Ivor Lewis procedures accomplish.

Advantages and Disadvantages

Each of the previously described procedures has certain pros and cons which are summarized later in discussion in **Table 2**.

Postoperative Complications and Follow-up

Esophagectomy for tumor is associated with high rates of morbidity and mortality. Esophagectomy is routinely considered as one of the most morbid operations performed worldwide.[12,13] The complication rates vary across the world with a range of 16% to 50%. All centers offering surgery should also be prepared to deal with the complications that will inevitably arise. Aside from the usual complications of any major surgery, those somewhat specific to esophagectomy include anastomotic leak or stenosis, conduit leak or necrosis, recurrent laryngeal nerve injury, and chylothorax.

Anastomotic leak

This complication generally occurs 3 to 5 days following surgery. Some surgeons routinely place a soft drain in the cervical incision in part to monitor for leaks. This was our routine practice at our institution for many years. However, we found that it did little to show us the presence of a leak and have as abandoned it. We are aware of no clear study in the literature documenting the efficacy of a drain in identifying an anastomotic leak. Generally, this is detected through careful monitoring of the patient's clinical status. Unexplained tachycardia, respiratory rate, or fever should generally be considered signs of anastomotic leak until proven otherwise. In our institution, we will perform diagnostic upper endoscopy for any postop esophagectomy patient who meets the aforementioned criteria. This should be performed by an experienced endoscopist as there is a potential for causing anastomotic damage with the scope, as the anastomosis is generally very close to the upper esophageal sphincter. This allows direct visualization of the anastomosis and the gastric conduit. Upper GI contrast studies should be considered as complementary to endoscopy in this situation, as small leaks can be difficult to visualize with a scope. If doubt remains, one should have a low threshold to open the cervical incision and directly inspect the anastomosis and the nature of fluid in the region. When small leaks are diagnosed, generally packing of the neck incision is the only treatment necessary, as these will usually close spontaneously. If a large leak is identified (which is a rare occurrence), consideration should be given to formal exploration in the operating room with possible strap muscle closure of the defect. This of course depends on the quality of the tissue and the overall condition of the patient.

Anastomotic stricture

This complication generally occurs later in the course. It may present as early as 2 weeks postop, but may not present until 3 to 4 months after discharge from the hospital. Most of these will respond to serial outpatient dilations. Rarely, a

Table 2
Comparison of surgical options for esophagectomy

Procedure	Advantages	Disadvantages
McKeown Esophagectomy	Radical resection possible Wide axial and radial resection margins Cervical anastomosis	Three separate incisions Longer operative time
Ivor Lewis Esophagectomy	Radical resection possible Wide radial resection margin	Intrathoracic anastomotic leaks can be devastating Primary tumor can be found to be unresectable after full abdominal mobilization
Transhiatal Esophagectomy	Wide axial margin No need for thoracotomy Single-stage procedure Cervical anastomosis	Limited radial resection margin Higher blood loss Not suited for patients with limited cardiac reserve
Minimally Invasive Esophagectomy	Radical resection possible No need for thoracotomy Anastomosis can be placed in the neck or the chest Faster recovery	Steep learning curve Highly equipment dependent
Left Thoracoabdominal Esophagectomy	Single-stage procedure Technically simpler procedure	Radial and axial margins are poor High rate of postop reflux Suited only for very distal lesions Postop pain can be significant

patient may require endoscopic electro-incision to manage an anastomotic stricture.

Conduit leak or necrosis

This complication occurs in a location distal to the anastomosis, and generally involves a leak from the suture or staple line of the gastric conduit. This will often present with enteric or bilious fluid in the chest drain. Endoscopy is again helpful in identifying the extent of leak or necrosis. In the case of a small leak from a portion of the gastric suture line, it is possible to repair this surgically if found early via a right thoracotomy. True conduit necrosis is the most feared complication. It must be recognized early to save the patient's life. Emergent right thoracotomy is required to resect all nonviable stomach and divide the anastomosis. Laparotomy and cervical exploration is then required to replace the remnant stomach in the abdomen and place a gastric drainage tube, with a distal jejunostomy tube for feeding. The esophageal remnant must be brought out in the cervical region as an end esophagostomy. If the patient survives this complication, plans can be made 4 to 6 months later to attempt to reestablish GI continuity by means of a colon interposition conduit.

Chylothorax

Chylothorax generally occurs following esophagectomy due to unrecognized injury to the thoracic duct within the right chest or at the level of the diaphragm. It generally becomes readily apparent when the patient starts on enteral feeds, at which time the chest drain output increases significantly in volume and turns milky appearing. Confirmation of the diagnosis can be made by measuring a triglyceride level in the chest drain fluid. A triglyceride level greater than 110 mg/dL is generally considered diagnostic. Visualized microscopic chylomicrons in the fluid are pathognomonic. Treatment of this complication is often termed "surgical" or conservative. Surgical therapy involves mass ligation of the thoracic duct as low in the right chest as possible. All tissue between the spine and the aorta is included in ligature, and this can be accomplished either by open thoracotomy or thoracoscopic ligation. It is particularly helpful to have the enteral tube feeds running at the time of going to the operating room, as the actual site of leak can often be identified with this maneuver. Conservative therapy involves feeding the patient exclusively with total parenteral nutrition (TPN) and allowing time for the low-pressure leak in the thoracic duct to seal.

The time to sealing is quite variable, with a mean of 16 days, but may go beyond 4 weeks.[14] Use of oral medium-chain triglycerides has been used in the past. However, this only results in a reduction of Chyle production and are not as effective as TPN. Octreotide has also been variably used in conjunction with TPN. Lymphangiography with the embolization of thoracic duct leaks has also been reported but is generally available only in very advanced centers with significant experience.

Given the lack of TPN in many centers in resource-limited environments and the extended length of stay, surgical intervention is often the treatment of choice. In our experience, when a chylothorax is diagnosed, the patient is prepared for surgical thoracic duct ligation as soon as possible. It is generally a very short procedure with little morbidity and mortality. Early recognition of this complication and intervention generally leads to very good outcomes, while failure to recognize chylothorax can lead to very high mortality rates. Conservative treatment with TPN has been reported to have mortality rates as high as 30%.[14]

Recent data showed that facilities carrying out esophageal cancer surgery in resource-limited settings have higher 90-day postoperative morality rates despite having a similar anastomotic leak and complication rates compared with other centers globally.[15] Given the severity of potential complications, it should again be emphasized that esophagectomy should only be carried out by experienced surgeons in centers with the appropriate intensive care staffing and full-time endoscopy. Postoperative patients must be rigorously assessed regularly during the postop period.

Unresectable Disease

Unfortunately, the larger percentage which is more than 90% of patients currently present in our setting with unresectable disease due to metastases and/or local invasion.[16] For these patients, palliation is the goal. Dysphagia and weight loss are the predominant symptoms at this point. The mainstay of care involves the palliation of dysphagia for nutritional support and pain relief. Many of the patients presenting at this stage are usually frail and may not withstand larger operations. Therapeutic modalities include the placement of esophageal stents for palliation, placement of endoscopic feeding tubes if tumor is nonobstructing or can be stented open, and in some cases operative placement of feeding tubes including gastrostomy and jejunostomy tubes. Tube feeding supplies are not available in some LMICs, so establishing luminal patency with stents is preferred. Due to the morbidity associated with operative approaches, endoscopic placement of SEMS has become the standard of care in resource-limited settings. SEMS placement can be conducted as a day case procedure with just light sedation and has also been placed with no sedation especially if the frailty index is high.[16] Palliative radiotherapy is also now more available and is also an option. However, palliation of dysphagia via radiotherapy takes time for the effect to be observed and needs multiple sessions, whereas the SEMS provide immediate relief of dysphagia. There has also been some data available on the role of palliative esophagectomy. Given the cost of care and low impact on prognosis and survival this is not as common in resource-limited settings like ours.

Financing Care for Esophageal Cancer

Provision of treatment of esophageal cancer is costly. Diagnostic and therapeutic endoscopy has a significant cost and has been listed as one of the barriers in these settings. In addition, surgical resection as well as chemotherapy and radiotherapy is also costly. The average cost for surgical resection at Tenwek Hospital in Kenya varies from $1500 to $5000 USD. This is quite a significant expense and has been a key barrier to the uptake of surgical resection. Not all countries provide these services as part of the National Health insurance schemes and patients have to foot the bills themselves. In addition, whenever there are complications, this also leads to prolonged hospital stay and this will ultimately lead to higher hospital costs. There are currently no screening programs for this cancer- and the few in existence are focused on high incidence areas such as China.

Key Lessons From Our Experience With Esophageal Cancer Treatment

Facilities that can carry out esophageal cancer care

Esophageal cancer care is very resource and labor intensive. Therefore, sites that aspire to provide care have to also put in place the required personnel and facilities. The core components of these are ICUs, Operative theaters, and having the human personnel needed including surgical and nursing staff. The presence of an adequate ICU or high dependency unit (HDU), and experienced nursing staff cannot be over-emphasized if an institution desires to undertake major esophageal surgery. Esophageal surgery should also be domiciled in centers that have a fairly high volume of cases. While this number may not be comparable to numbers reported in high resource settings, it may be reasonable to have it conducted in centers that perform cases at least weekly. Furthermore, it is essential to have 24-h endoscopy capacity in order to appropriately care for potential postoperative complications. Often simple things are overlooked, such as enteral feeding formulations. Most patients with esophagectomy will require enteral feeding (generally through a surgically placed jejunostomy) for 7 to 14-days postoperatively. Most surgeons begin oral feeds on postoperative day 5 to 10, at which time jejunostomy feeds are progressively decreased. Many centers in developing countries have difficulty in maintaining a steady source of enteral feeding formulations. This must be addressed before initiating a program in esophageal surgery.

Training, capacity building, and research

There is a need for increasing the number of trained specialists who can offer care for patients with esophageal cancer who require esophageal surgery. This includes multidisciplinary team members including nurses, surgeons, anesthesia, oncologists, and radiologists. Local capacity building is key for sustainability. The surgical training can be in 2 main categories. In the first pathway, surgeons who have prior experience in esophageal surgery can visit high-volume centers for additional exposure. In the second, ly, surgeons may train specifically to specialize in thoracic surgery. The College of Surgeons of East, Central, and Southern Africa (COSECSA) has been active in this area and now has subspecialty fellowship training in cardiothoracic surgery. The surgery trainees live and work at the facilities that train them. From prior research, we have also shown that the graduates from the COSECSA training are more likely to remain in their region and also to practice in areas that are considered more rural. The gradual building up of this pool of specialists will ultimately translate to care being more available as well as improve outcomes in the region.

Research goes hand in hand with the provision of care. Tracking the outcomes of these patients through registries and prospective studies will provide much-needed data from these resource-limited settings that will also drive policy change. There has also been research into screening and early detection of esophageal cancer and its feasibility in resource-limited settings.[17]

Creation of bundles for care/protocols for intensive care units and postoperative care

One of the key lessons that we had from our facility is the introduction of care bundles and protocols. Prior to this, the postoperative orders and other necessary investigations would be conducted as they were needed. There were some standard postoperative care items but even these would sometimes not all be conducted. To standardize care and also to standardize the process, protocols were introduced. These came with a set of orders that were simply attached to the patient's file. This meant that even the nurses were able to identify and follow-up on missing items. In addition, these proved to be important when newer trainee surgeons were involved in the care as they would simply follow the orders on the chart. This made both patient care and handover processes much smoother. We also found that having patient rounding lists greatly improved this process. The switch to electronic medical records also greatly enhanced patient care. Currently across the world, there is utilization of Enhanced Recovery After Surgery (ERAS) Protocols that are designed to achieve early recovery after surgery. These can similarly be translated to resource-limited settings but will need each site to look into how they can adapt them and begin their use.

SUMMARY

Despite the challenges faced, care for esophageal cancer is changing across the continent. With advances in technology, there have also been efforts to embrace newer techniques including minimally invasive surgery, which may be feasible if the disease can be detected earlier. There remains a need for the right equipment, expertise, and facilities in-country to implement these changes. Currently, most of the efforts to advance esophageal cancer care in less-resourced settings are toward improving outcomes after treatment, increasing the number of patients that are diagnosed earlier, and increasing the pool of health workers that are able to offer care.

CLINICS CARE POINTS

- Despite vastly improved therapeutic options in recent decades, esophageal cancer continues to be a very difficult malignancy to manage with a curative result.
- Esophagectomy for malignancy continues to be one of the most morbid surgical procedures performed.[18]
- In general, esophagectomy for malignancy should be performed in high-volume centers whereby complications can be recognized early, and appropriate intervention

performed to prevent disastrous outcomes. In fact, this ability to recognize complications and rescue the patient seems to be one of the most important factors influencing differences in mortality rates between various institutions.[19]

- While early endoscopy following esophagectomy was once considered unsafe, we now feel strongly that when a complication is suspected, early endoscopy by an experienced endoscopist is key to achieving good outcomes.[20]
- Increased availability of neoadjuvant and adjuvant therapy in resource-constrained areas will likely improve outcomes in esophageal cancer.
- In patients who are not surgical candidates, we feel strongly that endoscopic stenting with self-expanding metal stents is the most effective means of palliation.[16]

DISCLOSURE

The authors have no disclosures to declare.

REFERENCES

1. Sung H, Ferlay J, Siegel RL, et al. Global Cancer Statistics 2020: GLOBOCAN estimates of incidence and mortality worldwide for 36 cancers in 185 countries. CA Cancer J Clin 2021;71(3):209–49.
2. Arnold M, Ferlay J, van Berge Henegouwen MI, et al. Global burden of oesophageal and gastric cancer by histology and subsite in 2018. Gut 2020;69(9):1564–71.
3. Codipilly DC, Qin Y, Dawsey SM, et al. Screening for esophageal squamous cell carcinoma: recent advances. Gastrointest Endosc 2018;88(3):413–26.
4. He S, Bergman J, Zhang Y, et al. Endoscopic radiofrequency ablation for early esophageal squamous cell neoplasia: report of safety and effectiveness from a large prospective trial. Endoscopy 2015;47(5):398–408.
5. Dawsey SM, Fleischer DE, Wang GQ, et al. Mucosal iodine staining improves endoscopic visualization of squamous dysplasia and squamous cell carcinoma of the esophagus in Linxian, China. Cancer 1998;83(2):220–31.
6. Mwachiro M, Mitchell E, Topazian HM, et al. Esophagectomy in patients with human immunodeficiency virus and acquired immune deficiency syndrome: a viable option. Semin Thorac Cardiovasc Surg 2018;30(1):116–21.
7. Mwachiro M, Topazian HM, Kayamba V, et al. Gastrointestinal endoscopy capacity in Eastern Africa. Endosc Int open 2021;9(11):E1827–36.
8. Rodrigues RL, Schneider F, Kalinke LP, et al. Clinical outcomes of patient navigation performed by nurses in the oncology setting: an integrative review. Revista brasileira de enfermagem 2021;74(2):e20190804.
9. Ma Z, Yuan M, Bao Y, et al. Survival of Neoadjuvant and adjuvant therapy compared with surgery alone for resectable esophageal squamous cell carcinoma: a systemic review and network meta-analysis. Front Oncol 2021;11:728185.
10. Buckle GC, Mahapatra R, Mwachiro M, et al. Optimal management of esophageal cancer in Africa: a systemic review of treatment strategies. Int J Cancer 2021;148(5):1115–31.
11. Yeheyis ET, Kassa S, Yeshitela H, et al. Intraoperative hypotension is not associated with adverse short-term postoperative outcomes after esophagectomy in esophageal cancer patients. BMC Surg 2021;21(1):1.
12. White RE, Parker RK. Oesophageal cancer: an overview of a deadly disease. Ann Afr Surg 2007;1:33–47.
13. Birkmeyer JD, Siewers AE, Finlayson EV, et al. Hospital and surgical mortality in the United States. N Engl J Med 2002;346:1128–37.
14. Seow C, Murray L, McKee RF. Surgical pathology is a predictor of outcome in post-operative lymph leakage. Int J Surg 2010;8(8):636–8.
15. Oesophago-Gastric Anastomotic Audit (OGAA) Collaborative: Writing Committee, Steering Committee, National Leads, Site Leads, & Collaborators. Mortality from esophagectomy for esophageal cancer across low, middle, and high-income countries: An international cohort study. Eur J Surg Oncol 2021;47(6):1481–8.
16. White RE, Parker RK, Fitzwater JW, et al. Stents as sole therapy for oesophgeal cancer: a prospective analysis of outcomes after placement. Lancet Oncol 2009;10:240–6.
17. Mwachiro MM, Burgert SL, Lando J, et al. Esophageal squamous dysplasia is common in asymptomatic kenyans: a prospective, community-based, cross-sectional study. Am J Gastroenterol 2016;111(4):500–7.
18. Sakamoto T, Fujiogi M, Matsui H, et al. Comparing Perioperative Mortality and Morbidity of Minimally Invasive Esophagectomy Versus Open Esophagectomy for Esophageal Cancer: A Nationwide Retrospective Analysis. Ann Surg 2021;274(2):324–30.
19. Abdelsattar ZM, Habermann E, Borah BJ, et al. Understanding Failure to Rescue After Esophagectomy in the United States. Ann Thorac Surg 2020;109(3):865–71.
20. Carr SR. When pigs fly: Early endoscopy after esophagectomy is safe. J Thorac Cardiovasc Surg 2017;154(3):1159–60.

Minimally Invasive Thoracic Surgery for Low- and Middle-Income Countries

Yihan Lin, MD, MPH[a], Dominique Vervoort, MD, MPH, MBA[b], Bibhusal Thapa, MBBS, MS, PhD[c], Ranjan Sapkota, MBBS, MS, MCh[d], John D. Mitchell, MD[a,*]

KEYWORDS

• Global surgery • Global health • Thoracic surgery • Minimally invasive thoracic surgery • Video-assisted thoracoscopic surgery • Lung cancer • Lung surgery

KEY POINTS

- Access to thoracic surgical care is limited and variable across low- and middle-income countries worldwide.
- Minimally invasive thoracic surgery can shorten hospital lengths of stay, may reduce health care costs, and can facilitate faster return to work.
- Select low- and middle-income countries have successfully introduced minimally invasive thoracic surgery.
- Increased financing, expanded surgical training, and more efficient surgical supply chains are necessary to facilitate scaling of minimally invasive thoracic surgery across the globe.
- Professional societies, academic institutions, policymakers, and industry have key roles to play and ought to collaborate to ensure efficiency.

BACKGROUND

Respiratory and upper-gastrointestinal diseases are among the leading causes of morbidity and mortality worldwide.[1] This burden is expected to continue to grow as a result of an aging population, air pollution, and the epidemiologic transition of low- and middle-income countries (LMICs) away from communicable diseases and toward noncommunicable diseases.[2,3] In particular, cancers of the airway and lung affect an estimated 3.21 million people worldwide, with 2.26 million new diagnoses and 2.04 million deaths each year.[1] In LMICs, tuberculosis remains prevalent, despite having been contained in high-income countries in recent decades.[4] Moreover, a considerable portion of respiratory and upper-gastrointestinal pathologies are amenable to surgical care for diagnosis, treatment, or palliation.[5] **Table 1** summarizes the global burden of thoracic and upper-gastrointestinal disease.

Despite the large and growing burden of disease, access to safe, timely, and affordable surgical care varies widely worldwide with 5 billion people lacking access when needed.[6] Access to thoracic surgery is even more limited in rural areas in high-income countries and in LMICs, although this is still poorly quantified.[7,8] Inequities persist

Funding: None.

[a] Division of Cardiothoracic Surgery, C-31012631 E. 17th Avenue, Aurora, CO 80045, USA; [b] Institute of Health Policy, Management and Evaluation, University of Toronto, Toronto, Ontario, Canada; [c] Thoracic Surgery Unit, Division of Surgery, Northern Health, Epping, Victoria, Australia; [d] Department of Cardio-Thoracic and Vascular Surgery, Manmohan Cardio-Thoracic Vascular and Transplant Center, Institute of Medicine, Kathmandu, Nepal
* Corresponding author.
E-mail address: john.mitchell@cuanschutz.edu

Thorac Surg Clin 32 (2022) 405–412
https://doi.org/10.1016/j.thorsurg.2022.04.003

Table 1
Global burden of thoracic disease partially amenable to surgery (per 100,000 population)

	High-Income Countries		Upper-Middle-Income Countries		Lower-Middle-Income Countries		Low-Income Countries	
Disease Group	**Deaths**	**DALYs**	**Deaths**	**DALYs**	**Deaths**	**DALYs**	**Deaths**	**DALYs**
Airway and lung cancer	57.46	1141.98	38.86	894.22	9.12	238.10	4.85	127.62
Mesothelioma	1.46	27.50	0.26	7.18	0.14	4.05	0.09	2.73
Esophageal cancer	7.26	152.06	11.52	262.19	2.55	69.49	3.51	97.47
Stomach cancer	15.05	269.46	21.29	497.71	5.58	151.80	4.99	138.62
Tuberculosis	1.32	28.41	3.70	142.32	24.96	965.16	38.46	1726.80
COPD	43.98	1001.39	50.93	1023.73	40.23	1002.76	17.63	482.27
GERD	N/A	87.05	N/A	74.99	N/A	81.16	N/A	58.70

Data obtained from the Institute of Health Metrics and Evaluation Global Burden of Disease Results Tool.[1]
Abbreviations: COPD, chronic obstructive pulmonary disease; DALYs, disability-adjusted life-years; GERD, gastroesophageal reflux disease; N/A, not available.

within LMICs because of variable socioeconomic development. For example, in Brazil, Russia, India, China, and South Africa (the BRICS countries), rapid socioeconomic, technological, and medical development comparable with high-income countries in the more affluent parts of the countries are countered by gaps in care akin to low-income countries in poorer parts of the countries.

In this review, we discuss the historical and contemporary trends in minimally invasive thoracic surgery (MITS) worldwide, summarize some of the literature documenting MITS experiences in LMICs, and present challenges and opportunities to scale MITS across variable-resource contexts.

MINIMALLY INVASIVE SURGERY SUCCESS STORIES IN VARIABLE-RESOURCE CONTEXTS

There are many examples of successful use of minimally invasive surgery in LMICs. In general surgery, minimally invasive surgery has been found to be feasible in many low-resource settings. A recent systematic review of the literature identified 18 examples of the use of laparoscopy in LMICs.[9] As one of the most commonly performed procedures in the world, laparoscopic cholecystectomies are now considered standard of care in high-income countries and is also becoming increasingly common in lower-resource settings. One of these examples includes the use of laparoscopy for cholecystectomy country-wide in Mongolia.[9] Mongolia is an LMIC in East Asia, where the first laparoscopic cholecystectomy was performed in 1994. Since then, a coordinated effort involving increased surgical capacity building and targeted training efforts have resulted in most cholecystectomies now being performed laparoscopically.[10,11] Studies have also shown that these surgeries are cost-effective from a patient and societal perspective[12] as a result of improved outcomes.[13] Additionally, there are many examples that describe sustainable training programs to ensure that these programs continue.[14]

In obstetrics and gynecology, the advantages of minimally invasive hysterectomies for benign conditions have been well documented in high-income countries.[15] Laparoscopic and robotic hysterectomies are preferred over abdominal hysterectomies because of reduced pain, shorter hospital length of stay, and improved operative outcomes. A hospital in Nairobi, Kenya, found excellent outcomes in patients undergoing these procedures, highlighting the feasibility to introduce this technology in LMICs.[16,17]

GLOBAL TRENDS IN MINIMALLY INVASIVE THORACIC SURGERY

Minimally invasive surgery was first introduced in the early twentieth century in Sweden and Germany.[18] Since then, minimally invasive techniques have been adopted by nearly all surgical specialties, including but not limited to obstetrics and gynecology, urology, general surgery, and thoracic surgery. MITS was first introduced in Stockholm, Sweden, in 1910 by Hans Christian Jacobaeus.[18,19] MITS most commonly refers to video-assisted thoracoscopic surgery (VATS) or medical thoracoscopy (pleuroscopy), each with distinct characteristics and indications (**Table 2**). More recently, robotic-assisted thoracic surgery has also had a significant increase in use in high-income countries around the world.

The benefits of MITS techniques include decreased surgical complications and reduced

Table 2
Minimally invasive thoracic surgery techniques

	VATS	Pleuroscopy
Anesthesia	General anesthesia, double-lumen endotracheal intubation, single-lung ventilation	Local anesthesia, conscious sedation
Indications	Stapled lung biopsy, pulmonary nodule resection, lobectomy, pneumonectomy, pericardial window, esophagectomy, parietal pleural biopsy, drainage of pleural effusion or empyema	Pleural cavity exploration, parietal pleura biopsy, pleurodesis, chest tube under direct visualization

Adapted from Lee P, Mathur PN, Colt HG. Advances in thoracoscopy: 100 years since Jacobaeus. *Respiration*. 2010;79(3):177-186.

intensive care and hospital lengths of stay. For example, in Brazil, a national propensity-matched analysis showed that MITS for anatomic lung resection was associated with significantly reduced major cardiopulmonary complications compared with open thoracotomy approaches.[20] This, in turn, allows patients to return to home faster, which in LMICs is an important metric: time off work is a major opportunity cost, especially in individuals that may be one of the only breadwinners for a family. Moreover, the reduced invasiveness of procedures can improve postoperative quality of life of patients and patient care satisfaction.

MITS has been shown to be a safe alternative to thoracotomy for multiple procedures. Some surgical societies and the National Comprehensive Cancer Network have identified it as a "strongly recommended therapy" for early stage primary lung cancer.[21,22] Current numbers of cases that are minimally invasive in high-income countries continue to grow.[23] A recent study comparing databases of the Society of Thoracic Surgeons and the European Society of Thoracic Surgeons found that 62.5% of lung resection were performed via VATS in the Society of Thoracic Surgeons database, compared with 21.8% in the European Society of Thoracic Surgeons database.[24] However, the penetration of MITS is still much lower in LMICs compared with high-income countries. Uptake varies from a complete absence in most LMICs to some of the highest institutional volumes in the world (eg, China, India) but with significant domestic variation.[25]

Although the published literature remains limited, the successful use of MITS has been reported in various LMICs. A center in India reported their series of video-assisted thoracoscopic lobectomies, which showed successful use in benign and malignant lung pathologies.[26] MITS has also been reported in Nigeria.[27] In South Africa, thoracoscopy was introduced for retained posttraumatic collections, and a 3-year review found this safe and effective.[28] Several other published studies include the experience in the Caribbean,[29] Philippines,[30] and Central and South America.[31] One of our authors here is shown assisting with a successful minimally invasive lobectomy in Nepal (**Fig. 1**).

CHALLENGES OF MINIMALLY INVASIVE THORACIC SURGERY IN VARIABLE-RESOURCE CONTEXTS

Despite the growth in MITS, several challenges prohibit rapid scaling across variable-resource contexts (**Table 3**).

There is an insufficient number of thoracic surgeons worldwide, although the exact number

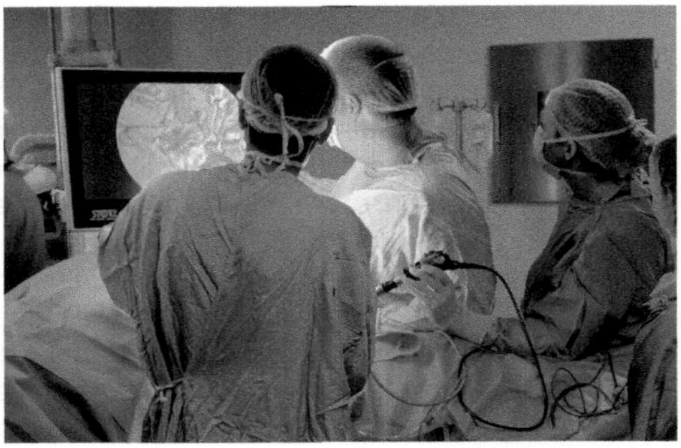

Fig. 1. Minimally invasive lobectomy in Manmohan Cardio-Thoracic Vascular and Transplantation Center, Kathmandu, Nepal.

Table 3
Challenges and opportunities for MITS in LMICs

Area	Challenges	Opportunities
Workforce	Insufficient thoracic surgical capacity Limited or no MITS experience/ training	Simulation training Virtual workshops Teleconsultations Opportunities for in-person training
Infrastructure	Limited or no MITS infrastructure Power outages Fragmented supply chains	Train/hire biomedical engineers Leverage local or regional industry
Financing	Limited financial risk protection for patients (high out-of-pocket expenditure) Limited to no government funds to acquire MITS equipment Proportionally small industry presence in LMICs	Industry partnerships Understand cost-effectiveness of MITS in local context to drive reimbursement decisions
Service delivery	Learning curve vs small thoracic surgical volumes Predominance of inflammatory pathologies presenting some of the most hostile operative fields, which potentially hamper learning curves and skills transfer Long surgical waiting lists	Regionalization to increase surgical volumes, improve outcomes, and reduce costs Improve surgical outcomes and facilitate timely hospital discharge
Information management and technology	Lack of electronic health records Few or no clinical registries	Mutual learning through international and national registries Virtual education and conferences Social networks
Governance	Limited prioritization of surgical care in LMICs Few LMIC-based thoracic surgical professional societies Political instability leading to procurement disruptions	Integration of surgical care in national health plans (eg, NSOAPs) Global surgical advocacy momentum Establishment or expansion of thoracic surgical societies into LMICs

Abbreviation: NSOAPs, national surgical, obstetric, and anesthesia plans.

remains poorly defined.[32] In LMICs, surgical specialization in thoracic surgery is less frequent, with a large proportion of thoracic cases performed by general surgeons. Few local training programs outside BRICS LMICs have sufficient, if any, MITS capacity. Correspondingly, training programs in these settings often do not have minimum case requirements or clinical milestones for MITS. This commonly requires surgeons to seek specialized training in the BRICS countries or in high-income countries. Even after receiving adequate training, however, surgeons still need minimum case volumes to feel comfortable performing these surgeries safely. One study showed that the highest proportion of surgeon respondents stated that at least 26 to 50 cases were necessary to safely perform these surgeries via VATS.[23] Other important staff, including operating room personnel and maintenance personnel, may also be few and far between, further exacerbating the workforce problem.

Challenges of infrastructure also contribute to the expansion of MITS. Centers with MITS capacity or capable of initiating MITS may be constrained by fragmented surgical supply chains or power supplies.[33,34] MITS equipment is often made outside of LMICs, with limited regional offices of the respective industry suppliers, which contribute to distribution delays. Regulatory and licensing guidelines could further complicate uptake in a region. Finally, political instability in LMICs may cause significant disruptions in procurement or deployment of industry personnel for support.

In addition, the cost of MITS equipment may be prohibitive. Many MITS companies based out of high-income settings are designed for single-use systems, or are made with materials that are not easily available in the local context. MITS companies based out of high-income settings generally do not offer reduced pricing for LMICs, whereas few MITS companies exist in LMICs. Many of the equipment require a constant supply of consumables. Distribution of companies in these low-resource settings remains scarce, with few offices and representatives available. This further leads to a lack of a constant and reliable supply chain whereby stockouts of surgical consumables and disposables frequently occur in LMICs.[33] Additionally, payment and reimbursement challenges exist, with a need for government buy-in to successfully launch a program and ensure affordability for patients, whereas out-of-pocket spending for surgical care is already large at baseline in LMICs[6] and the cost of cancer, including lung cancer, is known to be substantial in Nepal.[35] Similar to minimally invasive surgery and many other specialized surgical procedures in LMICs, these services tend to be centralized in private centers or require external (ie, no or limited government) funding.

MITS has had a measurable positive impact in the management of some common thoracic surgical problems. Thoracoscopic pleural biopsies have made it easier to attain definitive histologic diagnosis in undiagnosed pleural effusions. This is often a major problem in LMICs, where tubercular effusions and advanced malignancy presenting as pleural effusions are common.[36] Additionally, thoracoscopic management of empyema, a common problem in LMICs, has transformed how this problem is dealt with. Early deloculation and decortication via MITS has allowed treatment durations, associated morbidities, and costs to be reduced. Separate to MITS lung resection procedures, widespread availability of these and similar procedures is likely to have the biggest impact on how thoracic surgery is practiced in LMICs. Improving training capability and infrastructure development are most likely going to be key in making MITS widely accessible to this population.

OPPORTUNITIES TO ACCELERATE AND SCALE MINIMALLY INVASIVE THORACIC SURGERY GLOBALLY

There have been significant strides in the use of minimally invasive techniques for thoracic surgery. However, significant discrepancies continue to exist, and adoption of these techniques requires coordinated efforts from multiple stakeholders.

Governments and ministries of health have a critical role in the success of minimally invasive surgery. Resource allocation and the stability of supply chains should be done at a high level to ensure sustainability of efforts in a country. Investment in infrastructure should include development of new centers and improvements of current centers with accompanying safety requirements and minimum standards. Regional centers should also be considered, to maximize access for patients and ensuring high volumes to improve patient outcomes.[37,38] Although initial costs are likely going to be high, government subsidies in the early phase could serve to increase volumes and thus decrease costs in the future. Once sufficient volumes are attained, MITS may be cheaper than open repairs. For example, in the United States, VATS lobectomies are, on average, 2% less expensive compared with open lobectomies.[39] Similarly, in Canada, minimally invasive esophagectomy was more cost-effective than open esophagectomy for resectable esophageal cancer as a result of lower costs and greater quality-adjusted life-year gains,[40] although results may not necessarily be generalizable to LMIC settings as a result of different contexts, surgical volumes, and equipment costs.[41] Moreover, financial risk protection must be ensured by ramping up health insurance packages, notably with the inclusion of surgical services.[42] For example, in Nepal, the government established *Bipanna Nagarik Kosh*, a basic health insurance package, in 2012 as commitment to help subsidize the costs of treatment for 12 high-burden disease groups, including all cancers.[43]

Surgical societies also have an important role to play. Education and training are critical to allow for continued improvement and learning of new technologies. Initially, training may have to be done by those from high-income country settings; however, as adoption increases, this should transition to local providers to ensure continued sustainability. In Brazil, a chest cavity simulator was used for these purposes,[44] which may be scaled or mimicked across settings.

Individual hospitals and providers must also take full responsibility for the progress. Monitoring and evaluation protocols are necessary throughout, not just in the early phases, to ensure that outcomes are closely followed. These should include not just initial morbidity and mortality data but must also focus on patient experience and cost markers to truly assess the clinical and financial effectiveness in these settings. Participation in national, regional, and international registries should be highly encouraged to continue learning from others and identifying areas for targeted improvement. Research and quality improvement initiatives should also be reviewed at set time periods.

Industry partners must be actively engaged with all of the previously mentioned partners. Equipment must come with training and servicing contracts. Pricing should be adjusted for these settings, with accompanying innovation and use of local industries and materials. Industry partners should no longer assume that there is no market in LMICs, as evidenced by the global burden of disease and cost-effectiveness data from laparoscopic examples that may drive further adoption. Instead, LMICs need to be viewed as an emerging market for industry, previously untapped.

In addition to the critical stakeholders mentioned previously, there have been other innovative efforts to increase technology and quality care in these settings. Biodesign teams have also shown success in creating such opportunities. For example, the University of Utah has an Extreme Affordability Conference, which leverages the idea of technologies in any resource setting that is highly affordable and appropriate for the context. The University of Utah has patented the Xenoscope, a first-of-its-kind disposable laparoscope that has the potential to disrupt markets in low-income countries but also has the potential to do this in high-income countries.[45] Similarly, in India, gasless laparoscopy has been adopted in rural settings, which has shown to be noninferior compared with conventional laparoscopy.[46,47] Furthermore, Stanford University offers a medical device innovation course, aimed at creating sustainable technologies for all settings. They also host a Design for Extreme Affordability program where students design products specifically geared toward use in low-resource settings. The program has resulted in various real-world innovations to improve access to and delivery of surgical care in LMICs, such as Nepal's first skin bank for allografts for major burn trauma.[48] These programs, informed by lived experiences, can serve as important incubators for future technologies.

SUMMARY

MITS remains underused in variable-resource contexts, such as LMICs, because of limited infrastructural capacity, clinical experience, and the necessary financing. Nevertheless, opportunities exist to reduce hospital lengths of stay, enabling patients to return home faster and minimize hospitalization costs, time away from family, and time off work. Strategic, collaborative efforts among health workers, institutions, academia, industry, societies, and governments are necessary to facilitate scaling and adoption of MITS across the globe and provide the best possible care for patients requiring thoracic surgical care.

CONFLICTS OF INTEREST

None.

REFERENCES

1. Institute for Health Metrics and Evaluation. Global Burden of Disease Results Tool. GBD Results Tool. 2021. Available at: http://ghdx.healthdata.org/gbd-results-tool%20. Accessed October 25, 2021.
2. Cohen AJ, Brauer M, Burnett R, et al. Estimates and 25-year trends of the global burden of disease attributable to ambient air pollution: an analysis of data from the Global Burden of Diseases Study 2015. Lancet 2017;389(10082):1907–18.
3. Bukhman G, Mocumbi AO, Atun R, et al. The Lancet NCDI Poverty Commission: bridging a gap in universal health coverage for the poorest billion. Lancet 2020;396(10256):991–1044.
4. Dheda K, Barry CE 3rd, Maartens G. Tuberculosis. Lancet 2016;387(10024):1211–26.
5. Debas HT, Donkor P, Gawande A, et al, editors. Essential surgery: disease control priorities, ume 1, Third Edition. The International Bank for Reconstruction and Development/The World Bank; 2016.
6. Meara JG, Leather AJM, Hagander L, et al. Global Surgery 2030: evidence and solutions for achieving health, welfare, and economic development. Lancet 2015;386(9993):569–624.
7. Pervez MB, Hashmi S, Jabeen M, et al. When surgeons are rarer than resources: our experience with improving access to thoracic surgery in an urban setting: a special report. J Pak Med Assoc 2019;69(Suppl 1):S77–81.
8. Eberth JM, Crouch EL, Josey MJ, et al. Rural-urban differences in access to thoracic surgery in the United States, 2010 to 2014. Ann Thorac Surg 2019;108(4):1087–93.
9. Wilkinson E, Aruparayil N, Gnanaraj J, et al. Barriers to training in laparoscopic surgery in low- and middle-income countries: a systematic review. Trop Doct 2021;51(3):408–14.
10. Wells KM, Lee YJ, Erdene S, et al. Building operative care capacity in a resource limited setting: the Mongolian model of the expansion of sustainable laparoscopic cholecystectomy. Surgery 2016;160(2): 509–17.
11. Wells KM, Lee YJ, Erdene S, et al. Expansion of laparoscopic cholecystectomy in a resource limited setting, Mongolia: a 9-year cross-sectional retrospective review. Lancet 2015;385(Suppl 2):S38.

12. Lombardo S, Rosenberg JS, Kim J, et al. Cost and outcomes of open versus laparoscopic cholecystectomy in Mongolia. J Surg Res 2018;229:186–91.
13. Wells KM, Shalabi H, Sergelen O, et al. Patient and physician perceptions of changes in surgical care in Mongolia 9 years after roll-out of a national training program for laparoscopy. World J Surg 2016;40(8): 1859–64.
14. Kang MJ, Apea-Kubi KB, Apea-Kubi KAK, et al. Establishing a sustainable training program for laparoscopy in resource-limited settings: experience in Ghana. Ann Glob Health 2020;86(1):89.
15. Perino A, Cucinella G, Venezia R, et al. Total laparoscopic hysterectomy versus total abdominal hysterectomy: an assessment of the learning curve in a prospective randomized study. Hum Rep 1999; 14(12):2996–9.
16. Parkar RB, Thagana NG, Baraza R, et al. Experience with laparoscopic surgery at the Aga Khan Hospital, Nairobi. East Afr Med J 2003;80(1):44–50.
17. Parkar RB, Kamau WJ, Otieno D, et al. Total laparoscopic hysterectomy at the Aga Khan University Hospital, Nairobi. East Afr Med J 2007;84(11):508–15.
18. Hatzinger M, Kwon ST, Langbein S, et al. Hans Christian Jacobaeus: inventor of human laparoscopy and thoracoscopy. J Endourol 2006;20(11): 848–50.
19. Lee P, Mathur PN, Colt HG. Advances in thoracoscopy: 100 years since Jacobaeus. Respiration 2010;79(3):177–86.
20. Tsukazan MTR, Terra RM, Vigo Á, et al. Video-assisted thoracoscopic surgery yields better outcomes than thoracotomy for anatomical lung resection in Brazil: a propensity score-matching analysis using the Brazilian Society of Thoracic Surgery database. Eur J Cardiothorac Surg 2018;53(5):993–8.
21. Yamashita SI, Goto T, Mori T, et al. Video-assisted thoracic surgery for lung cancer: republication of a systematic review and a proposal by the guidelines committee of the Japanese Association for Chest Surgery 2014. Gen Thorac Cardiovasc Surg 2014; 62(12):701–5.
22. Ettinger DS, Wood DE, Aisner DL, et al. NCCN Guidelines insights: non-small cell lung cancer, version 2.2021. J Natl Compr Canc Netw 2021; 19(3):254–66.
23. Cao C, Tian DH, Wolak K, et al. Cross-sectional survey on lobectomy approach (X-SOLA). Chest 2014; 146(2):292–8.
24. Seder CW, Salati M, Kozower BD, et al. Variation in pulmonary resection practices between the Society of Thoracic Surgeons and the European Society of Thoracic Surgeons general thoracic surgery databases. Ann Thorac Surg 2016;101(6):2077–84. https://doi.org/10.1016/j.athoracsur.2015.12.073.
25. Rocha MFH, Coelho RF, Branco AW, et al. A census of laparoscopic and robotic urological practice: a survey of minimally invasive surgery department of the Brazilian Society of Urology. Int Braz J Urol 2019;45(4):732–8.
26. Kumar A, Asaf BB, Puri HV, et al. Video-assisted thoracoscopic surgery lobectomy: the first Indian report. J Minim Access Surg 2018;14(4): 291–7.
27. Falase BA, Majekodunmi AA, Ismail S, et al. Video-assisted thoracic surgery in a Nigerian teaching hospital: experience and challenges. Niger J Clin Pract 2016;19(2):233–6.
28. Oosthuizen GV, Clarke DL, Laing GL, et al. Introducing video-assisted thoracoscopy for trauma into a South African township hospital. World J Surg 2013;37(7):1652–5.
29. Smith A, Ramnarine I, Pinkney P. Evolution of video assisted thoracoscopic surgery in the Caribbean. Int J Surg 2019;72S:19–22.
30. Danguilan JLJ. Clinical innovations in Philippine thoracic surgery. J Thorac Dis 2016;8(Suppl 8): S613–7.
31. Terra RM. Thymic minimally invasive surgery: state of the art across the world: Central-South America. J Visc Surg 2017;3:124.
32. Vervoort D, Meuris B, Meyns B, et al. Global cardiac surgery: access to cardiac surgical care around the world. J Thorac Cardiovasc Surg 2020;159(3): 987–96.e6.
33. Nazir A, Vervoort D, Reddy CL. From the first mile to the last: challenges of the global surgical supply chain. Am J Surg 2021. https://doi.org/10.1016/j.amjsurg.2021.03.033.
34. Mechtenberg A, McLaughlin B, DiGaetano M, et al. Health care during electricity failure: the hidden costs. PLoS One 2020;15(11):e0235760.
35. Khatiwoda SR, Dhungana RR, Sapkota VP, et al. Estimating the direct cost of cancer in Nepal: a cross-sectional study in a tertiary cancer hospital. Front Public Health 2019;7:160.
36. Shrestha UK, Thapa B, Sayami P. Diagnostic thoracoscopy in undiagnosed pleural effusion: our experience in Manmohan Cardio-Thoracic Vascular and Transplant Center. J Gen Pract Emerg Med Nepal 2014;3(4):13–8.
37. Chhabra KR, Dimick JB. Strategies for improving surgical care: when is regionalization the right choice? JAMA Surg 2016;151(11):1001–2.
38. Darling GE. Regionalization in thoracic surgery: the importance of the team. J Thorac Cardiovasc Surg 2020. https://doi.org/10.1016/j.jtcvs.2020.06.138.
39. Subramanian MP, Liu J, Chapman WC Jr, et al. Utilization trends, outcomes, and cost in minimally invasive lobectomy. Ann Thorac Surg 2019;108(6):1648–55.
40. Lee L, Sudarshan M, Li C, et al. Cost-effectiveness of minimally invasive versus open esophagectomy for esophageal cancer. Ann Surg Oncol 2013; 20(12):3732–9.

41. Yanasoot A, Yolsuriyanwong K, Ruangsin S, et al. Costs and benefits of different methods of esophagectomy for esophageal cancer. Asian Cardiovasc Thorac Ann 2017;25(7–8):513–7.
42. Reddy CL, Vervoort D, Meara JG, et al. Surgery and universal health coverage: designing an essential package for surgical care expansion and scale-up. J Glob Health 2020;10(2):020341.
43. World Health Organization Country Office for Nepal. Nepal – WHO country Cooperation Strategy: 2018-2022. World Health Organization; 2018.
44. Martins Neto F, Moura Júnior LG de, Rocha HAL, et al. Development and validation of a simulator for teaching minimally invasive thoracic surgery in Brazil. Acta Cir Bras 2021;36(5):e360508.
45. Assali SK, Szoka N. Xenoscope. SAGES. 2020. Available at: https://www.sages.org/publications/tavac/xenoscope/. Accessed February 21, 2022.
46. Mishra A, Bains L, Jesudin G, et al. Evaluation of gasless laparoscopy as a tool for minimal access surgery in low-to middle-income countries: a phase II noninferiority randomized controlled study. J Am Coll Surg 2020;231(5):511–9.
47. Aruparayil N, Gnanaraj J, Maiti S, et al. Training programme in gasless laparoscopy for rural surgeons of India (TARGET study): observational feasibility study. Int J Surg Open 2021;35. None.
48. Cai L, Long C, Karki B, et al. Creation of Nepal's first skin bank: challenges and outcomes. Plast Reconstr Surg Glob Open 2017;5(11):e1510.

9780323849791